Yoga: The Practice of Myth and Sacred Geometry

Rama Jyoti Vernon

LOTUS PRESS

Twin Lakes, WI USA

Editor: Kathleen Bryant

Illustrations: ©2014 Rama Jyoti Vernon

Cover design: Tonita Abeyta

Project manager: Ruth Hartung

ISBN: 978-0-9406-7626-8

Library of Congress Control Number: 2014954487

For information address

LOTUS
PRESS

Lotus Press
P.O. Box 325
Twin Lakes, WI 53181 USA
800-824-6396 (toll free order phone)
262-889-8561 (office phone)
262-889-2461 (office fax)
www.lotuspress.com (website)
lotuspress@lotuspress.com (email)

Printed in USA

Advance praise for

Yoga: The Practice of Myth and Sacred Geometry

"Yoga: The Practice of Myth and Sacred Geometry is for all of us who want to continue in the study of yoga's deep teaching and technical instruction. The wonderful diagrams and photos will clearly assist us as we learn and teach asana and pranayama while walking life's journey. Thank you, Rama, for sharing the heart, soul, and passion of your own practices, insights, and reflections, and for imparting your years of yoga experience, study, and teaching. This is a book I will treasure for years to come."

—Lilias Folan, PBS host and author of *Lilias! Yoga: Your Guide to Enhancing Body, Mind, and Spirit Midlife and Beyond*

"Rama floated into my life in 1992 with a 'presence of Self,' immediately touching my heart. When she teaches, asana becomes a dance of story, philosophy, subtle body knowledge, and basic safety. She interweaves the essence that makes yoga alive. In Yoga: The Practice of Myth and Sacred Geometry, Rama imparts this essence. She shares the precision of yoga practices while merging the stories behind the practices, marrying the practice with the heart of yoga. Her students learn to explore yogasana on the mat and in the world. Rama has been my guiding light. With this unique asana manual she offers, in a very accessible format, the spirit and the depth of yoga. Through teaching and living yoga, she makes a difference in the world!"

—Hansa Knox, Director of Training at PranaYoga and Ayurveda Mandala (Denver, CO), past president of Yoga Alliance

"Rama Jyoti Vernon unfolds the profound mystery of the practice of yoga while guiding the reader with practical skill. As practitioners journey through this book, they will experience the true sense of the word myth that will manifest as the sacred geometry of the body, mind, and consciousness."

—Vasant Lad, B.A.M.S., M.A.Sc., Ayurvedic physician, founder of The Ayurvedic Institute (Albuquerque), author of *Ayurveda: Science of Self-Healing* and other titles

"It's exciting and rare for me to come upon a modern-day writing that offers a fresh light, and breathes new life, into the ancient teachings of yoga. This is one such book."

—Richard Miller, PhD, author of *Yoga Nidra: The Meditative Heart of Yoga* and other titles

"Rama Jyoti Vernon has been a pioneer in bringing yoga to America and has inspired my own practice in innumerable ways. Her heart-centered wisdom as a teacher of teachers and of hundreds of thousands of students around the globe shines through in this book. Not only does Rama's understanding of the biodynamics of asana and breath make this a must read for everyone who aspires to serve others through the teaching of yoga, but the great value and humility she brings to the calling of yoga teacher—as 'servant' or 'fellow seeker'—lights the path through the darkness for countless fellow seekers, me included."

—Amy Weintraub, Founder of the LifeForce Yoga Healing Institute, author of *Yoga for Depression* and *Yoga Skills for Therapists*

Table of Contents

Author's Note

Oṃ Gaṃ Gaṇapataye Namaḥ

Gaṇeśa, the son of Shiva, who is the Lord of all Yogis, is invoked before any event, undertaking, or mantra. He is the favored deity of scribes and merchants, and he is associated with wisdom, good luck, successful enterprises, prosperity, peace, beginnings, journeys, building, and also with books and writing.

Gaṇeśa is the remover of obstacles, both spiritual and material. He is a protector, evident by the rattle that is heard before his darśana, or revelation. The rattle is to chase away the evil spirits that symbolize hindrances on the spiritual path.

In one hand, Gaṇeśa holds a bowl of rice and in the other, the Vedas. This symbolizes that one needs material fulfillment as well as spiritual nourishment. It is believed that when one is hungry, the mind cannot soar to loftier heights and becomes consumed with survival at the most basic level. Perhaps this may explain why Gaṇeśa is said to dwell in the first chakra, Mūlādhāra, guarding the chamber of the Inner Self, just as he is known to be the guard of his mother Pārvatī's chamber.

Gaṇeśa's huge ears symbolize the ability to hear all things, the ability to listen, and to listen compassionately. His small eyes symbolize shutting off the outside world to look within. His long trunk, which brings nourishment from the ground into his mouth, symbolizes discrimination, for it takes more time for food to reach his lips, allowing time for evaluation or re-evaluation of the action.

Gaṇeśa represents a vast universal energy, an energy that we can bring into all of our lives and our yoga practice.

With this book, I offer the wisdom of my many teachers. It is the labor of a lifetime, the culmination of sixty years of yoga study and teaching, and a decade of writing. I offer it with love to all my teachers and students, past, present, and future.

—Rama Jyoti Vernon

For more information about Rama Jyoti Vernon go to www.ramajyotivernon.com

FOREWORD

Rewind. It's 1973. I'm studying yoga at the Yoga College of India in San Francisco. A group of yoga students are visiting from the Institute for Yoga Teacher Education (IYTE), a school that Rama Jyoti Vernon has helped found.

Fast forward. It's 1976. I'm sitting in Rama's home, learning the art of pranayama with Rama as my teacher, with a group of fellow students from the IYTE, where I'm now taking classes to increase my studies in yoga.

Fast forward. It's 1977. I've just submitted my first article, Yoga for the Blind, to the Yoga Journal, the magazine Rama helped found in 1975.

Fast Forward. It's 1978. I'm attending numerous parties hosted by Rama in her home, where visiting yogis from around the world are sharing their knowledge and presence.

Fast forward. It's still 1978. I've just been invited to serve as the vice president of the California Yoga Teachers Association (CYTA), which Rama helped found several years earlier.

Fast forward. It's still 1978. CYTA has just agreed to spin off IYTE, which is to become the San Francisco Iyengar Yoga Institute, where Rama will continue teaching classes.

Fast Forward. It's 1979. Rama has invited me to host Ian Rawlinson, a senior student of T.K.V. Desikachar, for a series of seminars at my Marin School of Yoga. Ian will introduce me to the teachings of T. Krishnamachara, and I will subsequently fly to Madras to begin formal studies with Desikachar in 1980.

Fast forward. It's 1981. I've been invited by Rama to become a member of Unity in Yoga, an organization that Rama has founded to promote unity among the various international schools of yoga.

Fast forward. It's 1984. Rama has established the Center for Soviet-American Dialogue to help connect citizens of the United States with those of the Soviet Union. She later changes the name to the Center for International Dialogue in order to expand its reach into the Middle East, as well as into Ethiopia, Central America, and Africa, among other sites.

Fast forward. It's 1992. Rama helps found the Regional Women's Gatherings (RWG), an organization dedicated to providing women a platform to express their visions for peace in the world. RWG culminates in the 1994 Georgetown University Conference, Women of Vision (WOV): Leadership for the New World, which brings together over 500 women and leads to the formation of the Women of Vision National Network, which provides ongoing WOV Regional Conferences.

Fast forward. It's 1995. Rama is an NGO delegate to the Fourth UN Conference on Women, where she is focusing on empowering women in Africa.

Fast forward. It's 2004. Rama founds the International Yoga College (IYC), which offers educational opportunities for experienced students and teachers of yoga.

Fast forward. 2004-Present. Throughout these years Rama continues to travel throughout the world, bringing her expertise, teachings, love, and creative energy to helping people come together to resolve their conflicts, and promote peace in their lives and the regions where they live.

Suffice to say, Rama has deeply touched my life in countless ways, as she has the lives of countless others around the globe. Rama is a woman of vision, who leads a mission-driven life, exemplifying peace and action in every breath she takes. It's been a privilege to know Rama through the years, through her many adventures. From my first meeting with her, and throughout the years, I've experienced light, love, and authentic presence in her every interaction with myself, and those around me. It's therefore an honor for Rama to have invited me to provide this brief foreword to her new book.

It's exciting and rare for me to come upon a modern day writing that offers a fresh light, and breathes new life, into the ancient teachings of yoga. Rama's offering, Yoga: The Practice of Myth and Sacred Geometry, is one such book. And I would expect no less from Rama.

Rama writes with the authoritative autonomy of one who has truly traversed the entire breadth and depth of yoga, from marketplace to mountaintop and back again. Rama offers us timeless wisdom derived from her years of study, practice, devotion, and sitting with her many gifted teachers. She offers us sage advice and knowledge that is at once practical, philosophical, and heartfelt, delivered with passion and appeal from page to page and chapter to chapter.

I take great delight in knowing that I will be sharing Rama's book with my yoga friends and students for years to come, providing them with, as I have found, a treasure trove of sacred teachings that enables us to find equanimity no matter our circumstances.

Richard Miller, PhD
author of *Yoga Nidra: The Meditative Heart of Yoga* and *Yoga Nidra Meditation to Overcome Trauma* (www.irest.us.)
San Rafael 2014

Author's Preface

For years, I was reluctant to write about yoga, always feeling I didn't know enough. Even though those feelings are still present, after continual urging of students and yoga teachers, I now offer these pages as an organic unfoldment of my own practices, insights, and reflections. I hope you, the reader, will receive this offering as simply that.

These writings encompass over a half-century of blessings by master teachers and yoga's ever-expanding presence in all areas of life. Yoga and its tributaries continue to be a map of how to live life on this earth plane to the fullest extent while finding serenity in the midst of all changing endeavors and experiences. Yoga has been my guide and preceptor on journeys through the valleys of the dark night of the soul to the mountaintops of unveiled understandings.

As a householder and mother, I have had to find ways to integrate my children into my practice and my life, no longer seeing the family as separate from my spiritual life, but as the spiritual path itself. Mine has been a journey of integration that continues to reveal itself. As a householder and yoga teacher, I have found that the fullest expression of yoga is not just within a pose but within every aspect of life. Yoga exists within each action and every spoken word, and it is expressed through every thought.

Over the years, I've come to believe that a yoga teacher's inner experiences, combined with an understanding of the deeper significance of yoga, creates a vibrational frequency that attracts students of a similar resonance. I have found that as I changed, some students dropped away while others appeared. I also discovered it was not up to me to discern whether I taught a "good" or "bad" class.

Among yoga's blessings: We learn balance within the polarities of opposites. As we learn the art of bilateral integration within the body, we also learn the same in life. We do not seek approval or cower under disapproval, real or imagined. As teachers and as students, we learn to stay centered in the midst of attachments and aversions, praise or blame, criticism or compliment. Through āsana, we learn to give up goal orientation, to give our all to the present moment, and then to release it, as we learn to release in Śavāsana. We learn to let go of the past and come into the present moment within our classes and within our lives.

As a teacher, I found that if I took on many classes and responsibilities and did not have time to deepen my own practice, it was possible to become dry inside and weary in body, mind, and spirit. I was feeling that weariness many years ago, until Mr. B.K.S. Iyengar said: "Practice twice as much as you teach." As I began to implement his advice, I discovered a wellspring of love and a true desire to serve. These words arose out of the depth of my soul: "To love is to go on teaching forever without growing weary."

I taught only when invited and discovered that I taught not so much for others but for the refinement of my own evolutionary unfoldment. As my understanding of the practices deepened, they brought me into ever deepening layers of consciousness. During class, I found it was possible to convey the essence of yoga not only through the spoken word, but also by allowing the words to be used as a vehicle for the universal presence to guide and inspire. Words convey energy: The Śakti of the masters reflects through the spoken word as well as through the teacher's silent presence.

Now, however, I find it a challenge to convey this feeling through the written word. It seems difficult to crystallize in writing what is a continual organic unfoldment of the practices. I hope that my reflections will encourage readers to seek their own experiences through the practices that explore the vast universe that lies within. We are always in the flux of change; nothing is solid. This book is not an end, but only a beginning of Self and Universal exploration. For me, it is a reminder of the evolution and integration of yoga in our world of today.

What is presented here may at times seem different than traditional approaches. It is not meant to confuse but only to share personal experiential understanding. Even though there are yoga traditions that are eternal and unchanging, there are also evolutionary spikes and spirals occurring in the U.S. yoga community as we find new ways to incorporate yoga into our everyday lives. We no longer have to go to the mountaintops but can now find the mountaintops in the marketplace.

Held within each āsana is the mythology linked to its name and the geometrical patterns of the cellular structures of creation. Through the practice of yoga, we can let our hearts convey our love of all humanity and the Divine essence of all creation. We do this when we caress our feet upon the earth in standing poses, when our toes and heels reach for the center of the sun in inverted poses. We can let our love for the Divine reflect in the ceremonious offering of our upper to lower body in forward bends. Āsanas reflect the art and beauty of the communion of Self with the Universal. They help us release the impediments that shroud the light that is always shining. We are not "becoming One with" but realizing the Oneness that already is. This is the Union of Yoga.

Blessings and prānaṃs to you always.

—Rama Jyoti Vernon

A Message to Yoga Teachers

There are no teachers; we are all students, bound together in infinite expansion of growth and exploration. We are not teachers, and yet we teach—not with the attitude of a great yogi or yogini, but as a servant or fellow seeker joyously sharing with others the knowledge and training we ourselves have found.

Together we ascend life's ladder, reaching for the light within the darkness. Ladened by karmic burdens, some cannot climb as swiftly as others. Those on rung six may reach out to help those on rung four, at the same time embracing the guiding hands of those on rung seven. In this way we come to be of service to humanity in the ever-unfolding quest for peace and enlightenment.

Be fearless as a fellow-seeker. Joyously share with others the riches you yourself have found through Yoga. We are all perennial students of Yoga. Teaching is simply the outgrowth of our own experiences. There is always more to learn, more to remember, more to realize, and more to share.

In moments of doubt, do not dissipate the positive forces of energy in feelings of unworthiness, remorse, or self-pity. Remember, you are a necessary part within the cosmic machinery. Insignificant as this part may seem to you, without it, the machinery cannot function.

Transcend environmental obstacles. View them as a test of the Divine. Within the cosmic plan there is a reason for each and every opening of life's pathways. If you are led to the path of a teacher, then let go and let Divine will work through you; the barriers to spiritual expansion will drop away.

Place your heart and soul within the teachings. Teaching yoga is not a business, not even a profession. It is a privilege and a blessing. See the Divine within your students and let your teaching be the worship of their universal truth and beauty.

Avoid attachments to a desired result. Remember Kṛṣṇa's words from the Bhagavad Gītā (VI:1): "Whoever does the work to be done without resort to its fruits, they are the Sannyasin and the Yogin, not the one who lights not the sacrificial fire and does not the works." Think of the classes and your teaching as āsana. Once we leave an āsana, the posture belongs to the archives of the past. Move within it to the very best of your ability, but when it is over, let go physically, mentally, and emotionally.

Do not indulge in distorted proportions of overconfidence or power fantasies, nor concern yourself with spiritually enervating thoughts as to whether it was a good class or a bad class, or whether you are a good teacher or a bad teacher. You are an instrument of the Divine; be not affected by criticism or compliment, praise or blame. As we teach, so we will be taught. Again, remember the wisdom of the Bhagavad Gītā (XI:9): "Nor do these works bind me … for I am seated as if indifferent above, unattached to these actions."

When we follow a yoga path, we follow a designated practice that clears pathways for experiential knowledge of this universal truth. The networks, methods, and practices are numerous and at times appear to be in conflict with one another. Within the confusing framework of learning, consider that there are as many methods as there are masters and teachers. Be respectful to all those who have gone before and to those who are emerging as the future light bearers of Yoga. For our own light of remembrance, it is important not to condemn, ridicule or vehemently oppose any system. We all gravitate towards that which seems more in harmony and keeping with our inner nature. Those balanced on the outer rims of independence and individualism would surely be excluded if there was only one way, one method, one teacher, one pathway to Self and universal awareness.

Teaching is not an excuse to neglect your own practice. Rather, allow your teaching to be the outgrowth of your practice. Believe and practice what you teach and teach what you practice. As your practice deepens, so too will your teachings. If you neglect your own practice, your words and teachings may become ineffectual and your stagnation will result in spiritual dehydration.

Teaching yoga is a practice in itself, an offering. As teachers, we cannot take a student farther or deeper than we have gone ourselves. A teacher creates a mood or invokes a mantle that invites the invisible presence into the class to protect, guide, and inspire students to reach the fullest expression of yoga, not just within a pose, but within one's life and one's own Being.

Be secure within the knowledge that the cosmic intelligence is working through you. Remove your will so that THY will may be done. You are the instrument in the hands of the Divine. Allow this instrument to be moved with ease, harmony, and the graceful precision of love.

Introduction

The Hidden Meanings of Haṭha Yoga

In the West today, the practice of yoga is usually understood to mean physical movements or body postures. However, there are six major branches of yoga, each designed to evolve with man's—and woman's—needs, whether they be emotional (Bhakti Yoga), intellectual (Jñana Yoga), vital (Tantra Yoga), mental (Rāja Yoga), or physical (Haṭha Yoga).

Over the centuries, Haṭha Yoga fell into disrepute among yoga philosophers who feared it might create too much bodily preoccupation and spiritual distraction. However, rather than dismissing it as an exercise only for the body, ancient writings about yoga uphold that Haṭha, one of the earliest yoga traditions, evolved as a spiritual practice to meet the connubial needs of the householder. The legendary origins of its beginnings date back to the mythological time of the great God of the Hindu pantheon of deities, Lord Śiva. It was during a discourse by Śiva to his consort Pārvatī that Haṭha and Tantra Yoga are said to have emerged.

The Polarities

The practice of yoga is based upon the bilateral integration of polarities. It is finding the nexus of the equinox within. The back body is like the winter of Self and is equated with the seat of the subconscious mind, relating to the back brain or cerebellum. The front body is like the effulgent light of spring, represented by the frontal brain or cerebrum, the seat of the conscious mind. Yoga is meant to bring together the front and back, right and left, upper and lower polarities. The union of these polarities is known as Ha-Ṭha Yoga.

Ha means "sun," and *ṭha* means "moon." In this instance, the sun, progenitor of light and life, is compared to the projectile energies of male, and the moon to that of the receptive and spatial energies of female. The ancient scriptures are filled with symbolic names and meanings for the forces of sun and moon. This bipolar and magnetic relationship is representative of all opposing forces of creation, such as day-night, light-darkness, and positive-negative. It is even found within the dual balance of psyche-soma, logos-eros, yang-yin, and masculine-feminine.

The masculine principle of creation is known as *puruṣa,* meaning "to fill with the dawn." Puruṣa is spirit. It is the substratum of being and beyond time. It is the center within the body and in the universe that is unmoving, changeless, and eternal. The feminine principle is known as *prakṛti,* which means "to bring forth doing or action." Prakṛti is the element of time that manifests through our third-dimensional world of form. It is the silent convergence of day and night expressing itself through the seasonal changes and cycles of birth, life, and death. It is the evolutionary field of change and transformation that manifests in multiple forms of creation. It is the feminine principle of matter, nature, and form.

In the practice of āsana, we usually identify with prakṛti—the action or "doing"—which can be seen in the way the limbs unfold with each variation. We don't often identify with puruṣa, the bindu or seed point that is unwavering and unmoving. The bindu is the point at the center of all yantra and all āsana. If we can simultaneously identify with puruṣa and find the seed point or bindu within the body in each āsana, and allow the limbs to unfold from that center point, we balance the polarities of puruṣa and prakṛti. Then, no matter where the limbs are or what āsana variations we are in, we can experience the timeless state of being balanced between puruṣa and prakṛti, being and doing. This is the inaction within action that Śrī Kṛṣṇa speaks of in the fourth chapter of the Bhagavad Gītā. This is how we find the place of stillness no matter what is going on around us. This is the profound practice of "being in the world but not of the world."

Eastern and Western practitioners speculate that on a physiological level, puruṣa and prakṛti relate to the two hemispheres of the brain and their intellectual and intuitive correspondents, as well as to the balance between the two divisions of the autonomic nervous system (sympathetic and parasympathetic). The right side of the body carries the masculine solar energy that relates to the sympathetic nervous system and the left hemisphere of the brain. In the subtle body, this is known as *piṅgalā.* The left or feminine side of the body carries the lunar energy and relates to the parasympathetic nervous system (which is dilating and cooling like the moon) and the right hemisphere of the brain. In the subtle realm this is known as *iḍā.* It is the autonomic nervous system that brings about alternating changes in constriction-dilation, acid-alkaline balance, and the catabolic-anabolic processes of the body. Thus, Haṭha Yoga demonstrates the ultimate liaison between the central nervous system (the brain and spinal cord), and the divisions of the peripheral nervous system, which control the voluntary and involuntary functions. Since the yogi does not separate mind from body, this also shows the respective liaison between the conscious and subconscious reflexes of the mind.

Nature demonstrates the meeting of light and dark at the setting of the sun and the rising of the moon, and where one season silently merges into the next. In yoga, we find the same convergence where the brain's right and left hemispheres, the body's front and back sides, and the spine's top and bottom poles meet in the equalization of the polarities.

Yoga as Union

Yoga is one of the six philosophical systems of India. The word *yoga* can be interpreted from the Sanskrit root *yuj,* meaning to yoke, bind, or join together. As yoga would be a unifying force of the polarities of *ha* and *ṭha,* Haṭha Yoga would be a dynamic state of being in which there is complete equilibrium of the alternating and dualistic forces of creation. Hence, yoga refers not only to a state of unified oneness but also to the methods that can bring one to that state. As I often tell students, yoga is remembering that we are already one. How can we join anything that has never been separated? There is nowhere to go and nothing to do but to be and breathe and remember the oneness that already is.

Swami Satchidananda, founder of Integral Yoga and a disciple of Swami Sivānanda of Rishikesh, was once asked if he was a Hindu. He thought quietly for a moment and then answered slowly and pensively, "I like to think of myself not as a Hindu but more as an 'Undo.' " Instead of "doing" yoga, perhaps it would be more accurate to say we are "undoing" through yoga. What is our rush? There is nowhere to go, only to realize that we are already there. Our practices are meant not to create more division, separation, competition, and pain, but to undo the impediments that keep us from realizing that we are already One with the universal source.

All of creation emanates from the one universal source. When we once again reunite through the experience of oneness and union with all fellow creatures, we become established in Yoga (Union). Union is Yoga and Yoga is the pathway to Union or Reunion. Yoga is non-dogmatic. It is not a religion but is the essence of all religions.

Although the practice of Haṭha Yoga, from all outward appearances, seems to be involved with the body, the body's role is as an aid to understanding the mind. In the hierarchy of body and mind—as in the cyclic distinction between the chicken and the egg—it is difficult to tell which has the most profound affect upon the other. When someone is experiencing an ecstatic state of happiness, the body seems to remain relatively free from sickness and fatigue. However, when one is in a depressed mood, the body becomes easily tired and susceptible to varieties of viral influences.

As it is accepted and determined that the mind has a definite affect upon the body, in Haṭha Yoga, it is found that the reverse is also true: The systems of the body affect the mind. Haṭha Yoga is found to be a therapeutic aid to lessen the physical pains, stresses, and illnesses that can serve as a detrimental distraction of one's mind and dedication.

In application, Haṭha Yoga systems vary, but in general, they consist of five parts (1) *āsana* (postural movements), (2) *prāṇāyāma* (breathing), (3) *bandhas* (locks), (4) *kriyās* (cleansing processes), and (5) *mudrās* (seals and gestures). Each of these five steps has both an external and internal significance. The mudrās, for example, outwardly appear to be only ceremonious symbolic offerings performed with the hands. But, inwardly, on a more esoteric level, mudrās are experienced as the silent gestures of all Indian philosophy combined: They are the seal of the mind with the soul, and the mind expressing itself through the body. The external aspects of the kriyās can be seen in the physical processes designed to remove toxins and blockages from the system. Internally, the kriyās can arise in breathing, movement, and meditation.

The bandhas are not only muscular contractions of the anus, navel, and throat, but are also meant to draw and direct prāṇa from peripheral nerve channels to specified locations within the spine. The word *prāṇa* is often used as a synonym for "energy," but we can look to its Sanskrit roots for deeper meaning: *prā* means "to bring forth," and *ṇa* is the eternal cosmic vibration. Even though bandhas are used mainly in prāṇāyāma, they can spontaneously occur within some āsanas.

The Symbolism and Significance of the Spine

In Haṭha Yoga practices, whether they be kriyās, mudrās, bandhas, prāṇāyāma, or āsana, there is a great deal of emphasis upon the importance of the strength and straightness of the spine. On the physical level, proper alignment relieves compression of the spinal nerve roots. When we look beyond the physical, we learn that the spine is poetically called the *meru daṇḍa,* the mountainous staff. This refers to the spine as being the central axis of creation.

All Haṭha Yoga practices center around the spinal nerve currents and cerebral interaction. The steadiness and erectness of the spine is extremely important in meditation so that energy may flow unimpeded between the spinal cord and the brain. If our posture is lax and our muscles unable to hold the spine erect for long periods of time, meditation will be distracted or it can take diverse courses, one of which is sleep.

There is a thin line between sleep and Samādhi. In sleep, the mind *(citta)* withdraws, affecting the central nervous system, evident because the sleeper cannot hold himself erect and must lie down to rest. In Samādhi, the posture is a mudrā. This mirrors the mind within the body. When the body maintains a pose even though it appears that one is in a sleep-like state, this is considered Samādhi. *Sam* means "to sum it up" or become one with. *Adhi* means "to stick to" or to hold a state of consciousness without lapse. This Sanskrit verb is also the source of the English word "adhere."

Samādhi is a remembrance that we are already one with the source of universal life intelligence and with all of creation. There are different forms and stages of Samādhi. Sometimes during āsana and meditation we have glimpses and go into the beginning stages of Samādhi, and then we come back to experiencing separative consciousness. Eventually, we may linger longer in the universal state of oneness.

A Hindu story illustrates the effects the spine can have not only upon the body but also upon the mind. This is a timeless tale about the continuous battle between the gods and demons who symbolize the light and dark forces. When the gods saw that they were losing the battle, they went to Brahma, their creator, with the problem. "Make peace with the demons," he urged. "Together you shall churn the ocean of milk until it turns into the nectar of immortality."

Acting on the advice of the lord of preservation, Viṣṇu, they used the giant mountain, Mount Meru, as a churning stick and the massive serpent called Ananta, twisted three and a half coils around the mountain, to pull and turn it. As the gods and demons proceeded to churn the terrestrial ocean of milk, poison appeared on the surface. In the crisis of the moment, they turned to the great lord, Śiva, who found the only safe way to dispose of the poison was to swallow it himself, which he did. He held the poison in his throat so that it could not spread to the rest of his body. Thus, Śiva became known as Nīlakaṇṭha, the Blue-Throated One.

With the release of the poison, amazing things began to happen. Out of the depths of the ocean appeared celestial animals, vegetation, gems, goddesses of beauty and harmony. At the very end, the celestial physician appeared, carrying in his hand the cup of the moon and within it, the sought-after *amṛta,* or nectar of immortality.

Symbolically, the battle between the angels and demons at opposite ends of the churning stick represents that constant conflict between the opposing forces of negative and positive, light and dark, expansion and contraction that exists within us all. The ocean depicts the depth and infinite vastness of the unconscious mind. The churning of the ocean of the unconscious is done through the mountain, which is representative of the spine. The spine acts as the churning stick when Kuṇḍalinī (represented as a serpent coiled three and a half times at the base of the spine) awakens. The poison represents the unresolved conflicts that lie harboring within the unseen depths of the mind and cannot be released and disposed of until the churning begins. The fear of both demons and the gods is symbolic of our own fear to quit the game and to withdraw to a point where the conflicts do not appear.

When the poison or conflicts were disposed of after they were brought to the surface, then the gems and jewels—what psychologist Carl Jung would call "the collective unconscious"—emerge in glorious patterns of beauty and harmony. These are symbolic of seeing one's own unconscious. The celestial physician, who has come to heal the ills of humanity, carries in his hand the moon, a symbol of the well-rounded or balanced psyche. The nectar of immortality (amṛta) that is held within is symbolic of the spirit of transcendent wholeness.

This ancient story illustrates the effects the body can have upon the mind. Yoga can bring up what is stored beneath the surface of the milky ocean of the subconscious mind. In āsana, the spine is extended, hyperextended, flexed, and laterally rotated. The movements are designed to strengthen the spinal nerve roots of the physical body as well as open the nāḍīs or channels of the subtle body. This in turn acts not only upon the limbs but also on the brain. The brain, the seat of thought, perception, will, memory and imagination, manifests from the human consciousness known as mind. We could accurately say that each time we affect the body, we also affect the mind. Āsana and prāṇāyāma are designed to bring up impressions stored in the psyche to the surface of the conscious mind for their release and healing. There is a saying in yoga: The invisible must become visible before it can be eradicated and transformed.

The Deeper Meaning of Āsana

Ās means "to be" or "to breathe." *San* is from *sam,* meaning "to become one with," and *na* is the eternal cosmic vibration. In āsana, we are breathing and being One with the eternal cosmic vibration. Āsana is a vehicle between the physical and subtle body. If practiced with breath, āsana expands consciousness. If practiced without breath, there is a contraction of consciousness. When we approach each pose as a Divine communion, āsana is no longer an exercise but an "innercise" where the inner secrets of the pose begin to reveal themselves. In practicing āsana this way, one honors and respects the body as a vehicle for self-transformation, not as an end in itself. Yogāsana is a mudrā; it is the vehicle of mind expressing itself through the body.

The Yoga Sūtras were compiled some 2,400 years ago by the sage Patañjali, who is known as the father of yoga. Commentaries on Patañjali's sūtras refer to there being only one pose, Dhyanāsana, the pose of meditation. In this pose, the head, neck, breast, and tailbone are in alignment with one another. This alignment can be found in nearly every pose, not just a sitting pose.

The first sūtra that describes āsana is s*thira sukham āsanam* (II:46), commonly translated as "take any comfortable pose." It would be more accurate, however, to say "take any pose and be comfortable." The term *sthira* is from the Sanskrit verb *stah,* which means "to establish steadiness," or to stay unwavering and unmoving. And *sukham* refers to that which is sweet, pleasant, or comfortable. If we were to define āsana as "pose," this sūtra instructs us to establish comfort and steadiness within the pose. Just as yoga is a state of union as well as a method that can bring one to that state, āsana is a state of steadiness as well as a series of postural movements that can help one achieve a stillness of mind in the midst of movement.

There are eighty-four basic āsanas. Their names are significant in that they depict all cycles of evolution, from the lotus and the tree to the fish and the swan. Birds, such as the pigeon *(kapota)* and the eagle *(garuḍa),* and four-legged creatures like the dog *(śvāna)* and the camel *(uṣṭra),* can be duplicated in the way the yogi moves the body. Postures are named for such creatures as the cobra and the scorpion as well as for legendary heroes of the Hindu pantheon. Describing āsana's deeper revelations, Mr. B.K.S. Iyengar, in his treatise *Light on Yoga,* says: "Whilst performing āsanas the yogi's body assumes many forms resembling a variety of creatures. His mind is trained not to despise any creature, for he knows that throughout the whole gamut of creation, from the lowliest insect to the most perfect sage, there breathes the same Universal Spirit, which assumes innumerable forms. He knows that the highest form is that of the Formless. He finds unity in universality."

Āsana as Sacred Geometry

The āsanas also take the form of maṇḍalas and yantras, as can be seen by the designs of the postures in which the body assumes a variety of angles, triangles, circles, and half-circles. Sacred geometry involves the universal patterns existing in the design of everything in our reality. It is seen most often in architecture, art, geometry, mathematical ratios, and harmonics. It is found throughout music, light, and cosmology. Sacred geometry governs the structure of matter and the energy to maintain that structure. It expands from the center and radiates outward. It also acts as a filter for light energy to be harnessed and focused, creating a holographic resonance from the microcosm of the human body to the Universal macrocosm. Sacred geometrical patterns are the ethereal blueprint for the arrangement and rearrangement of matter, which implies order within a system and how that system interacts with other systems.

Since the human body is the finite within the infinite, sacred geometry manifests through organs, glands, and all other anatomical and physiological systems. Each organ consists of its own memory in the shape of a hologram. Trapped emotions can create pain, malfunction, and eventual disease, exerting an influence in the body as well as on mind and its thoughts.

According to yogic philosophy, all matter comes into existence out of a single point known as bindu or point bindu. This point is like a rapidly spinning disk, out of which all of material creation flows. The point bindu acts like a zero point in time, weaving together geometric patterns that assume the shape of matter.

On a subtle plane, auras and cakras are the primary interactive points within the human system that hold the bodily structure together, establishing the basis for all things to occur. The gravity of the cakras sustains the cellular structure of tissues and organs in neat vibrational patterns. These patterns, which keep us from being pulled apart, can be seen as sacred geometry. As sacred geometry, āsana creates ordered space for a disordered field. The effect is a sense of peace that is not usually found in exercise. The prefix "ex" means to project outwards; thus, yoga can be thought of as "innercise." Āsana increases the psycho-physiological coherence within our physical and subtle systems.

In āsana, our bodies assume geometrical forms of straight and diagonal lines, circles, squares, and triangles, all signifying an aspiration of convergence from duality to a unified field of consciousness. These patterns resemble yantras, symbols of deities as forms of increased vibratory frequency, more subtle than a picture or statue. Yantras contain the five elements within their corresponding geometric forms. Like a magnet, yantras draw consciousness from the outer to the inner world. When yantra is combined with mantra, it is defined as tantra. The sound and form bring balance to the visual and verbal or, respectively, the right and left hemispheres of the brain.

In each āsana that takes on the form of a yantra, there is a seed center or bindu. If we internalize the consciousness in āsana, we will find this bindu, out of which the āsana organically unfolds. The limbs extend out of this procreative seed point, creating spaces within the body's cellular structure. When we create a vacuum or space, light comes in to fill it. (Disease can be thought of as an absence of light.) In āsana, the geometrical forms or yantras that the body assumes are force fields of energy. The body becomes a hologram of light, displaying a variety of forms and designs. Each is a condensed, crystallized experience of the Divine.

Through his emphasis on the specific, systematic alignment of yoga poses, Mr. B.K. S. Iyengar has given the world a gift. In working with him for many years, I found that alignment within the poses is not only for the anatomical and physiological balance of the body, but also to realign the individual's bio-energetic field through the alignment of the molecular structure around the body as well as within it. In other words, in yoga āsana, we balance the auric field of the body while creating bilateral integrative alignment. Through their myriad of forms, āsanas create energy fields.

As I continued to practice, I realized that āsana not only honors all forms of creation, but also is an invocation to the Lords of the Universe that manifest through diagonal lines, squares, circles, and triunes of the heavens. The yantras can be a focal point of visualization, concentration, and meditation. But even more, yantra can be an entryway to expand one's consciousness from one dimensional field to another. The body in āsana becomes a living matrix invoking Divine presence through the yantras and their presiding deities. In other words, as sacred geometry, āsana is an intersecting point through which the individual can connect and commune with the Universal.

Baddha Koṇāsana, for example, may reveal the form of the star tetrahedron, which is based on Divine equilibrium. This form of a six-pointed star is seen in Judaism as the Star of David. In Hinduism, the star is Śrī Yantra, the intersecting balance of Śiva and Śakti. Matter cannot exist without this equilibrium and balance. The star tetrahedron of Baddha Koṇāsana is a planetary merkaba—a vehicle of light or living field that responds to human thought and feeling. In Hebrew, merkaba means "chariot of God" (*mer* is "light"; *ka,* "spirit"; and *ba,* the body). The merkaba is composed of two opposing tetrahedrons spinning in opposite directions. In ancient Egypt, merkaba referred to rotating fields of light that could take the spirit from one dimension into the next.

The star tetrahedron is one of an infinite number of forms on earth and in the cosmos. The same energetic forms that pervade our planet reveal themselves in Āsana, which honors them through *nāmarūpa* (*nāma* = name, *rūpa* = form), from the humblest insect to the loftiest sage. Divinity can even be found in the word āsana: *as* is "to be" or "to breathe"; *sam* is "to bring it together with" or "to become one with"; and *na* is "the eternal cosmic vibration." In āsana, we are breathing and becoming (or being) One with the eternal cosmic vibration. This definition suggests that prāṇāyāma is actually embedded within each of the postures.

Indeed, breathing within āsana is vitally important. Breath restores energy to what we refer to as the aura or the light body. When we breathe in, the aura contracts or pulls in. When we breathe out, it expands. Individual consciousness limits the degree of expansion and contraction of the auric field and in turn limits the bandwidth of our experiences in life. Yoga expands consciousness. When we practice the yantras within āsana, it is important to move with the breath (especially on the exhalation). The breath is the subtle, invisible link between mind and body and between the gross physical plane and the planes of light, where yantra as sacred geometry originates.

Inaction Within Action

The yoga of equanimity is the doctrine of poise in action. This is what Kṛṣṇa terms the "inaction within the action" during his advice to Arjuna in the Bhagavad Gītā. Arjuna, the great warrior, is about to enter the battlefield that represents life, when Kṛṣṇa tells him: "It is the idea 'I am the doer' that binds one to Saṃsāra. If one is a silent witness of their activities, feeling as if 'it is done through me. I am a non-doer,' we free ourselves."

If we identify with the actionless self, no matter what work or how much of it is done, the action become no action at all. This is the inaction within the action. Through such a practice one's own karma loses its binding nature.

On the other hand, I may sit quietly and do nothing outwardly, but if I am thinking that I am the doer, I am then always in action, even though it appears I am sitting quietly. This is action within the inaction. The restless mind is doing the action even when the body is still and motionless. Actions of the mind are considered to be real actions. Nor can anyone even for one moment remain truly actionless, for we are driven to action by the forces of nature.

Kṛṣṇa says in the Bhagavad Gītā (IV:20), "Having abandoned attachment to the fruits [results] of the action, ever content, independent and needing nothing, we do nothing even while engaged in action." This is a form of śauca, the first niyama. In śauca, which means purity, our actions have no motive; they are done for their sake alone. This too is inaction within the action.

Śrī Kṛṣṇa continues, "The sage who has the knowledge of the Self knows the oblation, the fire and the instrument by which the melted butter is poured into the fire and that he himself has no existence apart from that of Brahma; does no action even if he performs actions" (IV:24).

It is believed that when the mind is in inaction while the body is in action, we work out past karmas, positive or negative, and do not accrue present or future karma. In āsana, if we can make the spine rajasic (active) and the head tamasic (inactive), the body and mind become sattvic (serene). We no longer "do" the pose; the pose is done through us. That is the inaction within the action.

As we learn the doctrine of action/inaction through the practice of āsana, the knowledge begins to spill into the actions of our lives. It can lead to purity of heart, absence from motive, and freedom from cycles of birth and death. This way of performing āsana helps us develop a balanced and peaceful state of mind even in life's most challenging times. In other words, the way we do the pose is the way we do our lives.

The Path of Perfection

In the Yoga Sūtras (II:47), Patañjali says *prayatna śaithilya ananta samāpattibhyām,* meaning that it is through relaxation of effort and meditation on the Infinite that āsanas are perfected. In this instance, perfection refers to steadiness, non-vacillation, and a sense of comfort. Even though the posture may not look to all outward appearances to be a relaxed position, inwardly there is an equalization of tension, which creates a dynamic relaxation. Although the frame of the body is firm and non-wavering, there is a feeling of physical as well as emotional lightness and well-being. This is what is meant by the inaction within the action and "meditation on the Infinite."

But is there really such a thing as the perfect pose? As the student delves deeply into the practice of āsana, the idealized image of how the posture should appear or even feel dissolves into the spontaneity of the moment. The conception that āsana is only for the sake of physical health and stamina gives way to doing the posture for the sake of doing it. We may begin the practice in hopes of getting somewhere or getting something from it, such as the release of tension or excessive weight. We may want a high or to awaken the Kuṇḍalinī Śakti. However, in the course of doing the posture for the sake of that alone, within that movement and that moment, a spontaneous state of meditation can transcendentally unfold. Without experientially grasping or striving, it simply happens.

Consider, as an example, one of the standing poses. Standing poses represent the vertical ascension of consciousness from the earth to the heavens. If the practitioner can feel at one with the earth while at the same time extending into the space beyond the body, and be at one within that space, then consciousness can distribute itself equally into every cell. Then the bodily awareness is not just on one or a few parts; it is everywhere. With just a devotional press of the heel into the earth or an inspirational extension of the finger to the sky, an ecstatic wave of energy can sweep through the entire system, bringing a tidal wave of bliss that wants to burst into an infinite sea of timeless joy. This is contentment that exists for its sake alone, not as a result of needing or wanting something one thinks will bring happiness. The experience of contentment is *santoṣa,* one of the internal practices (niyamas) described in the second chapter of the Yoga Sūtras.

On a more mundane level, we find that through the postures, we can learn in a compressed period of time to cope with a variety of circumstances. This can be done by continually exploring new postures and their variations so that there is a continual movement from that which is comfortable and familiar to that which is uncertain. One example of this would be learning to stand on the head or on the hands. For those whose feet have rarely left the ground, many hidden as well as obvious fears must be overcome to do a headstand. But, as one becomes increasingly familiar with moving through space and feeling secure in that suspended state, it becomes easier to let go of unnecessary support (such as the ground beneath the feet).

As one great yogi said, "learning to move from the known to the unknown in āsana is like learning to let go of the body gracefully at the end of one's life." At the root of our fear of the unknown is *abhiniveśa,* what Patañjali referred to in the Yoga Sūtras (II:9) as the clinging to life and the fear of death. Here, death represents the ultimate unknown.

To the yogi, the mind and body are not separate realities. In the most esoteric sense, āsana is a reflection of the mind manifesting through the body. Even though it's not actually possible to see the mind, its operative functions can be seen and monitored through bodily actions and reactions. For this reason, there are said to be a thousand variations on each posture. A thousand is an Eastern symbol for infinity. We could assume that this means that there are infinite ways in which to gauge, express, and explore oneself through āsana. As we learn to progress from one variation to a less familiar one with fluidity and ease, this skill cannot help but develop a new spatial relationship that spills over into our lives, giving greater flexibility as we move from one situation to a less familiar one.

It is also possible to see attitudes of aversions, inhibitions, fears, strivings, and desires for achievement in the way the body responds to an āsana. In other words, it is possible to see by our practice just how we live our lives. Excessive indulgence, transgression of the physical needs, periodic rigidity in the mental and emotional attitudes may show in the way the body moves or, perhaps, doesn't move. For instance, assuming a forward bend by bringing the head aggressively to the knees before the stomach is humbly brought to the thighs may indicate inward striving and eagerness for results. In conceptually trying to get to the finished point of the posture, we forsake its precision for its range.

The basic standing posture, Tāḍāsana (Mountain Pose), provides several examples of how the mind reveals itself through āsana. When the weight is distributed more toward the ball of the feet and the toes, the posture reveals eagerness and anticipation of the next moment. When the weight is heavier on the heels, the posture indicates a reaction or holding back, the attempt to recapture that which is behind. If the shoulders are rounded and the chest concave, the posture suggests fear or a defensive attitude. (It is thought that perhaps the weight of responsibilities, commitments, and even guilt is carried upon the shoulders and upper back.) The position of the head when standing can show whether we are oriented toward the future or the past. Ideally, the head is balanced over the base of the spine and the feet so that the body is aligned to the pull of gravity. If the head is forward, it indicates projection into the future, and if the chin is pulled tightly into the throat and the back of the neck is firm and taut, this might indicate withdrawal or retraction to the past. Thus, when practiced with precision and awareness, āsanas are condensed aids in learning how to set aside, both physically and mentally, preoccupations with actions of the past and future, allowing one to find greater energy within the spontaneity of the present.

Although āsana provides all the external bodily benefits that most exercises do, yoga poses are also physiologically capable of regulating such things as glandular imbalances, neuromuscular tension, and cardiovascular disturbances. Because āsana is combined with rhythmic breathing, it is a tranquil way of rejuvenating the body and refreshing the mind. This is one of the key differences between āsana and most forms of exercise. As the word "exercise" suggests a projecting out and away from oneself, an āsana may be thought of more as an "innercise." During innercise, it is possible to momentarily withdraw, whether through action or non-action, to that innermost core within one's Being to commune equally with body and mind through their link, the breath.

Though traditionally āsana is considered to be a prerequisite of prāṇāyāma, I have found the two are intertwined, and can be related to the practice of the other six limbs of yoga: *yama* (universal conduct), *niyama* (individual discipline), *pratyāhāra* (sense withdrawal), *dhāraṇā* (concentration), *dhyāna* (meditation), *samādhi.* All the yamas and niyamas—such as *ahiṁsā* (non-harming) or *tapas* (discipline)—can be experienced in āsana practice. So too is prāṇāyāma found in each āsana. Each of the limbs can be found in a single āsana. And every āsana becomes *dhyanāsana*—the pose of meditation. In Paścimottānāsana (seated forward bend), for example, we offer the upper body to the altar of the lower body. The upper body is the subject, and the lower body the object. When subject and object are separate we experience dhāraṇā. But as the upper body bows forward, there may be a feeling that subject and object fuse into one; this is dhyāna. If this state can be sustained, dhyāna flows into samādhi.

The Primal Power of Prāṇāyāma

Prāṇāyāma is comprised of two words, *prāṇa* and *yama.* In Sanskrit, *yama* means "to restrain." Yama is also the name of the god of death, and death is the ultimate restraint. The word *prāṇa* is often simply defined as absolute primal energy. But as all sciences and systems of yoga are centered on the knowledge and understanding of this substance, prāṇa is regarded as the sum total of all energy manifest within the universe. Prāṇa displays itself as motion, force, gravitation, and magnetism. It maintains the universal macrocosm as well as the microcosm of the body, giving movement and force such as growth, repair, circulation, nerve impulses, digestion, elimination, and respiration. As the most obvious manifestation of prāṇa in the human body is the motion of the lungs, prāṇāyāma is commonly interpreted as a restraint or pause in the movement of the vital breath. Looking more closely at the roots of the word, *prā* means "to bring forth," and *ṇa* is the eternal cosmic vibration. In practicing prāṇāyāma, we are bringing forth the eternal cosmic vibration, retaining it within our being. That is a very powerful thing.

When we breathe consciously, the act of breathing becomes prāṇāyāma. You can feel the difference: When you practice conscious, slow breathing, your cells vibrate at a different frequency. You experience a shift of renewed cellular energy when you convert the breath into prāṇa.

In referring to the relationship of breath with the body and mind, there is an analogous description found in the great Indian epic, the Rāmāyaṇa, where the sage Vaśiṣtha says: "For the motion of the chariot, which is the physical body, the creator has created the mind and prāṇa (vital breath) without which the body cannot function. When the prāṇa departs, the mechanism of the body ceases and when the mind works, prāṇa or vital breath moves. The relation between the mind and prāṇa is like that between the driver and the chariot." As both appear to exert motion, one upon the other, the sage continues by saying, "The wise could study regulation of prāṇa or vital breath if they desire to suspend the restless yearnings of the mind and to concentrate. If there is any doubt that the breath is an invisible link between the body and the mind, we have only to observe its altered patterns when angry, fearful, asleep, or in meditation. When angry, the breath accelerates, when fearful, it stops momentarily. When sleeping, it is considerably slower and deeper and when in meditation, the breath is subtle almost to the point of nonexistence."

In the second chapter of the Yoga Sūtras, Patañjali speaks about prāṇāyāma, the fourth of the eight limbs of yoga. It is said that if you can hold the mind still for twelve breaths, you can enter into different stages of yoga practice, such as pratyāhāra, or sense withdrawal. If you can hold that for twelve breaths, you enter dhāraṇā, or concentration. If you are able to concentrate on an object for twelve breaths, you enter dhyāna, the state of meditation. And if that state is held for twelve breaths, you go into samādhi. It sounds simple, but it is actually quite difficult to hold the mind steady for those twelve breaths or for twelve seconds. The more we slow down the breath, the more we slow down the waves of the mind. If the breath speeds up, the waves of the mind become hyperactive and agitated. It is the state of mind that is the essence of yoga. Prāṇāyāma practiced with a restless mind increases restlessness.

It is more difficult to slow down the circuitous wanderings of the mind than it is to slow the breath, but by slowing the breath, it is believed possible to slow the rapidity of one's thought waves. Through gentle rhythmic cycles of inhalation and exhalation, it is possible to bring about energetic tranquility of thought as well as action. This is the foundation of yoga, encapsulated in Patañjali's second sūtra: *yogaḥ cittavṛtti nirodhaḥ.* Yoga stills the fluctuations, storms, disturbances, noise, or confusion that arises in the field of the mind. I believe that yoga is not the joining or yoking of the individual soul (Ātman) with the universal (Brahman) but, rather, a methodology that releases the impediments that keep us from realizing that we are already one.

The Integration of Breath

Although my early approach to teaching yoga emphasized form and structure, I felt a need in later years to move to a more organic, integrative approach to the postures, emphasizing the breath above all. This approach, relying on the breath to lead the movement, allows the gentle and natural unfolding of each pose, in which the student discovers a state of inner poise within any dynamic posture.

In the classical yoga tradition, one inhales when moving away from the midline of the body and exhales when closing the midline. This makes logical sense because the diaphragm drops down to expand the lungs on the inhalation and rises on the exhalation to expel toxins from the lungs. However, particularly in our culture today, people tend to focus more on the front part of the body. This is why most people associate their lungs only with the front body as opposed to the back and sides. The front body represents futuristic thinking. When we identify with the front body, the mind is always on the next moment in anticipation of the future. This keeps us in reaction rather than action. In yoga, we learn to *act* out of clarity rather than *react* out of confusion.

I saw how this relates to breathing patterns one day in 1969, during a class from Jean Bernard Rishi and Karin Stephan, also students of Mr. B. K. S. Iyengar. The way that they guided the breath impressed me. They placed their hands on students' backs while they were practicing Child's Pose and asked the students to breathe into their hands. As I did this for students, I found that when I lightened my touch as they breathed in, it was almost as though I could pull their backs up toward my hand. And then, as I progressively adjusted the pressure of my hands downward along their spines, they could expel more from the lungs. During this practice, the students became very calm and quiet, as if in an altered state of consciousness. They weren't so front-brain oriented, which is the way most of us live, in the frontal lobes or thinking part of the mind.

We access the conscious or thinking part of the mind whenever our eyes are open. When our eyes are closed, we access the subconscious, the unseen recesses of the mind, the intuitive parts of self. Yogis relate the back brain, the cerebellum, to the posterior nerves of the spine and to the subconscious regions—the involuntary, the parts we cannot easily access. The back body in yoga has always been known as the intuitive part that we can't see. In yoga, it is known as Paścima, referring to the Lord of the West, the side of the setting sun. This is the root of the pose known as Paścimottānāsana, the pose of the West side or back of the body, where the sun sets. And when the sun sets, there is darkness: We cannot see, so we must feel.

Yogis relate the frontal lobes of the brain to the anterior nerves of the spine, the part we can see, represented by Pūrva, the Lord of the East. When the sun rises in the East, we can see. The āsana known as Pūrvottanāsana is the stretch from the front side of the body, representing the presiding deity of the East and the rising sun.

This ties in with Ha and Ṭha, the sun and the moon, the light and the dark, and all the polarities that we balance through our practice. While we often think of polarities of right/left and top/bottom, rarely does a person think of the back. When doing this style of "back breathing," I experience a sense of deep inner peace. I feel like I am dropping into a region in the back body, a place so highly intuitive it borders on prescience. I realized that this was the way to access the subconscious, the hidden part of mind we cannot see. And I understood: This is one of the most powerful practices in yoga.

Back Breathing

I introduced this breathing exercise into my own classes. As I worked with students, I saw that I could take this style of breathing into āsana. Many years later, around 1980, I was studying with Angela Farmer in England and Greece. She too had come into working in this way, emphasizing the breath and bringing it into the precise alignment of the Iyengar method. The result was to allow the pose to evolve organically from the breath.

Angela said that if you observe an infant sleeping on his stomach, you can see the spine rise and fall, indicating that the child is breathing into the back. So I watched my own infant daughter, and sure enough, she was breathing into her back.

When we begin by breathing into the back and then take this breath into a pose, we bring the full force and totality of being into that pose. We find basis for this from medical and anatomical studies, even from language. *Phreno-,* the Greek root that refers to diaphragm, is the root of the words "frenetic" and "frantic." The term schizophrenic literally means "split diaphragm." Researchers have found that people with schizophrenia rarely, if ever, breathe below the diaphragm into the abdominal cavity. They tend to focus the breath above the diaphragm in the front upper regions of their chests. Yet when we breathe frontally, we create more freneticism and franticness—more of this hyper-energy that our culture is known for. I believed that slowing the breath—lowering it below the diaphragm and emphasizing the back body—could calm the mind, slowing down the *vṛttis,* the mind waves. Once I dedicated myself more deeply to this style of breathing and started to incorporate it into the poses, I found that every pose became a moving meditation, and I could experience a true, deep, inner stillness no matter what the body was doing. According to the Yoga Sūtras (I:2), this is the essence of yoga, to still the mind.

Angela said something in class one day that particularly resonated with me. She said: "Inhale, do nothing, and let the breath spread horizontally across the back." Practicing this way, I found that all of a sudden my shoulder blades were like the wings of a bird, carrying the arms out like the extension of the wings. I felt as though I were stretching across the plane of the earth with my consciousness. When it was time to exhale, instead of dropping into myself on the out-breath, I lifted up and allowed the spine to elongate on the exhalation.

We have a tendency to inhale while lifting the shoulders and exhale while collapsing the spine. What I found was that I could inhale and simply hold the space, creating an awareness of the horizontal movement of my back—from my shoulders, to the lower ribs, to the hips, moving laterally with the in-breath. Instead of collapsing as I exhaled, I elongated vertically to grow up out of the space the inhalation created. When I breathed this way, the waves of the mind stayed very still, no matter what I was doing. Whether I was sitting, walking, eating, or practicing āsana, I could keep the mind still just by visualizing the horizontal expansion and vertical ascension of this breath, like an eagle taking flight.

From here, it was easy to go into that meditative state. The breath was the link. In yoga, breath is known as the invisible link between the mind and the body. It is a bridge. If we practice āsana without the breath, the mind becomes agitated. The way to still the mind is through the breath. The breath is a grosser manifestation of mind. When we breathe into the back, we give space for the breath to open the unseen parts of the mind that allow us to find dhyanāsana, the pose of meditation, in every pose.

Moving From the Exhalation

Realizations often come to me while teaching and practicing. From my Sanskrit lessons, I learned that *ahaṁ* means "I am" and *kāra* (from *kri*) means "to do" or "to act." Therefore, *ahaṁkāra* is the word for ego, and it means "I am doing." My wonderful Sanskrit teacher, Dr. David Teplitz, helped me make these associations. The inhalation is ahaṁ, meaning "I am." The first time a fetus takes a breath, it becomes a human being. On that first breath, the child's individuated consciousness, which is its ego, is established. This is the first moment we experience our separation from Source.

In Āsana, it is on the inhalation that the ego, ahaṁkāra, asserts itself. If we inhale as we move into an āsana, then the ego is guiding us into the pose. On the exhalation, the ego relinquishes itself. Thus, if we move on the exhalation, we move without ego into the pose. We do not accentuate the ego, and we are not moving with self-will but instead let divine will move us. Moving from the breath creates a fusion; Divine will and personal will come together to do the pose. It is as if āsana is being done through us rather than from us.

In the Yoga Sūtras (I:34), Patañjali gives one of the many ways to create stillness of the vṛttis or mind waves: *pracchardana vidhāraṇābhyāṁ vā prāṇasya,* or "By exhaling and restraining the breath, the mind is calmed." He never mentions the inhalation. In more esoteric commentaries on the Yoga Sūtras, it is said that it is on the exhalation that the ego unravels itself. As we move into āsana on the out-breath, it appears we are not giving power to the separative consciousness of the ego.

Years later, I understood this was Angela's meaning when she said, "Inhale, do nothing." The inhalation is a time for us to take in spirit—inspiration—while the back body, which is intuitive, opens to the universe. On the exhalation, the spine elongates, offering the back body to the front body, uniting the seen with the unseen. This is a very powerful duo. When we move into a pose with the awareness of the back body as well as the front body, we create that mystic union between the cerebrum and cerebellum, the pituitary and pineal glands, respectively relating to the front and back brain. This is the convergence of the polarities that constitute this world. In the ancient classical teachings, it was said that in the moment when Śakti awakens, the prāṇa moves through the system, and the prāṇa moves the body spontaneously in the pose. By emphasizing the back breath, we can come into conscious awareness of allowing the prāṇa, which manifests through the breath, to bring us into an organic unfoldment of the pose. We can be like the rishis—the adept yogis—awakening Śakti through the breath and allowing it to carry us into āsana.

According to yoga philosophy, every conscious experience becomes a subconscious impression or *saṁskāra.* One aim of practicing yoga is to bring the subconscious impressions up to the surface. One of my yoga sūtra teachers said that the invisible must become visible before it can be eradicated—or as I prefer to say, transformed. This is one of the most powerful benefits of yoga. However, if we do the postures without emphasis on breath, it is difficult to bring the subconscious impressions (saṁskāras) up to the surface of the conscious mind where they become visible. As a result, we press them down, repress them, compress them, and embed them more deeply into the psyche.

So even though we practice yoga to bring saṁskāras to the surface, the nature of our practice can instead create more repression. When we relive these experiences in our practice, we are free of them. They do not manifest again. This is why Śrī Aurobindo Gosh calls yoga "compressed evolution." We don't always get the impressions out by the roots, however, and that's why the breath is so important to bring us into these deeper layers of self.

Some of our pain can be emotional pain that manifests as physical pain. When we get to the root of the emotional pain, it is possible for the physical pain to disappear. It is the moment when, as the Yoga Sūtras (I:3) say, *tadā draṣṭhu svarūpe avasthānam,* or "When the seer and the seen abide in his or her own form." We realize that we are already one with the eternal cosmic vibration. We have only to release the impediments and obstructions that keep us from realizing this oneness. There is nowhere to go, nothing to do, only to be. That's why we inhale, do nothing. It allows us that state of being, and on the exhalation we hold that state of being even in the doing. This becomes the inaction within the action. We can move deeper into the pose because the impediments that have held us back for so long dissolve away. The breath is the guide that takes us deep into the hidden chambers of the inner self.

Ujjāyī Breathing and Āsana

One of the great yoga breaths is *ujjāyī. Uj* means "upward," and *jāya* means "victory." Ujjāyī can be translated as "victory over oneself." This is another reason for moving and extending the spine on the exhalation. In the first chapter of Yoga Sūtras (I:12), Patañjali says one of the many ways in which to still vṛttis, the mind waves, is a*bhyāsa vairāgyābhyāṁ tannirodhaḥ. Abhyāsa* refers to checking the downward pull. *Vairāgya* means "dispassion" or, as it is usually translated, "nonattachment." One of the ways to learn dispassion or nonattachment is to breathe in, remain unmoving, and observe from a place of neutrality. If we give ourselves that space each time we inhale, we start to become less attached to having to go somewhere or get something out of a pose. We do the pose for the sake of the pose alone, and this spills into the rest of life. So if we are moving upward to victory (jāya), we are transcending the lower self or checking the downward pull (abhyāsa).

The ujjāyī breath, in which the glottis is partially closed, creates sound. It has a friction, creating a whispering sound like the wind in the trees. The mind becomes calm by listening to this sound. New research has shown that the ujjāyī breath tones the vagus nerve. This nerve, which originates within the base of the brain, interfaces with the cardiovascular, respiratory, and digestive systems. Through its effect on the parasympathetic nervous system, it is also responsible for peristalsis within the intestinal tract.

For people who exert a lot of physical effort in āsana, ujjāyī helps to keep the mind calm while the body is taking strong action. The sound helps them to hold to something, like holding onto a thread. For this reason, when I demonstrate āsana, I practice ujjāyī so that students can hear the breath.

Years ago, I was demonstrating this breath during a workshop on an island in British Columbia. It was a beautiful summer morning, and we went onto the deck overlooking the Pacific Ocean. As I instructed the class on ujjāyī breath during sun salutations, and amplified, primordial sound seemed to fill the air. I was impressed by the depth and power of the students' ujjāyī breathing, until I looked out to the ocean and discovered the sound was coming from a family of orca whales swimming by. That day, the whales became our teachers of ujjāyī, reminding us of the tranquility we can find within ourselves.

In the third chapter of the sūtras, Patañjali said that if you focus on the trachea, hunger and thirst will be subdued, meaning that we can overcome cravings. Thus, when we practice ujjāyī, and the breath creates friction as it moves into the trachea, cravings are abated. This illustrates how breath can have a profound effect on the brain.

Breath and the Brain

Through my practice I discovered the co-creative relationship of the lungs and the brain. Their tissues are similar. Whatever affects one will affect the other.

If we want to access the higher, more expansive centers within the brain, we would use the breath. The brain requires about 20 percent of our total oxygen consumption when we are at rest, and it's obvious that many of us don't breathe adequately.

Some people think we should only breathe abdominally. Others say we should only breathe above the diaphragm, intercostally or holotrophically. Most don't even mention the back in connection to breathing, even though the lungs are located as much in the back body as they are in the front.

My mother, who studied to be a surgical nurse, worked in the field of natural healing her whole life. She said that if we unfold the lungs, they would equal the size of a tennis court. This analogy shows how many lobes and alveoli are in the lungs and how many cells may not receive the nourishment of the breath when we are not breathing to capacity. Each time we change position in āsana and breathe to our fullest capacities, the breath has the potential to move into different folds of the lungs, stimulating and creating new neurological pathways in the brain. If we oxygenate the brain through the breath, whether it is ujjāyī, back breathing, or another form of prāṇāyāma, it is possible to intensify awareness and experience more expansive states of consciousness.

Changing Our Lives Through Breath

The breath of most yoga practitioners tends to be in the front upper body when they are moving into a pose. By breathing into the back, we will fill the upper, middle, and lower lobes of the lungs—from the back to the sides and around to the front. In doing this, consciousness expands equally, bringing awareness to the back body as much as to the front body. For most individuals, the breath usually rushes to the front in anticipation of a future action or to get somewhere in a pose. Since the way we do a pose is the way we do our lives, this may reveal how we rush breathlessly from one moment to the next or from one activity to another. By learning to breathe into the back, we have time to reflect and observe. We can then stay calm and centered in āsana as well as within life's actions.

I think we can also relate the breath to what is said in the Tao: "Remain unmoving until the right action occurs." Being still on the inhalation gives us time to be unmoving, to center our minds, our bodies. And *then* when we move, we move from a center of greater equanimity and calmness of mind. We don't move from confusion. I see so many people taking action out of their own confusion, and this seems to create only more confusion. When we breathe consciously, our lives begin to change, and we become part of the solution to life's challenges rather than adding to the problems.

When people have difficulty breathing, it shows an accelerated short attention span. As a society, everything we have is in twenty-second sound bites—no wonder people find it hard to settle into the breath. The essence of yoga is to still the waves of the mind. The sūtras tell us that if we practice prāṇāyāma with a restless mind, we will produce more restlessness. Likewise, if we practice āsana with a restless mind, we will produce more restlessness. Slowing the breath shifts this pattern. Whatever we bring to the pose is what we accentuate. If āsana unfolds from a calm breath, the mind will also become calm and serene.

The Divinity of Breath

The greatest gift teachers can give to their students is to give them the awareness of their own breath because the breath is God. Consider again the Sanskrit roots: The energy that is in the breath, or prāṇa, is from *prā,* to bring forth; *ṇa,* the eternal cosmic vibration; *ya,* yes, intensifying the action; and *ma,* to measure. In prāṇāyāma, we are bringing forth the eternal cosmic vibration into the field of nature in this third-dimensional "reality." Not all breathing is prāṇāyāma. But when we focus the mind on the breath, we convert breath into prāṇa.

The word *haṭha* is sometimes translated as "force." The *Haṭha Yoga Pradīpikā* (dating to the mid-1300s) describes pranayama very differently than the way Patañjali described prāṇāyāma centuries before. The *Haṭha Yoga Pradīpikā* refers to inhalation as *pūraka* and exhalation as *recaka.* Patañjali used different terms for the breath, *bāhya-vṛtti* (exhalation) and *aṅtara-vṛtti* (inhalation). *Vṛtti,* again, refers to the mind waves. The distinction is more like allowing the breath, rather than forcing the breath.

As we can see by the words describing breath, prāṇāyāma is more of a meditative practice. Inspiration means to bring in Spirit. Expiration means to offer the Spirit to the space and the world around us. We take that breath in with sacredness. In today's fast-paced culture, how often do we honor the sacredness of the breath? In āsana, when we move with the Spirit of breath, the pose becomes sacred.

The breath is the one aspect of the self that is both voluntary and involuntary. When we practice prāṇāyāma, the breath is consciously controlled. The mind, for most people, is involuntary, while the yogin's mind is voluntary. A yogin can even control citta, the subconscious parts of the mind that are hidden in what I refer to as the back brain, the cerebellum. The idea is to make the involuntary become voluntary. Then we can change and transform. We can make thousands of affirmations a day, but we will never make a change if the subconscious is not aligned with the conscious. When the subconscious and conscious parts of the mind are aligned, then we can make those shifts.

Through the breath, the yogin learns to make the involuntary voluntary. Even the autonomic functions of the body become voluntary. In the early days of biofeedback, yogis proved that one can slow or even stop the beat of the heart and activate it once again. Yogis can also slow the mind waves from beta to alpha to theta, as shown on an encephalogram. Thus yogis have demonstrated that if we slow down the breath, we slow the waves of the mind and the beat of the heart. If we do not put stress on the heart, we lengthen our earthly years. It is said the yogis measure their lives not by the number of days but by the number of breaths. The monkey, who is short-lived, breathes thirty-eight to forty-two breaths per minute. Humans breathe, on average, seventeen to twenty-one breaths per minute. The tortoise, the longest-lived of all species, breathes approximately four breaths per minute. Through gaining mastery over breath, the yogi can increase his or her lifespan.

But not all people practicing and teaching yoga are yogis. Some people can control the body and create the appearance of the perfect pose, but can they control their breath and their mind? Some people can stop the breath, but can they stop the anger they project toward another? If the way we practice is to allow the breath to move us, to allow Spirit to do the practice, something magical begins to happen. A single inhalation can go on for minutes, as if opening to the universe. It transforms hearts and emotions and strengthens the neural pathways to receive the light that is always shining.

Practicing Svadharma in Āsana

An important concept for every yoga practitioner is *svadharma. Sva* means "one's own," and *dharma,* which is commonly translated as "law" or "duty," is from *dṛś*, meaning "to see." Svadharma, therefore, means seeing one's own nature, one's own place, one's own life's purpose. When we practice svadharma, we are seeing our own nature, our own place, or that which is right for us.

In the Bhagavad Gītā, Śrī Kṛṣṇa, the universal soul, teaches Arjuna, the individual soul, on the battlefield that represents the opposing polarities of life. Arjuna wants to run away from the battle, not out of cowardliness or fear but out of compassionate regard for his fellow countrymen, his relatives, and his teachers. He does not want to slay those who were once near and dear to him. In trying to help Arjuna perform and follow his dharma, Śrī Kṛṣṇa tells him: "One's own work done imperfectly is far better than another's done perfectly."

This is an important verse to apply to life's purpose and mission, to the practice of yoga, and to the practice of āsana. In āsana, each of us needs to ask: Have I gone to the edge of what is right for me today, at this moment, or have I over-reached in the pose, which may have consequences tomorrow? Have I trespassed my dharma in trying to compete with others in the class?

The continual vigilance of *dhāraṇā,* concentration, is key to practicing āsana. Injury is possible during āsana only when the student: 1) forgets to allow the breath to unfold organically within the pose, 2) tries to achieve the goals of others, and 3) pushes violently into a position beyond svadharma, what is right for them. When we go beyond svadharma, injury can occur.

Coming to the Edge

A student who is not over-reaching his or her individual dharma in a pose may be deriving even more results than a student who is intent upon attaining a goal far beyond his or her reach. Svadharma is the exploration of what is commonly referred to as "the edge" of a pose. In practicing svadharma, we stay on the precipice of the pose only as long as the breath is calm, which indicates that the mind is calm. If the breath becomes erratic, and we are successful in calming it, this means we can stay a little longer on the edge or go as far as our breath will allow.

Some students may push beyond svadharma, what is right for them, but the opposite may also occur. Sometimes, when we come to "the edge," or what we think is the edge, there is an impulse to stay in a familiar comfort zone for fear of exploring a new variation. This can represent how we approach new situations in life. When we hold to what we think is a comfort zone, we may linger there, afraid of "going beyond." There may be a tendency to stay where one is rather than venturing into unexplored areas that represent unexplored regions of oneself. By using the breath and the vigilance of a concentrated mind, we become more discerning, able to recognize if we are over achieving or under achieving. There is a thin line between comfort and complacency.

In the psychophysiology of āsana, we can observe this in relation to life. Are there areas in life where we "under do" and other areas of life where we "overdo"? Usually, this will become evident not only when we explore the edge of a pose, but within the pose itself. For instance, in Adho Mukha Śvānāsana (Downward-Facing Dog), the upper back may be over-stretching because the pelvis and sacrum are holding back and not initiating an upward movement. When this happens, the upper body compensates by over-stretching as the lower body under-stretches. This creates conflict within the spine, which reveals possible conflict in the mind, which may reflect as conflict in an area of one's life.

Different Students, Different Dharmas

Returning again to the words of Kṛṣṇa, "One's own work done imperfectly is far better than another's done perfectly." We may transgress svadharma by coveting another's āsana, trying to be there ourselves even if we are not ready. This is addressed in the Yoga Sūtras in the third yama, asteya. (For more about the yamas and aṣṭāṅga, the eight-limbed path of yoga, see the appendix.) Asteya can be translated as non-stealing or non-coveting, and it encompasses not coveting the qualities or accomplishments of another.

Those who have a competitive nature may want to be where someone else is and strive for what they view as the full expression of the pose, in turn transgressing svadharma. In striving, we may forget the most important aspect of the pose, the breath. To "get the pose," we may stop breathing while still stretching the body. As a result, instead of opening internal space, we begin to close it and open ourselves to possible injury.

While it is humbling to back off one's edge to recapture the breath, which is the spiritual essence of a pose, it is helpful to remember Patañjali's sūtra (I:22) that recognizes the differences among students. To paraphrase: Yogins are of nine kinds according to their methods of practice—slow, moderate, and speedy. These methods have again three degrees each such as gentle ardor, medium ardor, and intense ardor. It is believed that students with intense ardor achieve samādhi quickly. In this case, "ardor" means detachment and aptitude combined with a feeling of reverence in devotional practice. Ardor is also enthusiasm and energy.

The three methods of practice (mild, medium, intense) are each divided into three parts, described by Patañjali as 1) mildly mild, moderately mild, and intensely mild; 2) mildly moderate, moderately moderate, and intensely moderate; and 3) mildly intense, moderately intense, and intensely intense.

A mild student has been likened to green wood—all smoke, but does not quite light and catch flame. A medium student is sometimes compared to dry kindling, one who is enthusiastic about learning and bursts into flame, though the flame is not sustained but appears extinguished ... then may reignite and burst into flame once more. An intense student of yoga is one who has sustained faith, enthusiasm, energy, and an intuitive feeling for or remembrance of the teachings. Intense does not mean aggressive or goal-oriented. It is ardor or sattvic *śraddhā,* which is serenity and reverential faith. This is considered to be the quickest method and the best means of attaining *kaivalya* or liberation, which is the ultimate aim of yoga.

These three methods—mild, medium, and intense—can be compared to the three Guṇas. The tamasic (mild) student takes more effort, but eventually the wood dries and can catch the flame. The rajasic (medium) student has an overly enthusiastic, up-and-down nature that is difficult to sustain. As students of tamasic or rajasic states continue with their practice, they can shift into sattvic states of awareness.

Sattvic (intense) students are steady and consistent in taking the practice far beyond the mat into every aspect of life. They maintain a steady flame of quiet enthusiasm and inner knowledge that will not flare up and then die out. The sattvic student keeps burning without end, like an eternal flame that ignites the light in others. This is known as *darshan,* from the Sanskrit root *dṛś,* meaning "to see." The sattvic or serene practitioner does not so much hear the words as feel the prāṇa or energy behind the words. It's as though the teachings reawaken something within them, a remembrance of memories stored within the hidden depths of being.

It is not what we "do" in the practice of āsana. It is the way in which we do it that determines if we are in svadharma or not. The one who does less may receive greater benefits than the one who does more.

Ken Keyes, the author of *The Hundredth Monkey,* is an example of practicing to the edge of svadharma. When I met him, he was paralyzed and living in a wheelchair. He demonstrated how he practiced yoga. He inhaled as he turned his head to the right and stayed there for as long as his breath lasted. He exhaled and brought his head back to center before taking this movement to the other side. As I watched him make this simple movement, I felt a profound and peaceful presence descend upon the room. He was in svadharma, exploring what was the full expression of āsana for him.

We Cannot Do the Same Pose Twice

Dr. Haridas Chaudhuri, founder of the California Institute for Integral Studies, once asked his students, "Can you swim in the same waters of the Ganges twice?" When I returned from a trip to India, where I visited the swift-flowing source of the Ganges, I told him that after trying to swim from one shore to the other and being carried downstream, I realized that not only could we not swim in the same waters twice, but I doubted if we could even swim in the same waters once.

This experience relates to a saying about yoga āsana, that we can never do the same pose twice. Each time we come to the pose, it is different. We can lose the reverence of the pose with the conditioned reflex of expecting it to be the same as when we practiced it previously, by crystallizing the āsana into the way it "should" be or the way it "should" feel.

If we did not have a good experience in this particular āsana before, we may come to it with resistance that tightens both body and mind, not allowing the fullness of the pose to reveal itself. On the other hand, if we had a wonderful experience in this āsana before, we may approach it with expectation. And if the pose does not come with ease this time, we might spend the entire practice trying to recapture the past experience.

However, when we come to the pose with a sense of devotion for the body as the temple of God, regarding the body as an altar of the Self, we will find that the āsana opens new portals of consciousness.

Many years ago, a visiting Buddhist lama was asked, "What is enlightenment?" He answered, "Seeing things as they are." I sat in puzzled silence for a moment and then asked, "How *are* things?" He laughed and explained: "This means seeing something that you've seen many times before but as if you are seeing it for the first time." He used a an object in the room as an example, but I thought of my husband and children, and how I'd categorized and compartmentalized them, not coming to them as if seeing them for the first time with wonder and appreciation.

Can we apply this lesson to the practice of āsana? When we do, it means coming to a pose with no past memory, but as if we are experiencing it for the first time. When we learn this through āsana, we are able to apply it to the people in our life—no baggage from the past, no judgments, no expectations, just being in the moment. By coming to a pose with the innocence of a clear mind and following svadharma, the pose will reveal its secrets, opening our eyes to the vast Universe within.

Letting Breath Be the Teacher

There are no clocks in the true practice of inner yoga. The breath is the mechanism that tells us if we can stay on the precipice of a pose or if it is time to come out of that pose. If the breath is calm, it means the mind is one-pointed and we can explore the possibility of going deeper into the pose. If the breath becomes rapid or erratic, it means the mind is scattered or disarrayed and it is time to back off the edge or even to exit the pose. If we practice āsana with a restless mind, it creates more restlessness. The object of yoga is to quiet the waves of the mind.

Injuries may occur if the student is not moving with the breath, whether entering the pose, maintaining the pose, or coming out of the pose. When we do not allow the movement of āsana to unfold from the organic expression of the breath, we close down the inner space where spirit reveals itself and, in turn, there is a tendency to over-reach and transgress svadharma. Overstretching creates a rubber band effect on the body. Instead of opening gradually into the inner sanctums of the pose, the body snaps back and closes the channels that bring light and knowledge of the deeper layers and true experience of yoga. We also compress organs and contract rather than elongate muscles. We stay only on the surface in the practice and cannot penetrate the depths of being.

Since breath is the invisible link between body and mind, it becomes the teacher, instructing us whether to stay in the pose or go deeper. It tells us whether to back off the edge of the pose until the mind is focused and one-pointed. When the breath is calm and rhythmic, it is the sign that we can proceed deeper into the pose.

Breath and the Five States of Mind

As the link between body and mind, breath is how we can perceive the five states of mind (mūḍha, kṣipta, ekāgratā, nirodha). In the third chapter of the Yoga Sūtras, Patañjali explains the five states of mind in reference to dhāraṇā (concentration). I have found that these states of mind relate directly to the five ways in which the breath manifests. The chart on page 30 relates the breath to the vṛttis.

FIVE STATES OF MIND AND THE BREATH

Breath is an Invisible Link Between the Mind and Body.
Our State of Mind Reflects in the Way We Breathe.

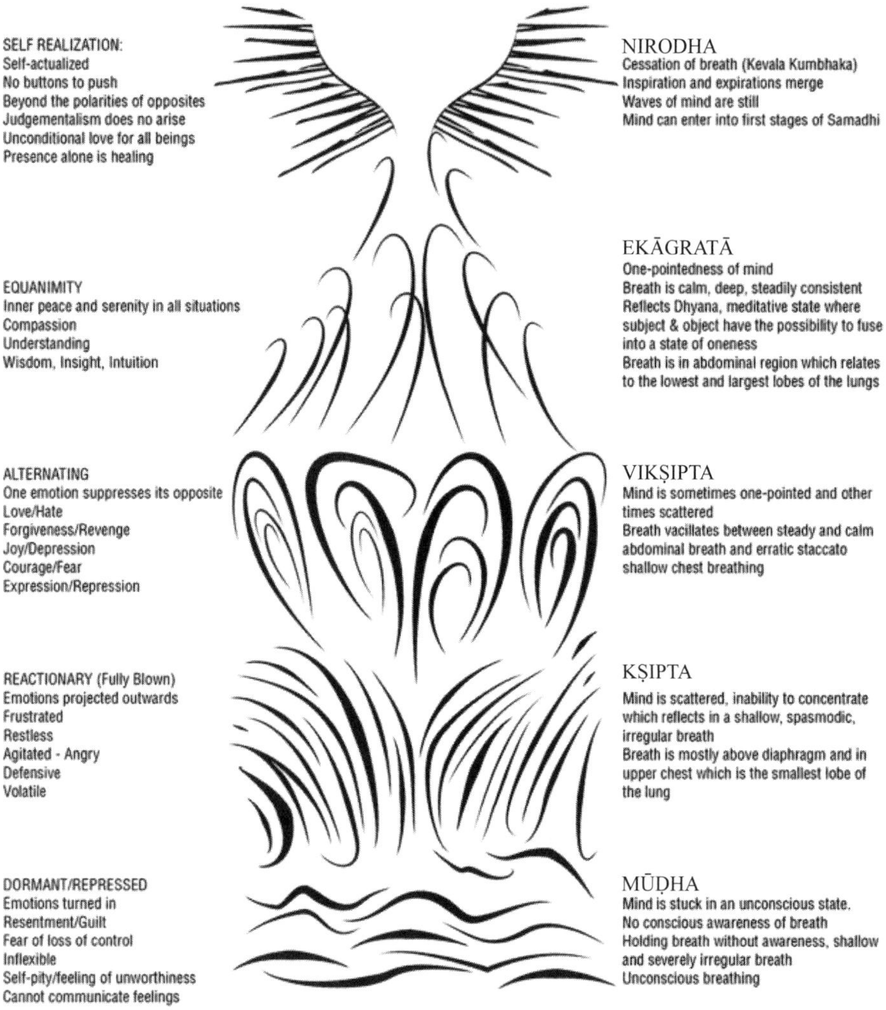
SELF REALIZATION:
Self-actualized
No buttons to push
Beyond the polarities of opposites
Judgementalism does no arise
Unconditional love for all beings
Presence alone is healing
NIRODHA
Cessation of breath (Kevala Kumbhaka)
Inspiration and expirations merge
Waves of mind are still
Mind can enter into first stages of Samadhi
EQUANIMITY
Inner peace and serenity in all situations
Compassion
Understanding
Wisdom, Insight, Intuition
EKĀGRATĀ
One-pointedness of mind
Breath is calm, deep, steadily consistent
Reflects Dhyana, meditative state where
subject & object have the possibility to fuse
into a state of oneness
Breath is in abdominal region which relates
to the lowest and largest lobes of the lungs
ALTERNATING
One emotion suppresses its opposite
Love/Hate
Forgiveness/Revenge
Joy/Depression
Courage/Fear
Expression/Repression
VIKṢIPTA
Mind is sometimes one-pointed and other
times scattered
Breath vacillates between steady and calm
abdominal breath and erratic staccato
shallow chest breathing
REACTIONARY (Fully Blown)
Emotions projected outwards
Frustrated
Restless
Agitated - Angry
Defensive
Volatile
KṢIPTA
Mind is scattered, inability to concentrate
which reflects in a shallow, spasmodic,
irregular breath
Breath is mostly above diaphragm and in
upper chest which is the smallest lobe of
the lung
DORMANT/REPRESSED
Emotions turned in
Resentment/Guilt
Fear of loss of control
Inflexible
Self-pity/feeling of unworthiness
Cannot communicate feelings
MŪḌHA
Mind is stuck in an unconscious state.
No conscious awareness of breath
Holding breath without awareness, shallow
and severely irregular breath
Unconscious breathing

The practice of āsana brings up kleśas, the afflictions or reasons for pain and suffering in life. These manifest as 1) *avidyā,* not seeing the nature of our Oneness; 2) *asmitā* or egoism, mistaking one thing for another (such as buddhi for puruṣa); 3) *rāga* or attachment; 4) *dveṣa* or aversion; and 5) *abhineveśa,* fear of death or clinging to life. When these painful mind waves rise to the surface where they can be healed and transformed, the breathing patterns change. Āsana provides an opportunity to calm the mind by calming the breath, even while practicing the more difficult poses, which reflect the more stressful situations in our lives.

The first state of mind that reflects in the breath is *mūḍha.* It is a dull state that is heavy, lethargic, or tamasic. I think of it as mud. When we are stuck in old obsessive patterns, it feels as if we are weighted down, unable to lift above or transcend the patterns. The breath reveals this state of mind by feeling stuck or appearing as non-breathing. The breath is held or even stopped at times, especially in stressful situations.

The second state of mind is *kṣipta. Keshe* means to throw out, scatter, or disarray. In this state, the mind is ricocheting from one point to another. The mind has a thousand thoughts and cannot focus. Fear, frustration, and anxiety are expressed through the breath, which is isolated to the clavicle region and the upper part of the torso. The breath stays mainly in the upper and smallest lobes of the lungs. The shoulders rise upward significantly on the incoming breath and drop on the outgoing breath. Large amounts of energy are expended with very little oxygen return. Extended periods of this upper chest breathing results in tension and fatigue to the shoulders and neck, respiratory diseases, and a chronically agitated mind. Like the mind, the breath is scattered and disarrayed, fast and shallow. If āsana is practiced with a restless mind, it produces more restlessness. During āsana, it is best to wait until the breath becomes calm before proceeding deeper into a pose.

The third state of mind is *vikṣipta. Vi* means to reverse, so *vikṣipta* means sometimes scattered and disarrayed and at other times more concentrated. Vikṣipta reflects as erratic breathing patterns in the upper parts of the lungs, while at other times, it may be calm, reflecting a one-pointed state of mind. The breath may move to the intercostal region of the torso and the middle lobes of the lungs, which are larger than the upper lobes. This breath pattern is usually seen when we are exploring a new āsana (or a new "edge" in a familiar āsana), when we are not quite sure where the pose may lead. Sometimes the breath is calm and one-pointed while at other times a kleṣa (such as fear) may arise, reflecting in the erratic nature of shallow and rapid breath.

The fourth state of mind is *ekāgratā. Ekā* is one and *gratā* is from *graha,* meaning "dwelling." Ekāgratā, which means "dwelling in oneness," is known as one-pointedness. It is a state of dhāraṇā (concentration), and it is the entrance to dhyāna (meditation), where there is sustained concentration and subject and object merge into one another. Ekāgratā is reflected in a calm, deep, and sustained breath. It can be felt as a sacral, pelvic, or abdominal breath, which activates the lowest and largest lobes of the lungs. This relieves pressure upon the heart and freshens the flow of circulation to the liver, kidneys, spleen, gallbladder, and stomach. Together with intercostal breathing, this breath massages the abdomen through the movement of the diaphragm. It has been used in asthmatic clinics and has been found effective in reducing high blood pressure and enlarged hearts. Breathing this way can calm and quiet the mind, and when practiced in āsana, it gives us the feeling that we can stay in a pose indefinitely. As long as this breath is prevalent during āsana, we can explore greater depth in any pose. This breath in āsana increases physical stamina, leading to greater confidence and trust in one's inner strength. It also strengthens and rebuilds nerve sheaths, which gives greater emotional stamina, and stabilizes the subtle body, organically opening channels for the light of illumination to reveal itself.

The fifth state of mind is *nirodha.* This means a cessation of the waves of the mind as one enters a samādhi state of awareness. Samādhi is when dhyāna (meditation) is sustained, leading to a total emergence with spirit. This state can be experienced within āsana when one enters the field of the yantra of the pose and communes with the presiding energy of that pose. There is a feeling of unification rather than separation, and the breath appears to be stopped. However, the breath of nirodha is a pole apart from the mūḍha breath, which is based on nescience and dense heaviness. In the nirodha breath, the incoming breath (ābhyantara-vṛtti) merges with the outgoing breath (bāhya-vṛtti). It is said that the breath stops in this samādhi-like state. Over the years, however, I have found that the breath doesn't actually stop. Instead, it is as if the incoming breath and outgoing breath are like rings of energy spiraling into one another, or as though the inhalation and exhalation are happening simultaneously as they spontaneously merge into one another. In this samādhi-like state, it feels as if we are no longer breathing ... but breath IS.

In the Yoga Sūtras (II:51), Patañjali refers to this state as *bāhya ābhyantara viṣaya ākṣepī caturthaḥ,* the fourth kind of prāṇāyāma that occurs during concentration on an internal or external object. This breath is known as *kevala kumbhaka. Kumbha* refers to retention, and *kevala* means isolated and absolutely pure. This is the breath in which the effortless retention is reflective of the stillness of the waves of the mind. Kevala kumbhaka brings consciousness into the first stages of samādhi. This can happen spontaneously within any āsana, demonstrating that wherever the mind goes, the prāṇa follows, and that breath and mind are inseparable. In the next sūtra, Patañjali continues that as a result of kevala kumbhaka, *tataḥ kṣīyate prakāśa āvaraṇam,* or "The veil over the inner light is lifted." The stillness of this breath reflects the stillness of the mind and fulfills the second and most important sūtra, *yogaḥ cittavṛtti nirodha,* meaning "Yoga is to still or quiet the waves or vṛttis of the mind."

The Methodology of Svadharma

We each have a different svadharma. What is right for one student at one time may not be right for another. What is right for us this day may change tomorrow. To stay in svadharma, we need to be vigilant and observant, and learn to be in the moment. The way to do this is through observing the breath, integrating prāṇāyāma into āsana.

When the body is aligned and we encounter pain in the pose, it is important to stop, stay in the pose and observe the breath. Is the breath calm and rhythmic or is it erratic and inconsistent? Can we breathe into the painful area and on the exhalation slowly spiral into the center to release the hardened outer layers that encircle the soft nuclei of the pain? Instead of plunging into the center of pain trying to deny or aggressively push beyond it, it is far more effective to circumvent pain by relaxing the surrounding areas. These areas may have built up psychological armor over time in order to protect their vulnerable core.

When you inhale, let it be a time of relaxation or doing nothing. The inspiration is a time to draw energies into yourself, to restore. On the exhalation, when the ego relinquishes or unravels itself, let the breath carry you deeper into the pose. Release a little more into the pose with each exhalation. As you come to an edge where pain arises, investigate its origin and its nature. Have you aligned the pose? What does this pain reveal to you? Why is it there? What does it need from you for its own healing?

On each exhalation, release more deeply into the pose and wait for a new understanding to reveal itself or a new door to open. If it does, on the next exhalation, enter into the opening that lies before you. As you practice the following āsanas, let the breath be your guru, the guide to lead you into the deeper labyrinth of the pose and the chambers of the inner Self.

The Postures
Āsana I sequence

Śavāsana

The Corpse Pose

Śava means "corpse."

Philosophical Introduction

One day many years ago, when B.K.S. Iyengar was staying at my home, a group of yoga teachers gathered for questions and answers. One of the teachers asked Mr. Iyengar why he practiced yoga. We expected a lengthy physiological response and were startled by the simple profundity of his answer: "So that I may die majestically."

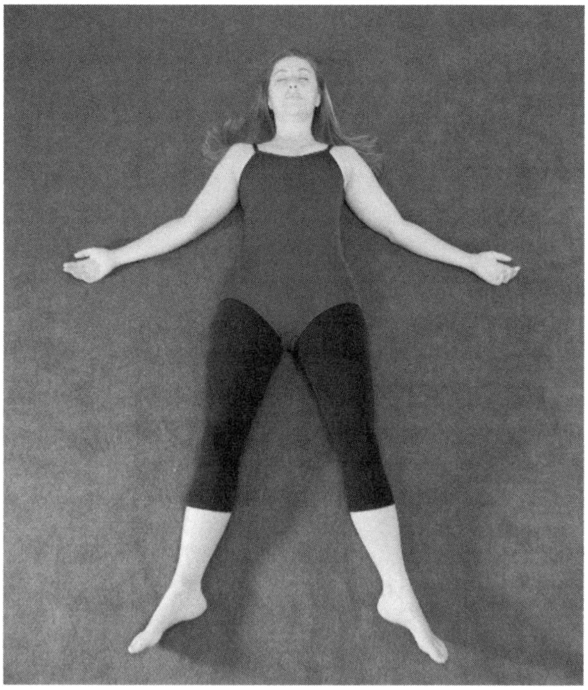

This statement reflects what yogis have said for thousands of years, that every day is a preparation for our last. According to Master Sivānanda Sarasvatī, "Our last thought determines our next birth." He elaborated that the last thought is determined by every thought that passes daily through the portals of one's mind. In yoga, it is believed that Eternal Life is not guaranteed, that we have to earn it. Śavāsana is a reminder that the end of one cycle is the beginning of the next. The pose also reminds us that energy can neither be created nor destroyed, only transformed.

Corpse Pose is one of the most difficult of all yoga āsanas. In it, we die before dying. It symbolizes letting go of the external phenomenal world. It is a form of pratyāhāra (one of the eight limbs of yoga), in which we withdraw the senses from the outer worlds and turn them inward to nurture the inner world. As our ego of the senses turns inward, we learn to die daily.

In Śavāsana, we withdraw from the dynamic activities of life and return to the bindu, the seed point present in all yantras (the sacred geometric patterns of existence). The bindu lies within the deep primordial central core of one's Being, where creation arises and returns. This is Śakti , or prakṛti, the feminine energy principal that gives momentum to life. During Śavāsana, Śakti retires within itself, returning to the seat of its own creation. Practicing pratyāhāra in Śavāsana is an opportunity to internalize the Śakti of the senses, which dart outwards as "doing," turning them back into a state of "being."

In the Tantra Śāstras, it is said that Śiva without Śakti is Śava, a corpse. In some manifestations, Śiva is depicted lying in Corpse Pose with the Goddess Kālī standing and dancing upon his body. (Kālī is also Kāla, referring to time, birth, life, and death cycles.) In this depiction, the corpse of Śiva is the resting place of Puruṣa, the timeless substratum of Being, the Immortal Self. As the corpse, Śiva—the immutable and instrumental cause of all creation—gives the foundation and impetus for consciousness to manifest into matter. Kālī is one of the forms of the Goddess Prakṛti, who manifests as the primordial cause of material existence. Prakṛti is the life force of the primordial dance of creation, the energy that is our heartbeat and breath, the prāṇa that moves digestion, reproduction, respiration, and elimination—the rhythms of all life.

The Corpse Pose is a pose of noninterference. This is a pose where we have removed the ego from disturbing the flow of prāṇa. When the prāṇas align themselves, the entire system can come into balance. Śavāsana is truly a time to relax, release, and let go, in body, mind, and spirit. It is a perfect pose to learn not only "how to die majestically" but how to live majestically and consciously in every aspect of our Being. If we can perfect Śavāsana, we perfect all poses.

Preparation

Śavāsana consists of several layers. As we learn to trust that the earth is there to support us, we learn to let go deeper and deeper with every outgoing breath, until the exhalation becomes much longer than the inhalation. Śavāsana becomes a time of surrender, and the outgoing breath carries us deeper into the center of Self. The incoming breath happens of its own accord.

There are times, however, when we cannot penetrate the first layer, and consciousness remains in the surface of our Being. We may even feel this as energy pulsating at the frontal brain toward the forehead. This may make it difficult to close the eyes. As we drop into the deeper layers, the prāṇa of the frontal cortex of the brain comes to rest upon the back brain (the cerebellum). When layers of protection and mistrust dissolve, consciousness sinks deeper into the mid-body. Eventually, as we learn to let go of the protective armor of lifetimes, we can let go into the back of the body and descend in consciousness ever more deeply until we fully surrender this body into the earth.

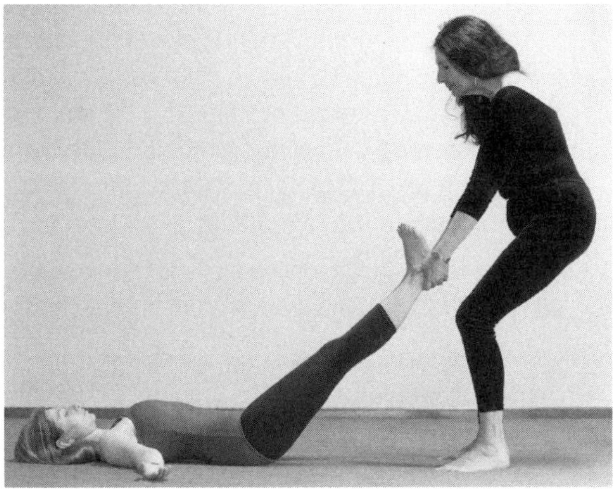

A teacher can assist students in preparing for Savasana by gently pulling on their heels to help them lengthen and relax the lumbar area.

Guidance

1. Lie supine on a mat on a level spot upon the earth or the floor. Hard surfaces reveal and release the tense areas and allow the body to relax. If you are lying on a soft surface, such as a bed, the surface will give way to tense areas of the body, which makes it more difficult to relax habitually contracted muscles.
2. Begin by bending the knees, placing the feet hip distance apart, and go into Setu Bandhāsana (page 91), Bridge Pose. This elongates the lumbar spine, which relaxes the frontal brain. Practicing Bridge Pose also helps flatten the sacrum to the floor, expanding the buttocks out away from the sacrum (meaning "sacred" bone).
3. Clasp the hands behind the head. Bring the bent elbows toward each other and, on the exhalation, lift the head, simultaneously elongating the back of the neck and the front of the throat.
4. Inhaling, keep the head lifted from the mat and feel the breath spreading across the back and widening the ribs. See if the breath will expand from the ribs to the hips, spreading out as much as possible across the back.

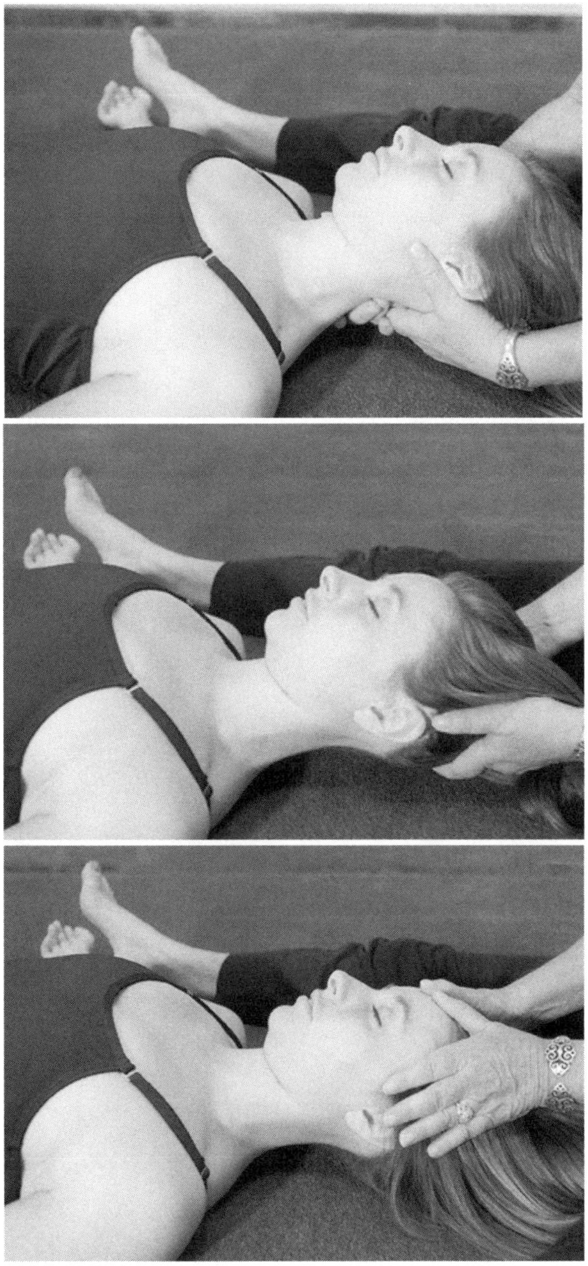

A teacher can gently lengthen the student's neck so that the base of the skull comes into contact with the mat, quieting the mind.

5. Exhaling, extend the neck a little more, and then rest the base of the skull (not the back of the head) on the mat. The hairline needs to be higher than the chin for the eyes to automatically close and draw inward, allowing the frontal brain to relax. If the chin is higher than the hairline, the frontal brain is active, preventing consciousness from deepening into the pose. If necessary, use a blanket to bring the hairline a little higher than the chin. Relax the frontal brain and bring energy into the cerebellum of the back brain, the seat of the subconscious mind. When the base of the skull rather than the back of the head is in contact with the mat, this quiets the mind and draws the sensory organs inward. When the head is in position, bring the arms to the side, turning the palms upward to receive the light
6. Inhaling, allow the breath to expand throughout the back of the torso, as this brings the breath into unused areas of the lungs.
7. Exhaling, keep the connection of the lumbar spine to the earth, as you slide one leg diagonally out and then the other (without lifting the feet from the mat).
8. Inhale and feel the breath widening the entire back of the body from shoulders to buttocks.

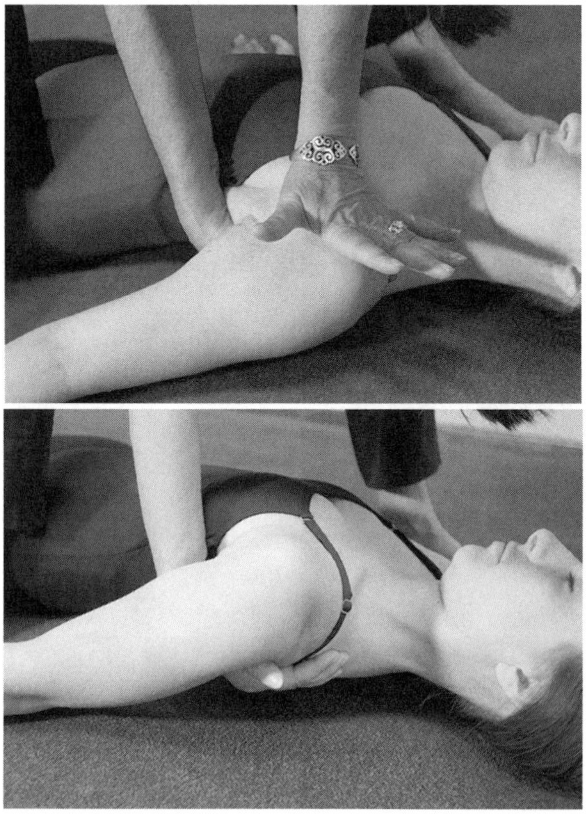

A teacher can assist by drawing the student's scapula downward while rotating the shoulder.

9. Exhale and allow the upper shoulders to descend, bringing the inner shoulder blades to the mat and widening the space between them. Now is time for the heart center, which is giving daily, to recede back into the center of the shoulder blades, as if sinking into the earth. Śavāsana is a time to receive and restore, not to give. Receive the energies of the heavens into the palms of the hands. Relax the fingers, which correspond to the five lower chakras (cakras), the five senses, and the sensory organs. Relax from the roots to the tips of the fingers.
10. Inhale and allow the breath to spread through the back body like wings.
11. Exhale and descend further into the earth, positioning the right and left shoulder blades and right and left buttocks equally upon the earth. Balance the back of the head, not from the alignment of the eyes, which can be deceptive because one side of the back of the head is usually flatter than the other. Instead, align the head by the way the breath feels in both nostrils. When the breath is balanced, keep the head in this position, and this will begin to balance the fluid in right and left hemispheres of the brain. Remember, the hairline is slightly higher than the chin throughout this process.
12. Inhaling, allow consciousness to soar horizontally across the earth plane with the back of the body.
13. Exhaling, relax the upper eyelid down to meet the lower lid without lifting the lower lid to the upper. Allow the ball of each eye to recede from the eyelids as if moving toward the back of the brain. Relax the lower jaw, letting it drop slightly away from the upper.
14. Inhale in such a way that the breath is gradually more refined. Eventually the inhalations become insignificant.
15. Exhale longer and deeper than the inhalations, giving the exhalation full attention. When exhaling, there should be no muscular contraction or tension. Exhalation is the act of allowing, rather than trying to make something happen.
16. Do not try to breathe in. Allow the breath to come in of its own accord, as if the Goddess Prakṛti, nature itself, is nourishing you with her own breath.
17. Let all the attention be on the exhalations, not trying to push the breath out but slowly allowing the breath to dissolve away. When you reach the

end of the breath, wait, watch, relax, and see if more space opens to let the breath descend more deeply into the inner sanctums of Self.

18. Inhale minimally, giving no attention to the incoming breath. Simply allow it to enter into the nostrils without friction, mentally moving the breath as close to the center of the nostrils as possible.
19. Exhale in a prolonged, deep, relaxed rhythm, allowing each breath to carry you deeper into the pose. Relax the sensory organs with every exhalation. Allow the eyes to descend toward the back of the skull. Relax the drum of the inner ears. Soften the breath as it flows from the right and left nostrils equally, without creating friction on the inner membranes. Relax the tongue from the tip to the base to the root. As you relax the head, brain, and sensory organs, the rest of the body follows.
20. Inhale to the center of the nostrils without touching the membrane of the circumference of the nostrils. This is the practice of ahiṁsā, nonviolence, when the breath entering into the body is so refined it doesn't even create friction upon these inner membranes.
21. Exhaling, disturb the molecules of air around you as little as possible.
22. Inhaling, bring the breath in as if it were already within you.
23. Exhaling, let the breath out as if there is nowhere for it to go.
24. As you relax the form, be aware of the space within and around the form. Be aware of the space between the sensory organs, between the arms and torso, between the fingers, between the legs, between the toes. Be aware of the space above and below the body. Allow each exhalation to lead you into the universal space within. Observe how far the outgoing breath will carry you into the deeper layers of the Self. (Remember, the ego dissolves on the exhalation.)
25. When it is time to come out of the pose, allow the incoming breath to lengthen gradually until it is equal to the outgoing breath. Allow the body to grow lighter, drawing in energy, light, lightness to every cell with the incoming breath. Grow even lighter with the outgoing breath as the subtle body lifts away from the gravitational pull and prepares itself for the activities of the day or evening.

Psychophysiological Benefits

It has been said that it is not in the pose but between the poses that we receive the benefits of āsana. In Śavāsana we receive the benefits from our practice at the deepest cellular level, and the pose is usually taken at the end of every yoga practice. If one gets up too soon after practicing without ample time in Śavāsana, the energy may drop later on in the day. If we spend fifteen or twenty minutes or longer in Śavāsana after practice, it will give a reserve of increasing energy.

Śavāsana can also be taken at the beginning of a yoga practice, preferably after Setu Bandhāsana or another pose that releases habitually contracted muscles. Śavāsana can be taken between poses that are done from a supine position, such as shoulderstand and Halāsana. It's especially beneficial after forward-bending poses ending with Paścimottānāsana. After āsana practice and between poses, practicing Śavāsana even briefly is an opportunity for the body to receive the benefits from the previous pose. Once habitually contracted muscles have released, practicing Śavāsana is an effective way for the brain and neuromuscular system to truly relax.

Śavāsana is one of the most difficult of all Yoga poses because it requires that we do nothing. Usually when we do nothing with our body, the mind remains active and restless. During Śavāsana, brainwaves are given every opportunity to slow down and rest so the body can repair and regenerate itself. It is important not to fall asleep in Śavāsana but to remain on the precipice of the relaxed alpha or theta brainwave states. (Theta is the state of hypnogogic imagery in which the collective psyche gives creativity and renewed energy). These brainwave states slow down the vṛttis or mind waves, which is the essence of Yoga and other spiritual disciplines. If the mind goes to sleep, however, the body wakes up, which is reflected in deep interior tensions. Tension in the body tightens the brain cells. When the brain cells are contracted, we cannot hear the Divine inner voice. When the senses turn inward and yet the mind does not go to sleep, we allow the neuromuscular system to relax and come to rest. When we let go, we open the channels, inviting the Universal consciousness to enter our Being.

As one goes deeper into Śavāsana, it can morph into Yoga Nidrā, the deep psychic sleep. In the deeper layers of Śavāsana, as in Yoga Nidrā, we learn how to drop into the deeper recesses of the unconsciousness and yet remain conscious. This is why it is important in Śavāsana not to fall asleep but to ride that thin line between sleep and Samādhi. This trains the consciousness to remain awake even while the body sleeps. Could this be what Mr. Iyengar meant when he said he was practicing yoga so that he may die majestically?

Śavāsana and the Kośas

In Śavāsana, consciousness moves to ever deepening layers within the kośas, the five sheaths of Being. As we unravel the tensions of annamaya kośa, the "food body" or physical sheath, the increase in sensitivity may unfold the prāṇamāya kośa, the pranic sheath of awareness of the subtle body. If we can relax even more deeply, we encounter the manomaya kośa, the mental and emotional sheath that allows latent impressions within the psyche to rise to the surface of the conscious mind and reveal themselves. With growing trust, the ego unravels itself a little more as we drop into the even subtler realms of the vijñānamaya kośa. This is a sheath or realm beyond the thinking or conscious mind, relating to the energy center of the heart, religious exploration, and devotional surrender to the Universal.

As the body dissolves into the deeper states of relaxation, it is possible to encounter the subtlest sheath or layer, the ānandamaya kośa, or bliss sheath, where consciousness is absorbed into a waveless sea of effulgent light. In this state, instead of growing heavier with each exhalation, the body begins to feel lighter with every outgoing breath. The body no longer feels inert, as if it's fixed to the earth, but may begin to feel like a void dissolving itself in infinite space where consciousness is as vast as the wide expanse of the sky. In this state, there is no boundary between skin and sky, earth and body, or finite and Infinite. All is One.

In Vedāntic philosophy, the mantra Tat Tvam Asi means, "Thou Art That, and That Is Thou." Śavāsana is a profound reminder that you are not this body. You are not this mind. You are not this passing personality. You are beyond the physical, astral, and causal bodies. You are the Supreme Self.

Śavāsana and the Breath

The karmic law of cause and effect is the law of giving and receiving. It is this ebb and flow that governs the flow of the universe as well as our breath. Some yogis have said that one's days upon earth are measured by the number of breaths one takes. At the end of life, all Divine energy given must be returned.

Breath is the invisible link between mind and body. It is the quickest way to understand the nature of the mind. We can't see the mind, but we can observe the functioning of mind through the breath. Śavāsana is an excellent opportunity to practice prāṇamāya, allowing students to get in touch with the breath. In Śavāsana, we focus on the exhalation rather than on the inhalation and in turn quiet the waves of the mind. The exhalation draws us away from the outgoing sensory stimulation of prakṛti into the vast inner realm of Puruṣa, the essence of our Immortal Self.

It is through exhalation that we discover the essence of prāṇamāya. Patanjali says, "By exhaling and restraining the breath, the mind is calmed" (I:34). Nowhere in the sūtras does he say that the mind is calmed through the inhalation. When we inhale, the cells of the brain have a tendency to inflate, which can at times inflate the ego, causing agitation in body and mind. In Śavāsana we emphasize exhalation, making the pose a time when the ego humbles itself.

When the exhalation is slowly released and we think we've reached its base, we wait. If space opens, we let the breath go even further as the body feels heavier and heavier, as if merging into the earth. As one drops further into the layers of Being, it feels as if the body is magnetized to the earth. We do not defy gravity but give over fully to the pull of gravity, almost as if the earth is molding to the contours of our back and limbs.

When we feel as though we cannot exhale any more, we may experience a sensation of panic. The fear of not being able to get enough breath may arise. This reflects the fear of not getting enough in any phase of life. It also reflects a fear of the unknown. Death is the ultimate unknown, but related are fears of change, of loss, of losing, of getting. When we deepen the outgoing breath, we can overcome internal subconscious fears and impressions (saṁskāras) by allowing them to rise to the forefront of the conscious mind, where we can see them and release them. Swami Jyotir Mayānanada, one of the great teachers of Rāja Yoga has said, "The invisible must become visible before it can be eradicated." In this way, Śavāsana with prāṇamāya can become an instrument of self-transformation.

In the Hindu scriptures, many stories depict great daring and heroism in battles fought against the demons, who are the archetypes of ego. Ego in this instance is the individuated consciousness that leads to separation, comparisons, and competition. The demons manifest as false attachments. One of greatest of these is abhiniveśa, which is the fifth painful vṛtti, or mind-wave. In the Yoga Sūtras, abhiniveśa is translated as the clinging to life and fear of death.

The fear of death relates to the fear of the unknown and other fears: the fear of lack (which leads to greed), the fear of not being good enough, the fear of not being loved. These are all the ego's attachments. Śavāsana unravels the grip of the ego. It dissolves the material constituents of the body and mind (desires) and helps us transcend the vast realms of the unknown. In Śavāsana we remove the ego from disturbing the balanced flow of prāṇa. When the prāṇas align themselves, the entire system can come into balance.

When we linger in the space between the outgoing and incoming breaths, we learn to be comfortable in the augmented state of non-resolution, the space between what was and what is yet to be. The state of suspension before we reach for the next incoming breath is a powerful revealer of what is already within us. In that state of suspension, old patterns may begin to drop away before the new begin to appear. If we are uncomfortable in this state of suspended animation, we may gasp and grasp for the incoming breath, which is reflected in wanting immediate resolution of a situation. We are not accustomed to the space between "what was" and "what has yet to be." With practice, we grow more comfortable within this space of non-resolution. We learn to trust and have faith that we are supported by something greater than ourselves.

According to many commentaries on the Yoga Sūtras, it is through the exhalation that we find the ultimate prāṇamāya, known as kevala kumbhaka, the retention of mind through the breath, a state in which we transcend the boundaries and limitations of our mortal coil. At this point, we are no longer breathing, but breath is present. It is as if the great Goddess Prakṛti, the Goddess of life and nature, is nourishing us with her own breath.

Even though this process of breathing can be applied to all āsana, Śavāsana is the pose in which we learn most easily to find comfort with the breath in a state of suspension. It is in this space that we can overcome fears and anxieties of the unknown to face life's challenges and changes more gracefully.

Śavāsana and the Cakras

The next time you teach or practice Śavāsana notice the hands. The hands are the extension of the heart center, and this is a very vulnerable point for some people. Closed fingers may indicate a fear of letting go and opening the heart. If the palms are turned down, this may signify the heart is not ready to open. Students whose palms turn upward to the light have described a sensation of opening in the cells of the brain. When the palms turn down, it feels as if the brain cells begin to contract and pull in. Even when the palms are turned upward to indicate "I really want to give," the fingers may inadvertently close, as if to protect the soft and vulnerable center of the palm.

The fingers and toes relate to various centers within the brain and the energy centers we call cakras. Cakra means "wheel" or "disk." Relaxing the fingers from the roots to the tips will relax the brain centers and, in turn, the sensory organs such as eyes and ears. Each finger relates to one of the first five cakras, its corresponding element (earth, water fire, air, or ether), and the corresponding sensory organ. For example, the thumb relates to the neck. Relaxing and opening the thumb joint influences the thyroid in the throat, which relates to Viśuddhi cakra, or the throat center. Viśuddhi relates to the element of ether and the sense of hearing.

The second finger relates to Anāhata cakra and is the element of air residing in the heart center, which is related to touch. The third finger represents Maṇipūra, meaning "the city of jewels," and relates to the element of fire and the sense of sight. The ring finger represents Svādhiṣṭhāna cakra and the water element in the procreative plexus, associated with the sense of taste. The little finger is the root cakra, Mūlādhāra, associated with the earth element, the coccygeal area of the spine, and the sense of smell.

In Śavāsana, when we relax the arms and hands that extend from our heart center, we open these subtle vortices of energy. We also open energy centers through the deep relaxation of the toes. The big toe represents the neck and throat cakra and the little toe (like the little finger), the root cakra. When one relaxes deeply enough into Śavāsana, it is possible to feel the sub cakras spinning, clockwise and counterclockwise, within the palms of the hands and the soles of the feet.

The tongue also relates to the cakras. The tip of the tongue relates to the root cakra, the very back of the top of the tongue to the throat cakra. If we can relax the root of the tongue, we open Viśuddhi, and the relaxation spreads out into the membranes of the throat down into the esophagus to the pharynx, into the bronchial tubes, and into Anāhata, the heart cakra. When the bronchial tubes relax, the breath becomes very calm. As the yoga sūtras (III:31) say, "Calmness is attained by saṁyama [concentration, meditation, Samādhi] on the bronchial tube." Commentaries on the sūtras elaborate, explaining that within the chest, below the trachea, is a tortoise-shaped tubular structure. By practicing saṁyama on this, one attains freedom from restlessness. Like a snake or an iguana that stays inert as a piece of stone, so can the yogin. If the body does not move, the mind can also be made calm.

Śavāsana in Āsana

Some teachers recommend practicing Śavāsana after every pose, saying that by doing so it is possible to enter a trancelike state where āsana becomes a flowing meditation. This is a powerful way to practice, but it is difficult to maintain this state in standing poses. Lying down and then standing up again interrupts the flow and jostles the nervous system.

I have found that when we learn to rest within each pose, we don't need Śavāsana after each pose. We find Śavāsana in every pose. We can even find Śavāsana during the standing poses. Look at how this relates to life. We may work ourselves hard and then collapse. But in yoga, we learn to rest while we are doing the work. We gradually develop the ability to relax within the action, whether in āsana or in life, cultivating a sense of being the "non-doer." In the Bhagavad Gītā (III:27) Sri Kṛṣṇa says, "He whose mind is deluded by egoism thinks, 'I am the doer.' "

In āsana, we don't have to push until we collapse with fatigue. When we become breathless and strained within a pose, it is time to come out and rest, breathe, and re-center the mind before taking the next pose. When we rush from side to side or pose to pose, the mind may become more restless rather than calm and one-pointed. Without synchronizing movement with breath, lactic acid can build up within the system, leading to fatigue. Yoga āsana is meant to eradicate fatigue, not create more. We learn to breathe and rest within the work. We learn to pull back from over-reaching, honoring what is right for us in the moment, not what others may expect of us. This is known as svadharma. (For more about svadharma in āsana, see the Appendix.) Shortness of breath or holding the breath reflects that one has gone beyond svadharma. When the breath is calm and prolonged, we may move a little further in a pose. Thus, the breath is the barometer telling us when to stay and when to exit a pose. (If, however, a student becomes tired and breathless during practice, he or she can lie down in Śavāsana or rest with the knees bent to retain the warmth and energy from the preceding āsana.)

We don't need to return to Śavāsana after each pose when we bring the principals of breath and relaxation into every pose. When the head and neck are relaxed and the spine active, this is relaxation within action or, as stated in the Gītā, "The inaction within the action." Why wait to curb the restless of the body and then sit cross-legged to curb the restlessness of the mind? The quiet mind we find in Śavāsana can be applied to every asana. We can create concentration (dhāraṇā) or meditation (dhyāna) within this and other more complex āsanas, which then gives us poise in more difficult situations of our lives. We can find the meditative seat in every position we take in yoga and in life.

Pavanamuktāsana

Wind-Relieving Pose

Pavana is the wind. *Mukta* means "to liberate" or "to free." Pavanamuktāsana is the wind-relieving pose that helps to balance and rebalance the pranic currents of the subtle and physical body.

Philosophical Introduction

This pose celebrates Vāyu, the Lord of the Wind. (Vāyu is a synonym for pavana, and both are associated with prāṇa.) In the Vedas, Vāyu is the deified wind, or the breath of the gods. He is the father of Hanumān, the devoted servant of Lord Rāma in the *Rāmāyana.* Hanumān, the great monkey, leapt from India to Lanka to help rescue Sītā (who represents Prakṛti or nature) so that she could be reunited with Rāma (who represents Puruṣa).

Hanumān symbolizes prāṇa and the freedom to move or travel as one wishes. He is able to fly through the air, timeless and boundless. He leaps above all material and spiritual obstacles, carrying those who have been lost in darkness upon his back. Hanumān represents that part of human nature that longs to be a *jivanmukti,* a liberated soul—no longer bound by the gravitational field of this third-dimensional plane, able to fly beyond or lift above past self-imposed limitations. This is the part of our nature that—even though caught in the cul-de-sacs of life's emotions and experiences—ultimately seeks its own spiritual liberation.

Guidance

1. Begin in Śavāsana. Breathe in and out in whatever way the breath chooses to flow.
2. On an exhalation, bring the right knee to the chest, clasping the hands around the front of the knee or the back of the thigh. Keep the head on the floor.
3. Inhale, allowing the breath to round the back, bringing it from the shoulders to the hips.

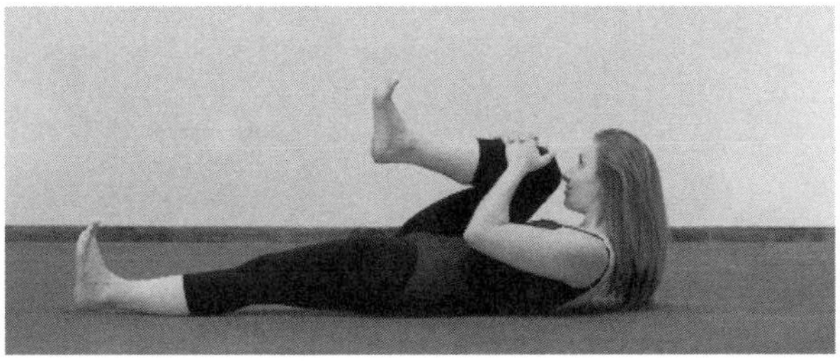

Relax the facial muscles as you bring the forehead toward the knee.

4. Exhale, and as you lengthen the front of the torso, elongate the neck. Relaxing the facial muscles, bring the forehead toward the knee.
5. Inhale and bring the breath into the entire spectrum of the back.

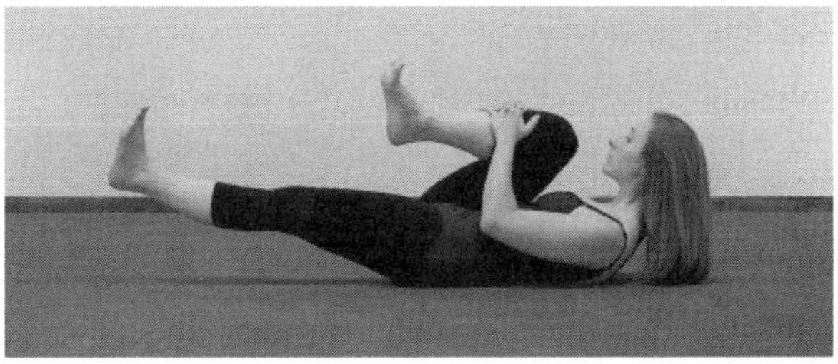

Pavanamuktasana, leg raised and neck extended.

6. Exhaling, bring the spine in like a backbend, elongating the front of the torso. Bring the left leg off the floor as far as possible without bending the knee. Continue to relax the face, neck, and shoulders. Assume an attitude of ease.
7. Inhale, and again round the back with the incoming breath, thinking of it as Vāyu, the breath of the gods.
8. Exhaling, bring the extended leg back to the floor, elongating the neck and bringing the base of the skull to the floor. Relax the arms to the sides of the torso.
9. Inhale and relax.
10. Exhaling, stretch the bent knee and foot to the sky and slowly extend the leg out, bringing it down to the earth.
11. Breathe and observe sensations before taking the pose to the opposite side.

Note: Moving deeper into the pose on the exhalation rather than on the inhalation helps the mind to become calm within the pose.

Psychophysiological Benefits

This pose not only releases flatulence and prevents vāta imbalance, it also is a good pose for strengthening the abdominals without putting strain on the lumbar spine. Pavanamuktāsana preserves hip flexibility and strengthens the neck. If the bottom leg is brought off the floor at the same time the head is lifted, it has an even deeper affect upon the core muscles of the torso. It can also act as a natural facelift—when the head is brought to the knee, the skin lifts counter to the gravitational pull.

In Pavanamuktāsana, we learn the importance of keeping the breath flowing and the mind focused to prevent the fluctuating currents of emotions that impact the physical body. When the mind and emotions remain in balance, or when they can be brought back to a state of equanimity when out of balance, the pranic currents realign, giving us greater physical and emotional strength, stamina, and stability.

Pavana and Vāyu are common synonyms for prāṇa. The five prāṇas are:

1. *prāṇa prāṇa,* which regulates the heart, lungs, and bronchial tubes
2. *apāna prāṇa,* the downward flow of gravity that carries waste matter from the system
3. *samāna prāṇa,* which is responsible for the digestion and absorption, regulating kidneys, adrenals, liver, gallbladder, spleen, pancreas, and stomach
4. *udāna prāṇa,* located in the throat and regulating the thyroid and parathyroid glands (associated with metabolism and calcium stasis); all-pervasive *vyāna prāṇa,* which unites all the prāṇas with the body and is associated with the nerves and muscles.

When we practice Pavanamuktāsana, we affect the pranic body, particularly the prāṇamāya kośa or energy sheath. The prāṇamāya kośa is the second of the five sheaths or layers that comprise the aura around the physical body (see page 245). This layer can't be seen, but it can be sensed throughout asana, prāṇamāya, and meditation. When the mind and emotions are scattered, the prāṇas can be thrown out of balance, and the disturbance may eventually sift through the kośas into the physical tissues, creating an opening for dis-ease. Yoga is a preventative because it keeps the five prāṇas or currents of the subtle body in alignment before any imbalance can manifest in the physical tissues. As a stabilizing āsana, Pavanamuktāsana not only increases core strength but also balances the prāṇas and gives us greater concentrative powers and quietness of mind in the midst of life's difficult moments.

In the *Bhagavad Gītā,* the great warrior Arjuna lamented, "O Kṛṣṇa! The mind is very fickle, powerful, wild, and stubborn. It seems to me that control of the mind is as difficult as catching the wind." The wind-freeing pose teaches us that, like Arjuna, we must continuously embrace change in this world.

Bālāsana

Child's Pose

Bālā means "baby" or "child." As is "to be" or "to breathe," *sam*, "becoming one with," and *na*, "the eternal cosmic vibration."

Philosophical Introduction

The name of this pose reminds me of Bala Kṛṣṇa, the baby or child form of Kṛṣṇa, the Lord of Love. Bala Kṛṣṇa was the Absolute in the form of an unassuming infant. When he was a small child, Kṛṣṇa had no boundaries and did not abide by limiting rules. His consciousness spread throughout the many layers of Universal existence. He was not bound by any one layer of existence but could expand from lunar to solar regions and beyond.

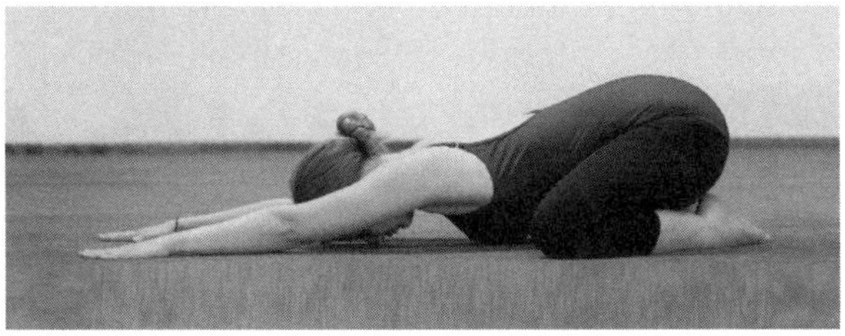

Bālāsana creates an opportunity to turn the senses inward.

Bālāsana reminds us to become innocent as the newborn babe, to be in this world but not of this world. Infants still hold an inner essence that remains soft and pliable in the early stages of transformation. The infant essence hasn't yet formed concepts, ideals, beliefs, judgments, and criticism of others. It accepts what is offered without complaint, criticism, or judgment.

Practicing Child's Pose is an opportunity to turn within and restore our energies, which are always darting outward through the senses and the sensory organs. Thus, Bālāsana is a form of pratyāhāra, the withdrawal of the senses when we temporarily pull away from the world into our womblike origins. According to commentaries in the Yoga Sūtras, "Wherever the mind goes, the senses follow. When a swarm of bees leave their hive for the construction of a new one, the queen bee leads the way. Wherever that large bee rests, the other bees also rest and when she flies, the others closely follow her course." The mind is like the queen bee and the senses are like the other bees, who follow wherever she may go.

In Bālāsana, the queen bee of the mind turns inward. We enter the pose by bending the knees, a symbol of humility, bowing before the earth and the heavens. We place the head gently upon the floor, as though offering the ego upon the altar of the earth. As we focus where the center of the forehead touches the earth, we are also recycling by drawing the earth's energy through Ājñā cakra, the forehead center, into our being. When we turn within, into the neglected inner worlds, this is an opportunity to soften hardened belief systems.

As children grow, they begin to assert their independence, wanting to do things for themselves that were once done for them by their parents. The child walks and then runs ... and runs playfully away from the parent, testing the boundaries. The child thinks she/he is separate and no longer dependent upon the parent, but all the while the parent is silently watching. If the child stumbles and falls and cries out, the parent rushes to embrace the child and soothe the wounds.

The parent/child relationship is similar to Bhakti, the devotional path of yoga. The universal mother and father are always with us. As we grow in life and assert our ego more, we think our actions come from us rather than through us. We forget to honor or rely on Source in our everyday actions. We stumble in life and at times fall. During these moments, the dark nights of the soul, we may silently cry out for help. "Oh God," may be our single cry as the Universal parent rushes to our side and holds us in the eternal embrace of love, reminding us that we were never separated, and that the Universal presence was always watching over us.

When we practice Bālāsana as bhaktins, who transform emotion into devotion, it is not enough to be a child. We turn the hands of time back even further and become as helpless as the infant who can do nothing for its separated self. We learn to rely on the guiding hand of an invisible source. Like kittens, we loosen the skin of our necks so the divine mother can pick us up and guide us into our life's purpose and right action.

Guidance

Bālāsana is one of the best postures for learning the three-part breath through the back body. The lungs are divided into three chambers. The upper lobes are the smallest, the middle are larger, and the lowest lobes are the largest. With the back breathing, we direct breath into the fullness of all three lobes as well as into the front, back, and sides of the lungs.

When the breath arises (usually in the upper body), it can become a guru or teacher to the lower parts, which are generally denser. Accept the breath wherever it arises, rather than chastising yourself if the breath doesn't start from the bottom. I learned that wherever the breath would arise, I could follow it and it would lead my consciousness into areas not yet explored. Wherever breath wanted to express itself first, even if it was in the upper clavicular region, rather than trying to push it down, I would allow it to arise and spread out and become a coach or teacher to the denser parts of the torso and lungs.

Each time we change position and use the breath, the breath expands into new areas within the myriad folds of the lungs. The breath can eventually be brought from the shoulders (the upper lobes of the lungs) to the middle lobes by breathing in and lifting the ribcage while expanding each of the ribs away from the synovial joints where they attach to the spine. Eventually, as one's lung capacity increases, the inhalation can be brought from the shoulders all the way down to the sacrum and even the base of the buttocks, which is a more dense area of the body and the most difficult to access.

Each incoming breath becomes the act of receiving. Each outgoing breath is the act of giving or surrender. Allow the receiving and giving to be equal to one another. You are the Bhakti Yogi, surrendering your offering of the Self into the pose.

1. Begin by kneeling on the floor. Rest the buttocks on the heels and open the knees so that the outside thighs are wider than the sides of the torso; this helps to lengthen the spine. Place the forehead on the floor. The hands may rest beneath the forehead, or you may relax the arms alongside the torso. With the next exhalation, elongate the neck.

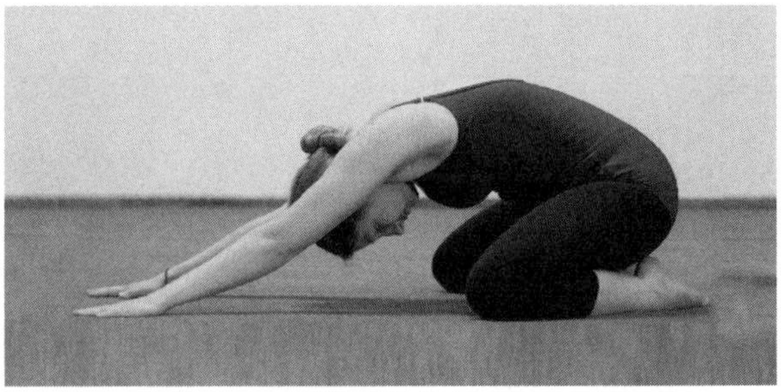

Bālāsana, expanding the back on inhalation.

2. On the next incoming breath, allow the breath to spread down into the shoulders, widening the space between the shoulder blades.
3. On the exhalation, relax the spine between the shoulder blades and offer it into the heart center.
4. The next incoming breath expresses itself in the back of the ribcage, widening the twelve sets of ribs away from the spinal column. This creates space in the synovial joints where the ribs attach to the spine. As you expand the back ribs, it may feel like you can take the breath into infinity.
5. Exhale, elongating the spine. Let it move like a crescent moon into the front of your torso.
6. On the next inhalation, slowly allow the breath to round the shoulders and back ribs, and then allow the breath to spread down a little further, into the sacrum and even to the base of the buttocks. The entire spectrum of the spine and back body is now feeling the breath. On the inhalations, as the back rounds, it is like the devotional offering to the heavens. On the exhalations, the offering is to the earth.

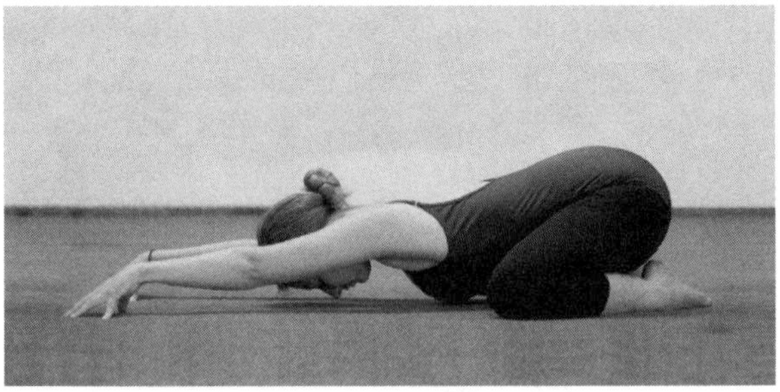

Bālāsana, exhaling and walking the fingertips out to find extension in the spine.

7. With each exhalation, keep raising the back ribs as you simultaneously elongate from the floating ribs and the base of the sternum. This creates a growing length in the front of the body and allows more prāṇa to flow through the spinal nerve roots and out into periphery of the body.

8. On the next inhalation, expand the shoulders upward with the breath and then move the breath from the shoulders down toward the middle and lower ribs, expanding them away from the spine. Allow the fullness of the breath to lift the spine upward to the heavens.
9. Exhaling, bring the spine in toward the heart and lengthen the neck, stretching it forward like a turtle reaching out from its shell.
10. Inhale and let the breath move upward from the shoulders and ribs and down to the sacrum.
11. Exhaling, draw the tailbone back as the base of the skull moves forward, fully elongating the spine. Keep the buttocks resting on the heels.
12. Inhaling, turn your attention to the feet and take the breath in as if from the pores on the soles of the feet.
13. Exhale, releasing any excessive energy from the head through the toes. Surrender with each outgoing breath, offering the spine into the front of the body.
14. When you are ready to leave Bālāsana, inhale and allow the breath to round the back as you sit up on the heels and simply observe the breath. If sitting on the heels is difficult, slide the hips to the side.

Psychophysiological Benefits

Even though this posture is referred to as a Child's Pose, it is more a pose of the infant. Newborn infants sleep on their stomachs with legs curled in the instinctual pattern assumed within the womb. As a child grows and unfurls the limbs, opening to this world, he or she rarely retakes the infant position. However, during moments of great anguish and grief, whether as children, teens, or adults, there is a tendency to curl into the protective infant pose, on the stomach, or on the side.

Bālāsana is often taken as a counter pose after Downward Facing Dog Pose or backbends. Even though our intention is to lengthen the front of the torso to be equal to the back during these poses, if they are not practiced appropriately, they can sometimes compress the posterior spine, especially the lumbar spine. Bālāsana helps release posterior compression in the lumbar area.

When practiced with the breath, Bālāsana opens the lungs and the intuitive back of our being like no other pose. Because the torso rests upon the thighs, Bālāsana massages the abdominal organs, including the stomach and intestines. It calms the mind and body because of its impact upon the parasympathetic nerves, which stem from the cervical spine and the sacrum and coccyx. It is an excellent pose in which to observe the breath as we return to the infant state of total surrender to the Universal Source, breathing once more as infants breathe, into the back from the shoulders to the hips.

It may take time to become accustomed to this style of breathing, lifting and expanding the back on the inhalation and allowing the spine to move towards the front body on the exhalation. Eventually, in all poses, you will begin to feel the breath moving into the back and then around to the sides and eventually to the front of the torso. There is a sense of total fulfillment in this cylindrical breath. It may be helpful to visualize the yantra of the circle, which reminds us to expand awareness from the inside. The breath begins to move from and into the center of our being, creating a mandala in which the whole is connected to its parts. If we can hold this space while exhaling, we begin to discover the vast Universe within, and the internal worlds become illumined by our own inner light.

Patañjali's Yoga Sūtras speak of the quietness and stillness of mind that manifests not on the inhalation but on the exhalation. It is during the exhalation, the sūtras say, that the ego unravels itself. By moving into the fullness of āsana on the exhalation rather than the inhalation, the breath helps the mind to become calm. We move in an egoless state, allowing the pose to come through us and not from us. This is a powerful breath to take into all poses and into the poses of life because it quiets the waves of the mind even in the midst of the action. This is the essence of yoga that Patañjali describes in the second sūtra: *Yogaḥ cittavṛtti nirodhaḥ*. "Yoga is to still the fluctuations that rise in the field of the mind."

Mārjāryāsana

Cat Pose

Mājārī refers to the cat.

Philosophical Introduction

Mārjāryāsana is commonly known as Cat Pose. It is a preparatory pose that usually precedes Adho Mukha Śvānāsana (Downward-Facing Dog), but it is powerful in its own right. A cat moves with stealth through time and space without disturbing the atmosphere around it. The cat's grace, agility, and fluidity of movement can mesmerize as well as mask a quality of fierce independence.

When breathing and elongating in Cat Pose, I think of the vehicle of the goddess Durgā. The vehicles of the gods and goddesses express aspects of their divine energy forms, and Durgā is depicted as riding a lion or tiger. Both of these big cats symbolize power, courage, and invincibility, like the great goddess herself. They are swift in their actions and can only be subdued and directed by one whose spiritual powers are greater than their instinctual will. Cat Pose invokes the courage, wisdom, and strength of the lion as well as the invincible qualities of Durgā, the goddess whose power and radiance was created from the gifts of the gods.

It is said that the gods created Durgā and armed her with their mightiest weapons because only she, a composite of all their great powers, could slay the demon who had unseated Indra, the lord of the Universe. None of the gods could vanquish the demon, who had obtained a boon that he could never be killed by man or god. When the demon came to the battlefield with Durgā, he fought sometimes as a buffalo, sometimes as an elephant, and sometimes as a lion. He fought from the earth and from space. Finally Durgā, radiating a great mantle of light, stepped off her lion, and with a beatific and compassionate smile, subdued the demon and took off his head with the swiftness of her sword. Their battle is symbolic of the struggle that goes on in the human experience between the demonic forces (anger, greed, pride, jealousy, envy, egoistic and separative consciousness) and Divine love, selfless service, and universal expansion of consciousness.

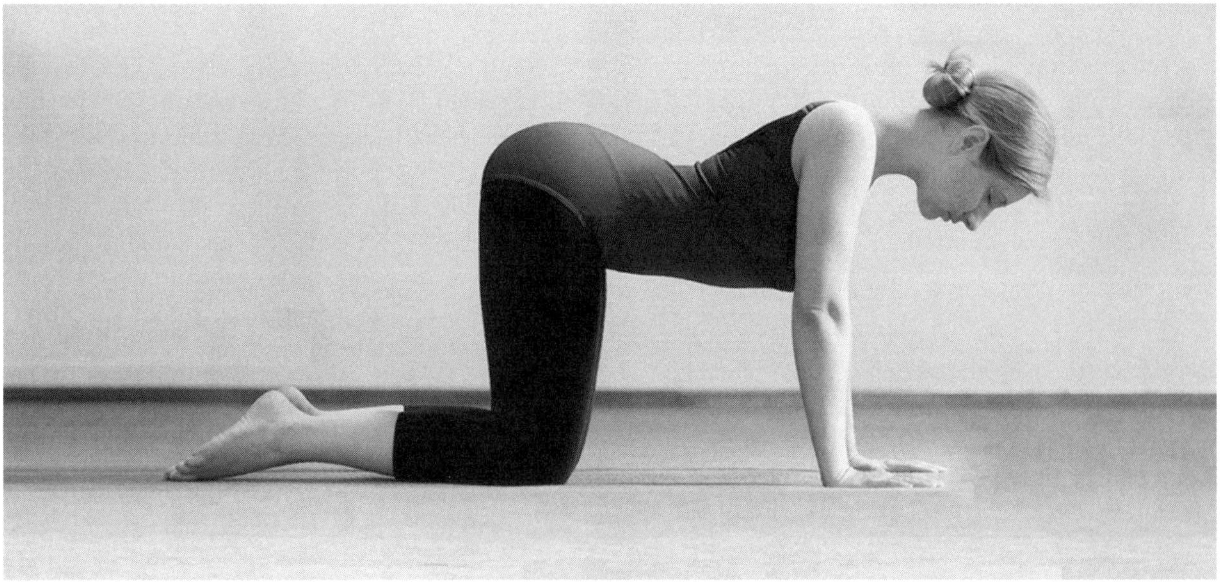

Mārjāryāsana, exhalation.

Guidance

The back breath learned in Child's Pose—inhaling and doing nothing, exhaling and taking adjustments or moving deeper—is the basis of the spinal movements in Mārjāryāsana. And Mārjāryāsana is central to all asana practice because it teaches how the breath can be taken into every pose without creating ripples or waves (vṛttis) within the field of the mind.

Moving only on the exhalation is, according to Patañjali's Yoga Sūtras (I:34), one of the important ways in which a practitioner can still the waves of the mind: "By exhaling and restraining the breath, the mind is calmed." Commentaries on the sūtras elaborate that the ego is disentangling itself from the body and the "feeling of self" in the core of the heart is moving on to the wordless, thoughtless state of concentration. This is possible only at the time of exhalation and not at the time of inhalation, which is why no reference to inhalation has been made in the sūtras.

On the inhalation, the ego asserts itself. On the incoming breath, when the ego asserts itself, we give it no power, only our observation. Thus, when we move on the exhalation, we are moving in an egoless state. From this way of breathing and moving, a growing feeling of happiness or a feeling of lightness may spread throughout the body. The breath fills new spaces, not just in the lobes of our lungs but in the cellular structure throughout our being.

1. Begin Mārjāryāsana on the hands and knees, placing the hands directly under the shoulders, balancing the weight equally on the inner and outer bones of the arms. With the middle finger facing straight ahead, create as much space between the thumb and the forefinger as possible, as if you were spanning an octave on the piano. Pay particular attention to the base of the thumb. This is the reflex to the neck. Neck tension reveals itself in the way the thumbs move. Spreading the fingers and pointing the thumbs toward one another helps release neck tension.
2. Next, press down into the Venus mound of the palm and the pad of the thumb. This strengthens the triceps and equalizes the pressure on the triceps and the biceps. The triceps represents the subtle body and the biceps, the physical body, so here we are giving equal attention to the physical body (annamaya kośa) and subtle body (prāṇamāya kośa).
3. Press down with the knees, resisting the inner thighs away from one another without moving the knees. When the inner thighs resist one another, the ischia (the bones of the buttocks) widen, stabilizing the sacroiliac joint where the pelvis meets the sacrum.

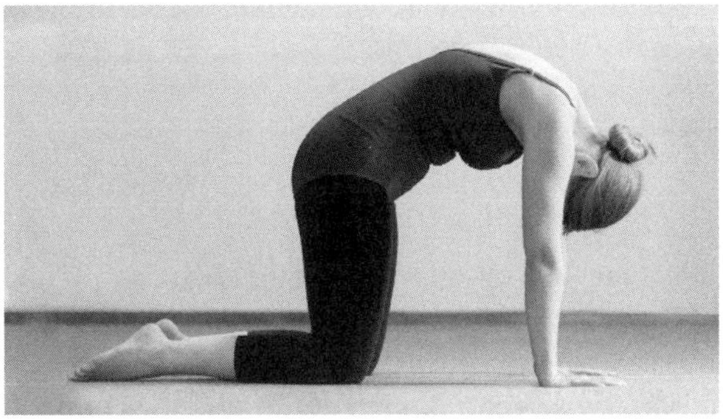

Mārjāryāsana, inhalation.

4. Inhale and allow the breath to round the back. Keep the navel passive. The inhalation spreads the shoulder blades, ribs, and hips away from the center of the spine. The head and neck are relaxed throughout the pose.
5. Exhaling, lift the sides of the torso up while allowing the spine to sink toward the center of the body, moving the tailbone back as the base of the skull moves forward. At the end of the exhalation, elongate the neck, bringing the chin up without compressing the back of the neck. (Do not lift the head.)
6. Inhaling, letting the breath widen the shoulder blades, widen the back of the lower ribs, and widen the sides of the entire back body, moving the kidneys away from one another. Feel the width of the hips as the breath comes in.
7. Then—holding the space created on the inhalation—exhale and move the spine inward to the front body and roll the shoulders down and back, moving the tailbone back to relax the navel. Keeping the navel passive while elongating from the top of the pubis to the navel will create a natural uḍḍīyāna bandha.
8. Continue to inhale and exhale. Lengthen with each exhalation, rolling the shoulders down the back, away from the earlobes, as the neck extends out even further. Allow the spine to drop in like

a saddle, pressing the knees down to move the tailbone back and up. When you roll the shoulders down on the exhalation, give space to the neck. Be very observant not to compress the neck or bend it too much.

9. When you are ready to complete the pose, exhale and bring the spine into the front body, then lower your hips into Bālāsana (Child's Pose), keeping the hands and arms where they are to give greater length to the spine.

Psychophysiological Benefits

Practicing Mārjāryāsana allows the student to ground and center, to find the inner wisdom of the cat. Thus, Mārjāryāsana is a good preparation for other poses. It can be sequenced at the beginning of a class or practice, or after breathing in Bālāsana (Child's Pose). The cat stretch is the ideal preparation for the breathing movements of Adho Mukha Śvānāsana, Downward-Facing Dog Pose. For students unable to kneel on the floor, the pose can be introduced standing with the support of a chair under the hands.

Mārjāryāsana is especially good for those with back problems and for pregnant women. Mārjāryāsana creates and preserves the flexibility of the spine and strengthens the erector spinae and rectus abdominus muscles. The stretch is helpful for releasing any spinal compression. It helps to remove or alleviate neck tension and releases excessive tension in the trapezius and the deltoid muscles.

The cat stretch also strengthens the biceps and triceps and increases bone density, preserving the health of the bones of the arms, hands, and thighs. Pressing the knees into the floor strengthens the hips, while moving with the out breath increases the flexibility of the hips. Any stagnant circulatory currents from the pelvis will flow freely through the lower limbs, and this may help prevent varicose veins.

Lengthening the spine and torso creates space for the procreative and digestive organs. The kidneys, adrenals, thymus, and endocrine glands are all benefited. As we stimulate lymphatic circulation, we also free up emotional impressions from the psyche.

On an energetic level, Mārjāryāsana helps us expand our consciousness to embrace two polarities simultaneously. We are aware of the crown of the head, and at the same time we are aware of the tailbone. As we learn to keep the navel passive, whether inhaling or exhaling, we unravel the blocked prāṇa at the navel center so that it can then flow upward to the heart center. This stretch allows prāṇa to flow from the base of the spine to the crown of the head, moving freely between the lower and upper cakras.

The dynamic of Mārjāryāsana represents the divine battle between the two poles of opposites. As the head moves forward, it wants to drag the entire spine with it. However, if the tailbone moves backward with equal tension, we find neutrality, honoring both the feminine as well as the masculine. As the spine lengthens, we create immense inner space for releasing emotions that have a tendency to get stuck in our cellular structure. By practicing Cat Pose, we bring growing strength to both the physical and subtle levels of being.

Adho Mukha Śvānāsana

Downward-Facing Dog

Adho means "downward," *mukha* means "face," and *śvāna* is "dog."

Philosophical Introduction

Household dogs are known to be loyal and unconditionally loving of their masters, reflecting our relationship to the divine. The sixth mārga (path) of yoga, known as Bhakti Yoga, is the path where emotion is transformed into devotion. The bhakta has her mind always fixed on God, seeing the presence of this divine form and obeying the heavenly commands and guidance. In the same way, the dog is ever watchful, giving loyalty and undying love and devotion to its master. It obeys commands and is sensitive to its owner's movements, whereabouts, and absences. Like the bhakta, the dog may even grieve if it cannot be near the one it loves, and it waits for the beloved to once more show his or her face. The love and devotion that the dog has for us draws us closer to it. Just so in Bhakti Yoga: Our love and devotion to the Universal is the cord that binds the soul to God.

The dog's playful bow, tail upraised, mirrors the geometrical form of this āsana, which is a triangle. In āsana, we use our bodies to create universal patterns known as yantras. *Yam* means "to support," "hold," or "contain." *Tra* means "in order to transcend." Its roots can be found in the word *trana*, meaning "to free" or "to liberate." Yantra, combined with mantra, forms the mārga or path known as Tantra Yoga.

In Vedic astrology, the angles rule the major domains of our life. Yantras are reflections of the myriad of ways in which the Divine manifests. Yantras, like āsana, are used to withdraw consciousness from outer to the inner worlds. When our bodies form geometrical patterns in āsana, the pose becomes an invocation for the corresponding celestial energies to enter into our field of consciousness through the cosmic gateways of yantra.

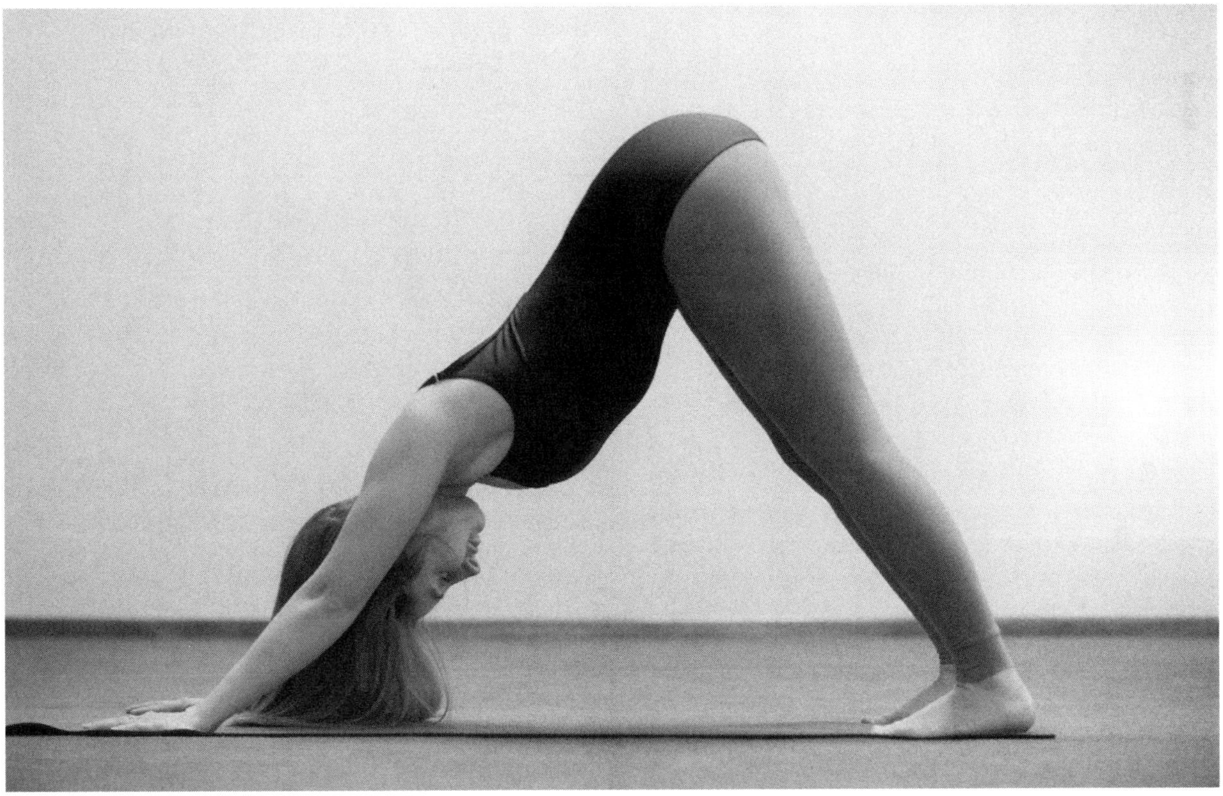

Adho Mukha Śvānāsana, final pose.

In the triangle (trikoṇa) formed by Adho Mukha Śvānāsana, the buttock bones are the apex, drawing light into the lower limbs as well as into the upper body. This sacred geometry represents the Holy Trinity found in many spiritual and religious traditions, such as Brahmā (the creator), Vishṇu (the sustainer), and Śiva (the transformer), or the Father, Son, and Holy Ghost. When the angles in this pose are aligned, one can enter into the energetic field of consciousness represented by the triangle.

When we offer the coccygeal plexus to the heavens, we invert the flow of apāna prāṇa, the downward pull of energy, and creating a natural mūla bandha without muscular contraction. *Bandha* means "to bind" or "lock." The bandha is not done by contracting the muscles in an attempt to pull the prāṇa up against the gravitational force. Rather, when the body is aligned appropriately, prāṇa automatically and effortlessly rises upward. When the tilt of the buttocks is in alignment with the heavens prāṇa moves up effortlessly to Maṇipūra cakra, the navel center. As this center is elongated through the concavity of the spine, the prāṇa flies up like a great bird into Anāhata cakra, the heart center. Uḍḍīyāna bandha is the name given to the movement of energy that rises from the solar plexus to the heart cakra.

For these bandhas to occur, however, the hamstrings need to lengthen, allowing the buttock bones to lift to receive the light from above. Mr. Iyengar used to say, "Your buttock bones are lying in darkness—lift them to the light and let them shine like the rays of the sun."

One day, I asked Mr. Iyengar why he didn't teach the bandhas. He simply replied, "The bandhas are in āsana."

As the buttock bones are lifted to the light of the sun, the navel must remain passive and relaxed for the prāṇa to pass through any knots or blockages in this area. Prāṇa can then flow freely with the gravitational pull to reach the heart center. When one becomes more adept in this pose, as the heart offers itself to the head, the neck will lengthen to bring the chin to the chest. This forms the third lock, known as jālandhara bandha. Jāla means "network" or "web," referring to our brain, and dhara means "to support." In the chin lock, which can happen spontaneously, the carotid sinuses and arteries are engaged, which helps to balance and regulate the blood pressure.

Adho Mukha Śvānāsana is one of the few poses that engages all three bandhas, creating the great seal, the mahā mudra, which is meant to contain prāṇa in the spine. In so doing, prāṇa is drawn into the suṣumṇā nāḍī, the central canal of the spinal cord, which awakens the Kuṇḍalinī Śakti .

Guidance

Adho Mukha Śvānāsana is the extension of Cat Pose. The only difference is that the knees are straight instead of bent. This pose combines a forward bend and backbend. On the inhalation, as we round the back, we offer the spine to the heavens. On the exhalation, we do a backbend, offering the spine to the earth. As in Cat Pose, the inhalation is a time to restore and renew, when the divine enters into our being. The exhalation is a time to give, offering the heart of our Being to the altar of the earth. This is the practice of Bhakti Yoga in āsana.

In Cat Pose, the goddess Durgā (symbolized by her vehicle of the lion) taught us to hold all perspectives simultaneously, and again in Adho Mukha Śvānāsana we learn to hold awareness of the sacrum and crown of the head, representing the two poles of the cosmos. As in Cat Pose, it is important to elongate the spine, creating space between each vertebra by dynamically moving the polarities away from one another on each exhalation. The Cat and Dog poses are ideal for beginning a class or practice because they establish moving with the breath, which can be carried into more complex āsanas.

1. Begin in Mārjāryāsana. The cat stretch is the prelude to Downward-Facing Dog. The hands and arms are shoulder distance apart. The knees are hip distance apart. The navel is passive and relaxed throughout every phase of the pose. The neck is extended and relaxed.
2. On an inhalation, draw the heart back, rounding the back toward the heavens. Turn the toes under, bringing the balls of the feet as close to the floor as possible.
3. Exhaling, straighten the knees and lift the buttocks. Allow the tailbone to lift the body into the pose by moving the tailbone back rather than coming forward onto the hands.

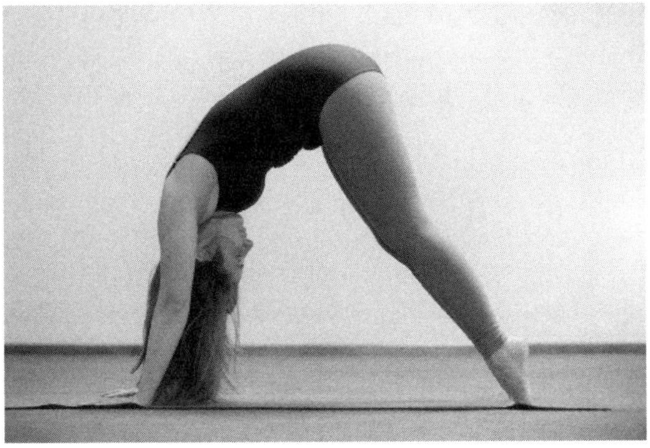

Inhaling, Round the back.

4. Inhale and remain still as the breath flows in, rounding the back.
5. Exhaling, come up to the balls of the feet, still lifting the tailbone and buttock bones, and then release from the calf to the heel. Lower the heels toward the floor, not to the floor, keeping the lift of the tailbone. We bring the heels down only to the point that we can preserve that lift.
6. Inhale, rounding the back to the heavens. Do nothing else.

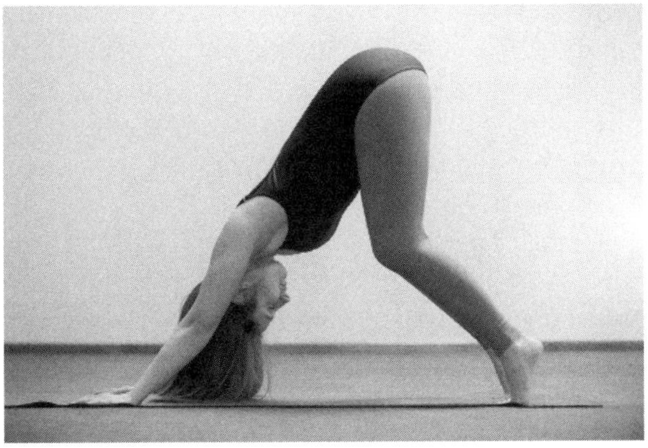

Exhaling, bend the knees to lift the tailbone.

7. Exhale and move the spine in like a backbend without losing the lift of the base of the spine. (Bend the knees if necessary to preserve that lift.) While lifting the heels, also lift the inner ankle and then roll to the ball of the big toe without dropping the inner ankle. As the heel bones are brought down—toward, not to the floor—the inner arch of the foot lifts up, as in Tāḍāsana.
8. Inhaling, lift the shoulders to the ears with an internal rotation of the arms. Widen the shoulders, rounding the back with the breath.
9. Exhaling, externally rotate the upper arms, bringing the shoulders down and back away from the ears as the spine moves into the front of the body in a backbend. Allow the neck to release with the gravitational pull, bringing the head closer to the earth.
10. Inhale as the skin of the back moves up to the shoulders, the shoulders lift to the ears, and the upper arm internally rotates. Rising up to the balls of the feet, fill the back from the shoulders to buttocks with the breath.
11. Exhaling, move the skin of the back toward the buttocks, externally rotating the upper arm as the inner shoulder blades descend with the spine into the chest wall. On the exhalation, the spine elongates. As it moves into the front of the body, the passivity of the navel will allow the prāṇa to be pulled in toward the spine and up behind the heart center in a natural and organic uḍḍiyāna bandha.
12. Inhaling, do nothing but fill the back with the breath.
13. Exhale. If the chest is lifted toward the chin, see if the chin is ready to offer itself—without effort—to the heart.
14. When you are ready to release, inhale, then exhale and bend the knees, keeping the elongation of the spine as you come down into Mārjāryāsana (Cat Pose) or into Bālāsana (Child's Pose).

Note: Students with tight hamstrings will need to focus more attention in this area to create length. It might be helpful to think of the tailbone as being the extension of the heels. On an inhalation, lift the heel bones. As the hamstrings soften and lengthen on the exhalation, raise the buttocks to the sky while the calf muscles relax toward the heels. If the heels are brought to the floor prematurely, this pulls the hips and tailbone down, and the pose becomes static rather than dynamic. The heels are to be brought to the earth only if the lift and offering from the tailbone can be preserved. The back of the knee is relaxed and neutral as the thigh skin moves from the top of the knee to the buttock and the calf skin moves from the knee to the heels.

Psychophysiological Benefits

Because there are so many details to consider when practicing this pose, Adho Mukha Śvānāsana requires focus and concentration. As we learn to expand our focus and hold the various parts and movement of the body in our field of awareness at the same time, there is an immense expansion of consciousness in the poses of our life.

The physical benefits of Downward-Facing Dog are similar to the Cat Stretch. Moving with the breath creates and preserves the flexibility of the spine and strengthens the erector spinae muscles. If practiced without holding tension in the neck, the pose relieves and even eliminates neck tension.

Adho Mukha Śvānāsana strengthens the bones of the arms and legs and the arch of the foot while lengthening the hamstrings and calf muscles. Because it is an inversion, it counters the effects of gravity on the reproductive and digestive organs and nourishes the brain. The stretch of the Achilles tendon influences the peristaltic activity of the intestines.

On an energetic level, Adho Mukha Śvānāsana frees the pranic flow between the lower and upper cakras. It leads to the mahā mudra, when all three bandhas are combined. Jālandhara bandha (chin lock) stimulates the thymus, thyroid, and parathyroid endocrine glands, while uḍḍiyāna bandha (abdominal lock) and mūla bandha (root lock) benefit the abdominal and pelvic organs.

However, we cannot define which cakra an āsana affects because so much depends on how one is practicing the āsana and how free or restricted the breath is. The effect in this pose would depend on the thoracic lift and on the lengthening of the spine with the breath. For instance, you can't say Adho Mukha Śvānāsana affects the first energy center, Mūlādhāra cakra, if the person's hamstrings are short and the pelvis is tucked and moving downward. The pose will not have the same affect as when the tailbone and buttock bones are lifted up. This is partly determined by the length of the hamstrings and by the lessening of the knots in the gastrocnemius muscle in the calf.

Many people bend at the waist in Downward-Facing Dog, chronically arching the back and creating anterior compression of the spine. They are not lifting the ribcage up off the pelvic region. When this happens, the energy becomes coagulated, not just in Svādhiṣṭhāna, the second cakra, but also in Maṇipūra, the third cakra, the center of will. If the navel center is tense or defensive, this may indicate that we want to make things happen. We may force rather than allow spirit to move through us. A hardened solar plexus may show lack of trust in an invisible power. This is why it is important to keep the navel center passive and relaxed during the duration of this pose and all yoga āsanas. In this way there is an equality of movement, allowing the prāṇa to flow freely from the base to the top.

In Adho Mukha Śvānāsana, we may also overstretch or overdo in one area, such as the shoulders, because another part, such as the pelvis, is not moving. It is humbling to not overreach in the areas of our greatest flexibilities while working on the part that is more dense and forgetful, but the more we overreach with our ambitious attempts, the more we block the energetic flow, especially in the navel center. We want to free this energy, and yet it is important that we also honor the self-will that Maṇipūra represents. Maṇipūra, the solar plexus, is the body's sun, the generator of personal energy that corresponds to the sun of our galaxy. It fuels the energy of the heart. When this energy flows upward to the heart center, we connect with Divine will and offer prāṇa to the Universal Source. When we do this, we are practicing Īśvara Praṇidhāna, the fifth niyama of Aṣṭāṅga Yoga according to the Yoga Sūtras (II:32). Then the āsana becomes an active form of remembering our creator and offering to that Source. In this state, we are not doing the pose … the pose is being done through us.

Śīrṣāsana Preparation

Headstand Preparation

Śirṣā means head.

Philosophical Introduction

It is not necessary to bring the feet off the ground to experience the benefits of Śīrṣāsana. When the head placement for Śīrṣāsana or this preparatory stage is at the triangular conjunction of the coronal and sagittal sutures of the skull, the cellular petals of the brain begin to unfurl one by one, like the lotus which only opens with the light of the rising sun. The crown of the head is the gateway to the solar region of consciousness. The Sanskrit name for this region is Sahasrāra or the Thousand-Petaled Lotus. In the East, "a thousand" means infinite. Think of the dessert pastry baklava, known as the "sweet of the thousand layers" because the paper-thin dough feels as if it is infinite both in the preparation and in the eating.

This center within the head is known to be the mystical dwelling place of the supreme Yoga, the Divine Union between Śiva and Śakti. In South India, ancient Yogis referred to this as the seat of Śivaloka, the world or dwelling place of Śiva, the timeless substratum of the universe.

Practicing Śīrṣāsana is said to awaken Kuṇḍalinī Śakti, who arises from her serpentine sleep. By inverting the prāṇas and creating a polar shift of the spinal subtle nerve currents, Headstand helps awaken this dormant energy, bringing clarity and light to the highest centers within the brain and in turn, the mind. As the Kuṇḍalinī or bio- or psycho-nuclear energy turns upward, and prāṇa rises through the sacral and coccygeal centers, the petals of the lotus within the head (which were drooping downward) are given new life and bloom upward. They unfold like the earthly lotus whose petals open with the light of the morning sun. The petals of the Sahasrāra unfold with the dawning of the Divine inner light.

Guidance

1. Begin in Mārjāryāsana, the Cat Pose. Elongate the spine with every exhalation. Bring elbows and forearms to the floor, shoulder width apart. Clasp the hands together at the root of the fingers, crossing the base of the thumbs and relaxing the fingertips.
2. On the exhalation, press down and anchor this pyramidal base with the bottom wrist bone and inner elbow.
3. Inhaling, let the incoming breath round the back.
4. Exhale and allow the spine to descend toward the earth while extending the neck forward and the tailbone backward.
5. Inhaling, allow the breath to fill the back the back of the body.

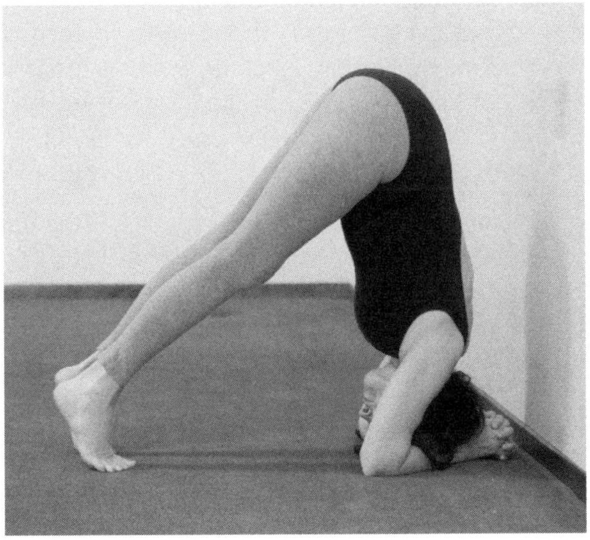

Using the resistance of the wall to help lengthen the spine in Śīrṣāsana preparation.

6. Exhaling, straighten the knees and lift, coming to the balls of the feet and bringing the buttocks to the sky.
7. Inhale and round the back with the breath.
8. Exhale and bring the spine in like a back bend while elongating the neck and lifting the tailbone. Do not bring the feet from the floor.

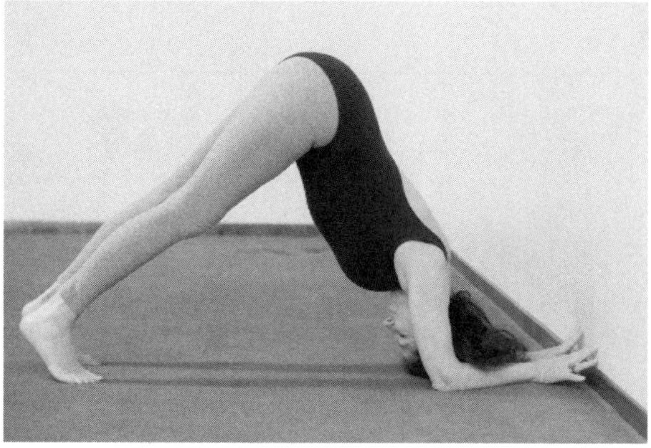

Focus on lifting the tailbone and creating a backbend during Śīrṣāsana.

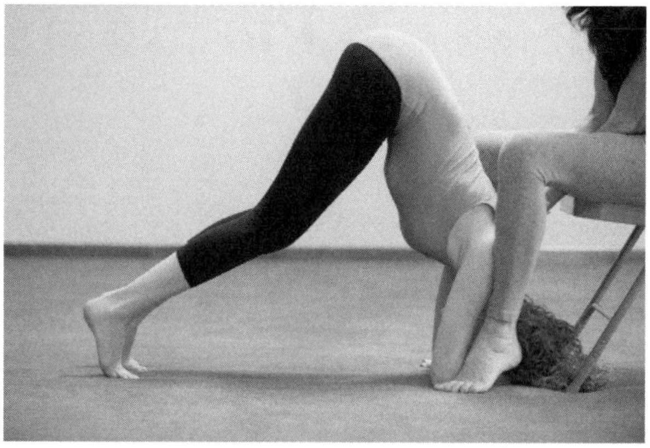

Continue lifting the shoulders as the student's head comes down toward the floor.

9. Stay in this preparatory position and breathe, lifting the shoulders away from the floor with every exhalation while pressing down with the inner elbows and bottom wrist bone. Keep elongating neck and extending spine on each exhalation. Raise the tailbone without lifting the feet from the floor. This helps lengthen the hamstrings, which relieves any resultant pressure upon the neck.
10. On an exhalation, lengthen the neck, lifting the shoulders. This time, allow the crown of the head to brush the floor. Continue to lift the shoulders to lengthen and alleviate any pressure upon the neck. Continue to lift the tailbone. It's important to move the armpits toward the legs to open the heart center and release pressure upon the neck.
11. When ready, exhale and bend the knees, bringing the buttocks to the heels.
12. Rest in Bālāsana (Child's Pose) and breath into the back, lengthening the spine.

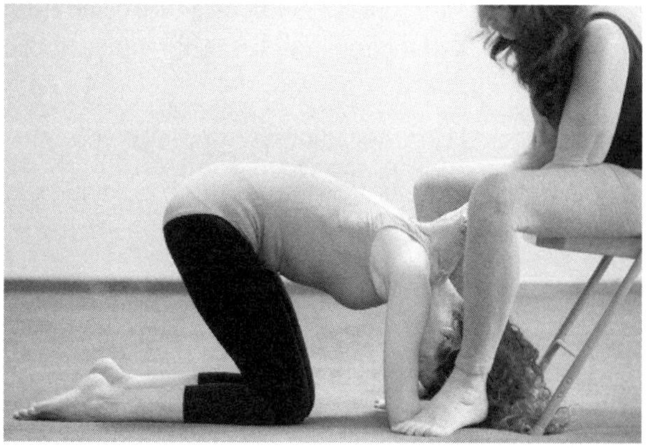

The partner supports and lifts the shoulders.

Assists: A partner or teacher can sit on the edge of a chair facing the practitioner as he or she takes arm and hand position for Headstand. The partner supports and lifts the shoulders as practitioner raises the hips into the variation of Downward-Facing Dog Pose sometimes referred to as Dolphin Pose. The head is not yet touching the earth as the shoulders are lifted. As the student walks in, the partner keeps lifting the shoulders and continues to do so even as the student's head comes down. The partner can use the side of his or her knees to gently press into the student's back. This is done to keep the armpits and chest from collapsing, which protects the neck.

Psychophysiological Benefits

In the preparatory stages of Śīrṣāsana, the student can focus on moving the thoracic spine from the back to front body on each exhalation and moving the forearms and wrist bones downward as if into the earth. Practiced this way, Śīrṣāsana releases rather than creates neck tension.

Śīrṣāsana affects the thalamus, located in the upper region of the brain, which holds the blueprint of every cell of the body. It also increases circulation to the hypothalamus, the master endocrine gland, helping to bring balance and equilibrium to the entire endocrine chain—including the pituitary, pineal, thyroid, parathyroid, thymus, adrenals, and procreative glands. It is an excellent pose for recharging brain cells, helps prevent memory loss and, if done appropriately, it balances the right and left hemispheres of the brain. It benefits the circulatory flow to the heart and the flow of cerebrospinal fluid to the brain.

Known as the King of Āsana, headstand has a stimulating effect on the sympathetic nervous system through the prefrontal cortex of the brain and the movement of the thoracic spine, which activates the adrenal glands. The adrenal glands secrete adrenaline, which prepares the body for "fight or flight," creating a heating and more constricting impact upon the system. Therefore, headstand is an excellent pose for those with low blood pressure. Those with high blood pressure can precede Headstand with twenty minutes of forward bends to dilate the blood vessels. In any case, it is recommended to follow Headstand or end a practice session with shoulderstand, the Queen of Āsana, to emphasize the parasympathetic flow, which dilates, cools, and calms the system. Traditionally, one would never practice headstand (the father or King of Āsana) without balancing it by practicing shoulderstand (the mother or Queen of Āsana).

The headstand represents a polar shift in the body. In reversing the poles of the body in relation to the magnetic poles of the earth, Śīrṣāsana recharges the system like a battery. Whenever one is fatigued, practicing the Headstand followed by the shoulderstand brings renewed energy and enthusiasm to body, mind, and spirit, helping one reconnect with the center of Being.

Headstand offers a new perspective, helping us to overcome individual and collective fears and their roots, including the ultimate fear of the unknown. This pose teaches greater flexibility by helping the practitioner adapt to any situation. It helps us to break free from old comfort zones, stuck patterns, and fixed belief systems to explore expanded perspectives.

The polar shift of headstand raises the feet from the darkness to the light and also inverts the spinal axis and the spinal nerve roots, which will resemble an inverted tree of life. This balances the pranic currents, giving a growing sense of lightness to body, mind, and spirit. It also shakes up old sediment in the subconscious. Practicing even the beginning stages of this pose becomes an opportunity for these latent impressions to rise to the surface of the mind, where suppressed and forgotten memories may be released, creating a growing cellular lightness. Once more, "The invisible must become visible before it can be eradicated (transformed)."

An Introduction to Standing Poses

In standing poses as in all yoga āsana, we create space in our body so Spirit can reveal itself. These poses are considered to be the salute to the Gods and Goddesses of the ten-sided Universe.

Philosophical Introduction

It is said that many moons ago, two *dānavas* (dark forces) performed difficult austerities to gain favor from Brahmā, the Creator. The boon they requested—to be unconquerable by any man—was granted. They then began conquering the three worlds, the Bhūloka (earth plane), Bhuvaloka (astral plane), and Svarloka (celestial planes). They drove the gods and sub-gods out of the celestial regions of the heavens.

Brahmā, Vishṇu (the preserver), Śiva (the destroyer or transformer), and the other gods met upon the banks of the great Ganges River. Knowing that no male or masculine energy could conquer these demons, they prayed to the Divine Mother, who answered their prayers by sending her ten Mahāvidyās, goddesses that manifest in different forms as consorts of Lord Śiva, the Lord of all Yogis. They also represent the ten incarnations of Vishṇu. It is interesting that the feminine outgrowth of the masculine is called upon to subdue the demons. In the story of the birth of Vīrabhadra, the invincible male warrior who arose out of the locks of Śiva's hair, Mahā Kālī was his feminine opposite. Together, they led Śiva's armies and were invincible.

The beauty of the standing poses is that they are like prayers calling upon the ten Mahāvidyās. They are an invocation of the great gods and goddesses of the ten-sided Universe. This is a poetic way to describe the art of standing poses. Within them, the body forms angles— the triune, squares, diagonals, et cetera—that also tie into the astrological constellations. In these poses we propitiate the Universal energy fields and offer ourselves through the angles, which are the visible and invisible universal planes of consciousness reflected in *yantras*. Yantras are the infinite energy fields of the divine essence of all Creation.

Psychophysiological Benefits

Our hips, thighs, knees, ankles, and feet are benefited from these poses. In turn, one's trust, faith, and sense of support is strengthened. Yoga practitioners don't have to waver, or lean heavily on others, or rely on others to reflect who they are. Standing poses help the practitioner find true inner core strength, the centeredness that reinforces the subtle body, producing amazing physical as well as emotional stamina. They strengthen the bones of the lower body, for bones grow along the lines of stress. Placing pressure on a particular area will increase circulatory currents to that area, helping to prevent porosity and increasing bone density. Practicing standing poses reduces high blood pressure, quiets the mind, and increases confidence in one's physical, emotional, and spiritual strength.

Standing poses require bending in the many directions of the Universe. They are prayers, and they offer the psyche the opportunity to transcend rather than sink into old patterns. In some poses the head drops toward the earth, a sign of humility, the humbling or transcendence of individual ego. In the standing poses, we use gravity to transcend gravity, lengthening and elongating the spine and stretching the limbs from the fullness of the bindu.

Tāḍāsana

Mountain Pose

Tāḍā is the mountain.

Philosophical Introduction

The Mountain Pose relates to Mount Meru in the bhūloka, the seen and unseen regions of the earth plane. Meru Daṇḍa, meaning "the mountainous staff," is a name for the spine in yoga. Meru Daṇḍa also means "the central axis of creation." Mountains in the earth plane, like our spine, are vortices of energy or energy fields. In Tāḍāsana, we emulate the strength and height of a mountain on the physical plane. We also honor the stellar regions that reach to the pole star.

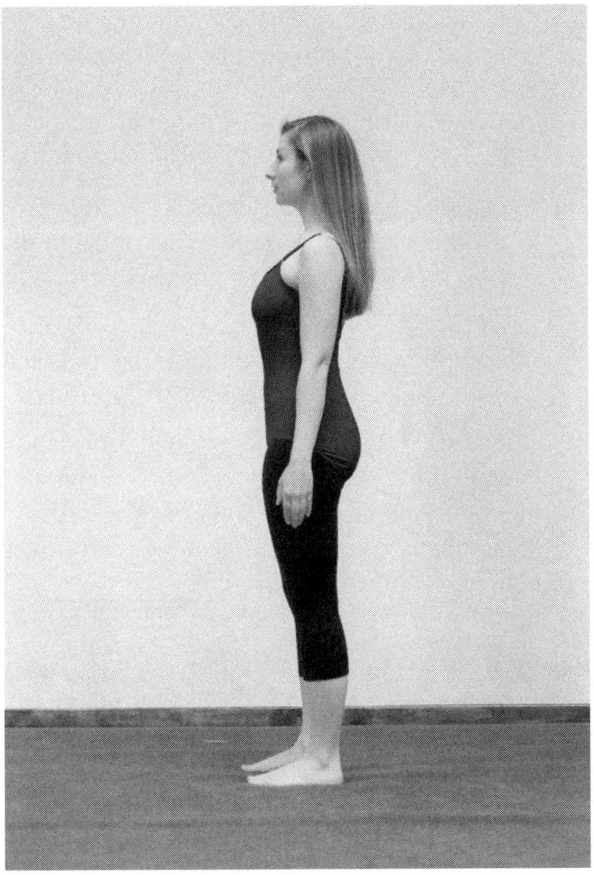

Tadasana is a standing meditation.

Tāḍāsana is the pose we begin and return to during a standing āsana practice. It is the centrifugal center of all standing poses, out of which they arise and to which they return. In Sanskrit, the letters D and T are interchangeable, so *Tad*-āsana could also be known as *Tat*-āsana. *Tat* means "that." One of the great mantras is Tat Tvam Asi, meaning both "Thou Art That" and "That Is Thou." Tat-āsana could be a time not of doing but of being. To be in the state of Thatness, one cannot be pulled into the future, which reflects as the body sways forward on the toes. The toes are the reflexes to the brain and sensory organs. It is important to keep them dynamically relaxed in Tāḍāsana, and in any āsana. We also move out of the state of Thatness when we pull back by locking the knees and tightening the neck in a stance of resistance. This reflects a withdrawal from the present moment to reach back into the past.

Tāḍāsana is a standing meditation where the weight on the feet is not moving into the future or the past. It aligns the right and left hemispheres of the brain by adjusting the weight equally upon both feet. It reaches through the pranic roots of the feet to caress the earth. It draws the earth's energies from the valley beneath our feet through the legs into the spine and up to the mountain peaks in the crown of the head. There are times we may feel as if we are in the valleys of our life. We cannot see or think clearly, making it difficult to get perspective on a situation. When we climb to the mountaintop in the outer or inner worlds, there is an unobstructed view with expanded clarity and realizations.

In the third chapter of the Yoga Sūtras, Patañjali discusses the placement of mountains and planets. Mountains are the vortices, places of convergence. The greatest deities are said to reside on the mountaintops and in the mountain caves where the sādhus go to turn their consciousness inward.

When practicing Tāḍāsana, I think of the goddess Pārvatī. Born as the daughter of Himavan, the Lord of the Mountains, Pārvatī is said to be the incarnation of Śiva's first love, Sāti. After Sati's death, Śiva withdrew to his abode on Mt. Kailāsa into a dark cave buried amongst the snows of the Himalayas. In his grief, he shut himself off from the outside world. In the meantime, demons arose from the underworld and drove the Gods out of the heavens.

The Devas met and came to the conclusion that only a son of Śiva could help them regain their celestial realm. But Śiva had no sons or daughters. The Devas then invoked the mother goddess, who appeared as Kuṇḍalinī, a coiled serpent. For the good of the world, she was determined to make Śiva her consort and father a child. This powerful Śakti took birth as Pārvatī, daughter of the Lord of Mountains. She came into this world to draw the ascetic Śiva out of his cave once more into the world of the Divine Līlā, into the play of life. After many failed attempts, Śiva finally took notice of her and eventually was beguiled by her charms.

Pārvatī, the Mountain Goddess, represents the part of us that creatively brings forth nourishment even in the midst of what appears to be rejection and disapproval. She is a reminder that there are no limits of possibilities when we use our energies in the pursuit of any spiritual goal. Pārvatī symbolizes the Eternal in her femininity, grace and beauty. She was ageless and, like Śiva, timeless. Pārvatī, the primordial prakṛti (the cause of all existing phenomena), balances Śiva in alternating poles of asceticism and eroticism, creation and dissolution. Theirs was a marriage of matter and spirit that brought order and balance once more to the Universe.

In Tāḍāsana, we create a zero point of neutrality between the two polarities: Śiva, representing Puruṣa (that which is unmoving and unchanging) and Pārvatī, representing prakṛti, the Divine Līlā, or play of life. Just as the mountain remains firm, steady, and stable, Tāḍāsana is gives us the same sense of firm steadiness and centeredness in the midst of the changing seasons of our life. Tāḍāsana is a reminder that a journey of a thousand miles—through valleys, caves, and the highest peaks of consciousness—begins where our feet stand.

Guidance

1. Stand with the feet hip distance apart.
2. Check that there is equal weight on both feet. The tendency is to lean on one leg more than the other. How we balance the weight on the feet determines the balance between the right and left hemispheres of the brain. More weight on the right side indicates more left hemisphere activity. Leaning more to the left indicates more right hemisphere activity.
3. Bring awareness to the toes. Are you leaning too far onto the toes? This implies going into the future, an indication that the mind is thinking ahead and planning what it will do next. Are you leaning too far back onto the heels? This locks the knees and creates tension in the neck, throat, and shoulders, and implies resistance or past repressions.
4. Roll the weight to the outer edges of the feet and, as you roll back across the balls of the feet, lift the inner arch and inner ankle.
5. Keep lifting the inner ankle as you lift the toes to feel the strength of the arch of the foot. As the arch and inner ankle lift, equalizing the weight on the heels and the balls of the feet, this brings the legs into a vertical or perpendicular alignment to the earth plane. Dropped arches can send pain through the whole body and has been related to heart problems. As we grow older, dropped arches may reflect prolapse within the internal organs. As we lift the arch, we strengthen these inner organs
6. Release from the roots of the toes to the tips of the toes.
7. Feel that you are caressing the earth with your feet. We honor the earth by giving to the earth and then drawing upon the earth energy for strength, allowing that energy to come into our being. This is how we become bhakti yogis in our pose.
8. Bring awareness to the knees. It is important to lift the kneecaps gently as the tailbone offers itself to the earth. This prevents locking or hyperextending the knees.
9. Inhale, allowing the breath to fill the back and the rarely used tissues at the back of the lungs.
10. Exhale and bring the spine into the front of the body to lift the heart as the tailbone and base of the buttock move straight down into the earth. As the lumbar spine lengthens and the heart center is offered up to the heavens, the crown of the head will align over the base of the spine. This prevents lordosis, overarching the back.
11. Inhale and let the breath fill the back body.
12. Exhale and grow down through the base of the buttocks, going into the circumference of the heels. Feel a lift in the abdominal organs. Take care not to squeeze the buttocks together, which compresses the solar plexus region.
13. Inhale and let the breath fill the back body, placing the hands on the tops of the hipbones.
14. Exhaling, press the hips down and lift the rib cage up off the pelvis. Move the pelvic rim down toward the earth and feel that deep strength and grounding.
15. Inhale and use the breath to lift the back of the rib cage.

16. Exhaling, press the hands down on the hips and keep strength of the lower body as you grow up through the upper body.
17. Inhale into the back body.
18. Exhale and slide the shoulder blades down, allowing the skin to move down the back as the sternum rises. This is the thoracic lift.
19. Inhale into the back body.
20. Exhale and draw the shoulders down, rolling the upper arms out. The palms relax, facing the thighs. Expand from the collarbones outward to the edge of the shoulders so that the arms hang freely. The arms lengthen like raindrops falling from the fingertips to the earth.
21. Inhale into the back body.
22. Exhale, bringing the base of the skull up off the axis of the neck. Lengthen the back of the neck without lifting or dropping the chin. This draws the energy from the front brain to the back brain and creates a balance between the two.
23. Inhale the breath into the back body.
24. Exhale, grow down into the valleys beneath the feet and raise the crown of the head to the unseen mountaintops within the heavens. Now you are connected to heaven and earth simultaneously. That's integral yoga.
25. When you are correctly aligned in Tāḍāsana, the mind comes into a thoughtless state of awareness, and the pose becomes a standing meditation.

Note: Beginners can start by pressing their backs into the wall with their feet approximately eighteen inches away from the wall and knees bent. Bring the outer edge of the shoulder blades to the wall while moving the inner edge of the shoulder blades away from the wall. This moves the spine toward the front body, lifting the heart center. Keeping the back on the wall, exhale and straighten the knees, feeling the skin move down the back and the neck lengthen. This brings awareness to the lengthening of the lumbar and cervical spine, which counteracts the tendency to compress the lower back.

The hardest thing for most people working on the details of Tāḍāsana is the breath. They need more abdominal breathing as they rise up and travel the path of the mountain, which represents our spiritual aspirations.

Psychophysiological Benefits

By practicing Tāḍāsana we gain steadiness of mind and body. The pose strengthens the stabilizing muscles of the abdomen and lumbar spine, as well as the arches of the feet, so that they do not succumb to the pull of gravity. In reflexology, the arches reflect the abdominal and pelvic organs. As we lift and strengthen our arches, we prevent prolapse of the corresponding organs. My mother, who was a reflexologist, used to say, "Your feet are the barometer of the body."

In Tāḍāsana, we create the perpendicular alignment of a straight line between the earth plane and heavens, representing a dynamic ascension of consciousness and our connection to the Creator. This alignment honors both the play of prakṛti (symbolized by Pārvatī) at the base of the spine, and the timeless and eternal state of Being within the crown of the head (symbolized by Śiva). Tāḍāsana unites these two polarities, coming into the center of neutrality between their magnetic poles. This is vairāgya—non-mood or nonattachment—which is one of the ways that Patañjali outlines for quieting the waves of the mind, the essence of yoga.

Practicing Tāḍāsana consciously—making adjustments to the feet, the knees, the rib cage, the shoulders and neck—helps us expand peripheral awareness and energize the corpus callosum, the connecting fibers between the right and left hemispheres of the brain. This brings balance to the feminine and masculine, the spatial and sequential sides of our nature.

Tāḍāsana prepares us for everyday life by teaching us to stand on our two feet. In practicing this pose, we learn how to stay within the center of Being, while at the same time interacting with the world around us. We gain strength of body, mind, and emotions so that we can aspire to the highest peaks without losing our connection to the earth. We find the mountaintop in the marketplace of life.

Tāḍāsana is the foundation of all standing poses. Preserve the feeling of Tāḍāsana as you move into all other āsanas.

Vṛkṣāsana

Tree Pose

Vri is to rise upward, as if transcending the ego in reaching for the light.

Philosophical Introduction

The tree represents the cycles of birth, life, and death and stands as a reminder of the immortality of the soul. Tree of Life symbolism is found in many cultures throughout the world, including Hinduism, Kabbalistic traditions, Aztec culture, the Brahmā Sūtras (Vedānta Sūtras), and the biblical Garden of Eden, in which grew the Tree of Life and also the Tree of Knowledge of Good and Evil. The tree is a magnificent symbol of staying centered in the midst of change. It represents the passing of time and the multitude of ways in which creation expresses itself.

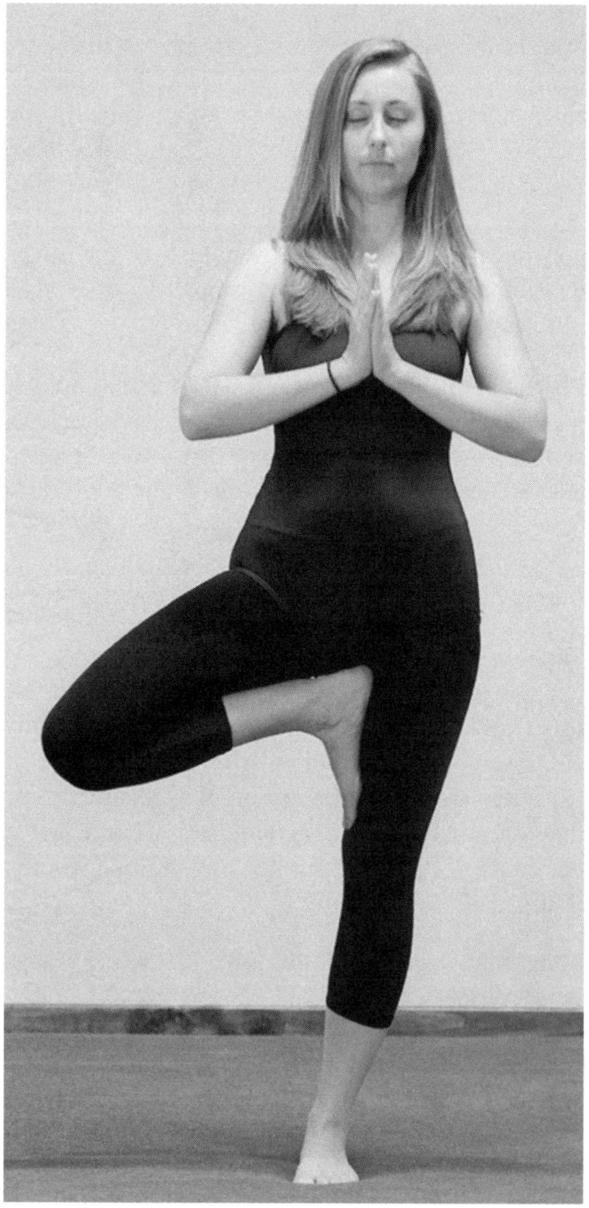

The tree is a magnificent symbol.

We live in a world of duality where the moon rises and the sun sets, where night and day are in contact with one another. In yoga, we attempt to balance these polarities of body and mind to bring us back to the center, where we reawaken from separative conscious and merge once more with the Creator. Both yoga and Āyurveda are based on Sāṁkhya, one of the six philosophical systems of India, which outlines a way to evolve from the plane of matter back to spirit. In Sāṁkhya, the dualistic nature of the universe is sometimes compared to an inverted tree springing from the roots of Brahmā, the creator, and branching into Puruṣa (masculine, consciousness) and Prakṛti (feminine, matter). Together, they gave birth to *Mahat,* the cosmic mind, and then to *Ahaṁkāra,* the ego. Thus the tree symbolizes the soul's journey from the Absolute into form and shows how we can evolve back into the Absolute, the original dwelling place of spirit. In this state, there is no separation of consciousness, no polarities of good and evil, day and night, masculine and feminine.

Ahaṁkāra, the sense of ego, or of "I am," is composed of three qualities, called *guṇas:* 1) *sattva,* the quality associated with lightness and subtle perception; 2) *rajas,* associated with fire, momentum, heat, and friction; and 3) *tamas,* associated with matter, darkness, and inertia. Material reality is perceived through the five senses (the *tanmātras*), leading to a concept of five elements (the *bhūtas*): sound/ether (*Ākāśa*); touch/air (*Vāyu*); sight/fire (*Agni*); taste/water (*Āpas*); and odor/earth (*Pṛthvī*). Creation as we know it descended from spirit into the density of matter, which is reflective in the play of life on the leaves of the tree. The essence of our yoga practice is to reawaken the remembrance of our source.

The tree also symbolizes free will and fate, the karmic cycle of creation. The vṛttis, the electromagnetic waves of the mind, give rise to desires (*kāma*) that lead to actions (*karma*). The result of actions lead to experiences (*bhoga*) that lead to impressions (*saṁskāra*) that drop into the subconscious field of the mind where most cannot be accessed consciously. In the *Bhagavad Gītā* Sri Kṛṣṇa tells Arjuna that the result of past actions is known as karma, and that portion of karma that gives rise to the present incarnation is known as *prārabdha karma.*

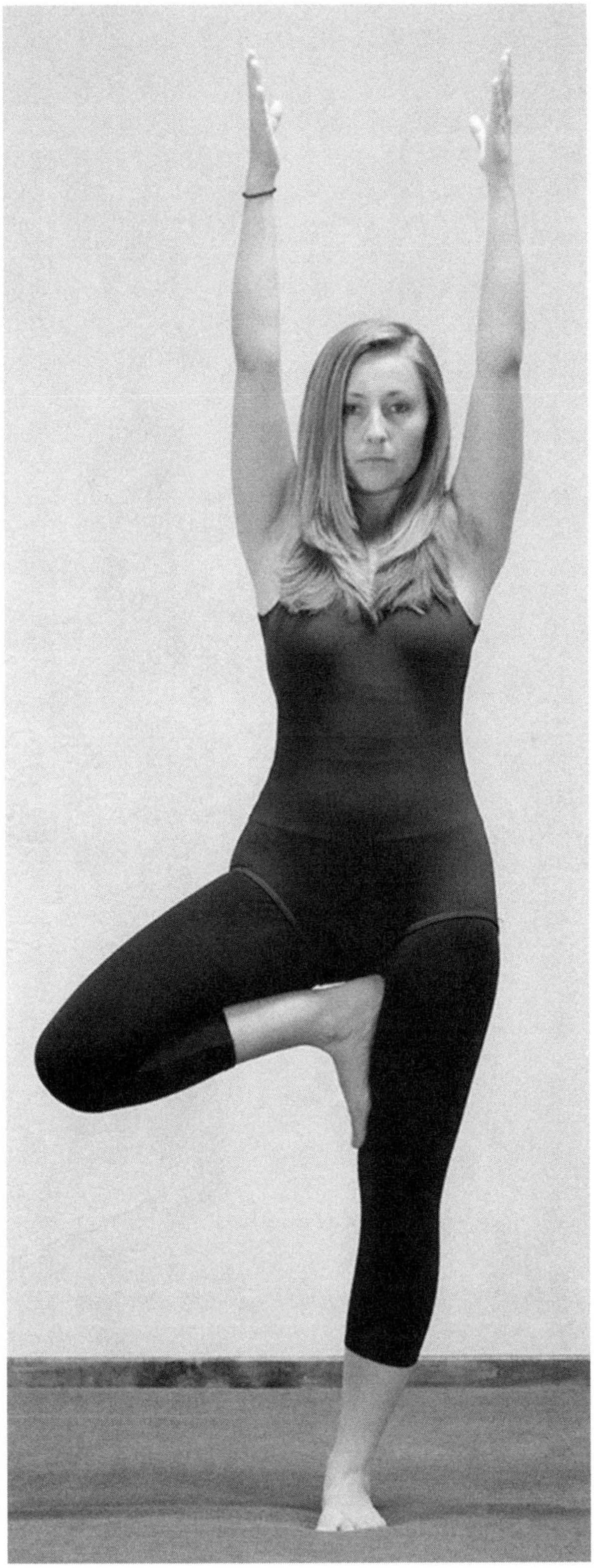

Release the shoulders downward as you raise the arms.

The trunk of the tree is prārabdha karma, grown from the seeds of past actions. The trunk, which some call fate or destiny, determines the origin and family of our birth. It establishes the place, time, and date of birth as well as the span of life. It represents our physical and spiritual inheritance and our destiny in the fulfillment of our life's purpose.

The branches represent *kriyamāṇa karma.* Kriya comes from *kar* meaning "to do" or "to act," and Mana from *man*, "to think," and *manas,* the mind. Some of these branches are the result of past actions, and others are being newly created. Free will is the outgrowth of the thinking mind. We are making choices in this moment that will influence our future destiny.

When the tree's fruit ripens and falls to the earth, reseeding itself, this is known as *saṇcita karma,* when the created karma goes back into a dormant phase. When the time and conditions are ripe, the seeds sprout up as a new tree. The Yoga Sūtras tell us that every conscious experience becomes a subconscious impression. Some are more deeply embedded in the layers of the subconscious, the unseen part of mind, while others may be closer to the surface, the conscious or pre-conscious mind. The ones that are deeper may not always come to fruition in a single lifetime.

Tree Pose, like other āsanas, can bring up subconscious impressions or saṁskāras. The subconscious impressions stored in the hidden depths of mind are like the seeds of *saṇcita karma* that have fallen into the earth beneath our feet. We cannot see them, therefore we dive into the earth with the sole of the foot to feel them while the upper body grows toward the light. Like the Tree of Life in the Garden of Eden, Tree Pose symbolizes our birth from the oneness of Brahman into the world of duality or matter. From this world of matter, we now aspire to return to the garden of the spirit.

Guidance

1. Begin in Tāḍāsana, the Mountain Pose, with the feet hip distance apart. If you need help balancing, stand with the back or the side next to a wall for support. Let the gaze of the eyes descend to a point on the ground about six feet in front of the feet. This can be a practice of *dhāraṇā* (focusing) or *ekāgratā* (one-pointedness). The point is like the *bindu,* the seed point of creation.

2. Keeping the hips level, grow down through the standing leg (the Tāḍāsana leg) and bring the opposite leg up. Place the foot on the inside of the thigh of the standing leg as high up as possible. The more adept can place the top of the foot on the opposite thigh in a half-lotus position. Draw the knee back with one arm while supporting the foot (if necessary) with the other. If the back arches, bring the leg a little lower on the thigh, or even down to the inner knee, calf, or ankle. It is better to keep the hips open and the lumbar spine elongated rather than bring up the leg prematurely.
3. Inhaling, bring the breath into the back, lifting the shoulders toward the ears.
4. Exhaling, grow down into the bottom foot, lifting the inner arch as the ball of the big toe presses into the earth. Relax from the heel to the tips of the toes. Draw prāṇa up the leg up from the earth to draw the top of the kneecap up, and then lift the hip off the upper thigh and elongate the spine, bringing the back spine into the front of the body, lifting the heart center toward the light as you relax the shoulders down. Elongate the back of the neck without lifting the chin.
5. Inhale and do nothing but breathe into the back, expanding it from the center of the spine equally to right and left sides.
6. Exhale and grow down through the bottom foot, lifting the arch and the kneecap. Lift out of the hip socket and elongate the spine, bringing the spine in like a backbend.
7. Inhale and bring the breath into the back from shoulders to hips.
8. Exhaling, bring the spine in and up toward the head without lifting the head. Extend the back of the neck on each exhalation without dropping the chin.
9. Inhale, breathing into the back.

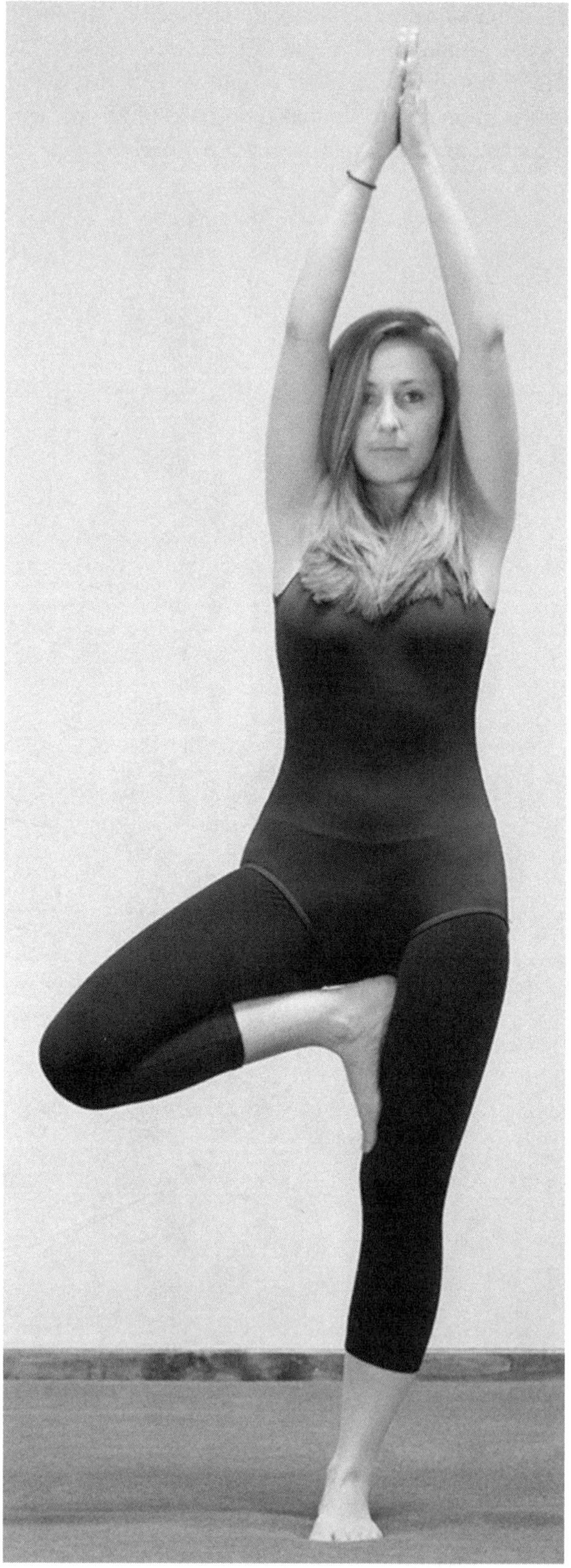

Eventually, the palms will join together.

10. Exhaling, release the shoulders away from the ears and let the arms grow like the branches from the trunk of the spine upward to the light. When raising the arms, be sure not to arch the lower back or lift the shoulders to try to bring the palms together. This creates neck compression. Instead, keep the arms parallel to one another, and with every exhalation, relax the tops of the shoulders down. Eventually the palms will meet. This relieves rather than creates neck tension.
11. Inhale, rounding the back with the incoming breath and relaxing the head slightly forward while lengthening the back of the neck.
12. Exhaling, grow down with the heel and ball of the foot, relaxing the toes. Lift the inner ankle, the tops of the kneecaps, and continue lifting up from the hips through the torso, elongating the spine and bringing it into the front body to offer the heart, along with the arms, up to the light.
13. Inhale and bring the breath from the shoulders to the hips.
14. Exhaling, reach out like the branches of the tree, creating space between the shoulder blades as the arms come down.
15. Inhale, do nothing.
16. Exhale, lowering the upper leg and returning to Tāḍāsana.

Note: If the arch of the standing foot drops, this collapses the adductors (the muscles of the inner thighs), and these muscles will not engage equally along the bones of the leg. Instead, establish your balance through the foot by lifting the inner ankles or the medial knee. If possible, make this adjustment even higher, from the side of the pubic bone, which will create openness through the sacral and pelvic plexuses.

Psychophysiological Benefits

Vṛkṣāsana strengthens the bones and muscles of the legs and increases hip flexibility, working on the gluteus medius and psoas muscles. As we lift the arms, the pose benefits the kidneys and adrenals above the kidneys. Tree Pose also centers the mind, aiding focus and concentration. In this and other balancing poses, we affect the inner ear and the pineal gland (the ancient "third eye"), a gland of receptivity that manufactures melatonin, which relaxes the brain and nervous system and aids in healing insomnia.

On an energetic level, Vṛkṣāsana balances the three doṣas (*vāta, pitta, kapha*) that comprise an individual's constitution according to the science of Āyurveda. A visualization for Vṛkṣāsana might be letting the roots go down deep beneath the earth because it is out of our roots that we find stability. When you describe the concept of "grounding" to students with dominant kapha doṣa (constitutions with more of the water and earth elements), they understand. They usually have their feet planted upon the earth. In fact, they may need to lift their arches because they sometimes have flat feet. When you instruct students with vāta doṣa (a dominance of the air element) to grow down through the feet, it may be harder for them. Practicing Vṛkṣāsana helps balance the doṣas by distributing prāṇa equally from feet to head.

Like a Bhakti yogi, we express our devotion through the sole of the foot as we caress and offer it to the earth. The arms lift, not from the shoulders, but from the base of the spine and the core stabilizing muscles: We are not reaching from the superficial, but from the deeper aspects of our Being. To reach upward, we must sink imaginary roots beneath the foot deeply into the ground. The deeper the roots of the foot, the higher the tree can grow and aspire toward the light. The leaves of the tree may blow about, but the trunk remains motionless in the center of life's storms.

Just as Vṛkṣāsana is a reminder to stay balanced in the midst of change—the seasons of life—it also reminds us to remain neutral and unattached within the center of the polarities of opposites: attachments and aversions, pleasure and pain, praise and blame, criticism and compliment, success and failure. The tree teaches us how to hold the unwavering center where we are not subject to the pull or sway of opposites.

Tree Pose is a more advanced variation of Tāḍāsana. It is Tāḍāsana on one leg. In Tāḍāsana, we learned to balance the polarities. Now in Vṛkṣāsana, we strive to find the same balance on one leg that we found on two. How does this relate to the balance of what we do in everyday life? Can we still hold the balance even though life may at times ask more from us in one area? Can we still hold the center (represented in Vṛkṣāsana by the spinal alignment and the hip opening) even when the storms of life swirl around us?

Naṭarājāsana

The Lord of the Dance

The Lord of the Dance is one of the many forms of Śiva, whose dances can be fierce or gentle, fast or slow. He dances in the evening twilight, and he dances to the music of the gods. He dances on the battlefield and before his marriage, showing that every moment in life is critical. His elations have all the rhythms found in the cosmos. As Natarāja, Śiva dances the world into and out of existence.

Philosophical Introduction

Śiva, the Lord of Yoga, is a contemplative hermit as well as the all-pervasive energy that dwells in all of Brahmā's creations, from the humblest insect to the loftiest sage. There are said to be 840,000 wombs of Lord Śiva and 84 basic Yoga Postures with 10,000 variations on each. These 840,000 postures represent the Infinite within the finite expressions of all created forms. Known to be the originator of the tradition of Hatha Yoga, Śiva was the guru of the first yogi, Matsyendra, the Lord of the Fishes. (Matsyendra's evolution from fish to man is described on page 195).

As Lord of the Dance, Śiva is most commonly depicted as standing with one foot on Apasmāra Puruṣa, the demon of ignorance and forgetfulness, while raising the other with toes pointing to the heavens. In this form of Naṭarājāsana, the pose resembles Śiva's mythic bow. One story of Śiva's bow is found in the Rāmāyana epic:

When King Janaka offered his daughter's hand in marriage to the one who could lift and string Śiva's bow, many princes gathered. Śiva's bow was so mighty that when it was brought to the court, it had to be transported by an eight-wheeled chariot pulled by five thousand soldiers. Seeing this, some of the princes fainted. None who tried could even lift it. The ten-headed demon king, Rāvaṇa, used all his might and the power of his twenty arms. The earth shook like a cradle as he struggled to lift the bow. When Rāvaṇa tried to string it, the weighty bow fell on his bosom and, if not for his karma written on his forehead, he would not have survived. It took five thousand men to lift the bow away from his body. In disgrace, the demon king flew back to Lanka in his aerial car, shouting to King Janaka, "When the right time comes, I shall carry away your beautiful daughter Sīta," and eventually, he did. Śiva's bow was the catalyst of the great epic of the Rāmāyana.

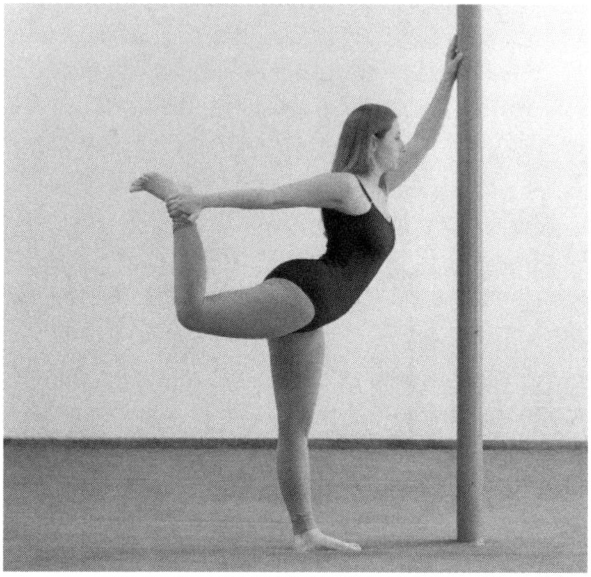

Maintain the upward lift of the torso in Naṭarājāsana.

In Naṭarājāsana, the bottom leg descends into the perpendicular alignment and gravitational pull of the earth. As we grow up out of the earth, like the mighty trunk of the tree, the bowed bend of the upper body assumes a lightness, representing Sīta's prayers to lighten the weight of the bow so her beloved Rāma could lift it. As one arm reaches for the ankle to emulate the stringing of the bow, the other arm reaches for the light of the heavens, as if sending the prayers to Śiva. Śiva must have heard Sīta's prayers, for Sri Rāma lifted the mighty bow as playfully as an elephant lifting a sugarcane.

While the upper body in the pose is light and playful, the lower leg and foot offer weight, strength, and devotion deep into the earth, as if to stamp down the contractive ego of forgetfulness. The other hand reaches above the clouds, where the celestial nymphs, knowing of Rāma's great feat, danced and rejoiced. Flowers showered down from the heavens as Rāma won Sīta's hand in marriage.

Guidance

1. Begin in Tāḍāsana, facing a wall with the feet approximately two or two and a half feet away from the wall. Place the palm of one hand on the wall, elbow straight. Maintain a strong foundation as you inhale into the back, spreading the breath across the back from shoulders to buttocks.
2. Exhaling, bend the knee, bringing the heel toward the buttocks and taking hold of the ankle.
3. Inhaling, relax the iliopsoas region from the core abdominal muscles to the front of the thighs. Relax the quadriceps muscle of the thigh.
4. Exhale, growing through the heel of the bent leg as you rise up out of the hip socket and extend the foot away from the hips.
5. Inhale, allowing the incoming breath to round the back as much as possible.
6. Exhaling, bring the spine in like a backbend, keeping the psoas region open and bringing the foot back as far as it will go, increasing the tension of the bow through the upper arm and the hand that is holding the ankle.
7. Inhaling, allow the incoming breath to round the back again.
8. Exhaling, bring the spine deep into the front of the body, lifting the heart center and lengthening the back of the neck upward as the skin of the back moves downward.
9. Inhale and breathe into the back.
10. Exhale and grow down into the earth with the bottom foot, lifting the top of the kneecap. Align the hips by lifting up out of the hip of the standing leg and lowering the hip of the rising leg.
11. Inhale and do nothing. It is a time to breathe.
12. Exhaling, elongate the spine as you move it into the front of the body. To prevent neck compression, do not lift the chin but elongate the back of the neck as the back skin moves downward. Flex the toes of the upper foot.
13. Inhale, pause, and on the exhalation come back to Tāḍāsana.
14. When you are ready, change sides. On an exhalation, bring the opposite foot up. Be sure to give equal length and attention to both sides.

Note: Students with knee injuries must take care not to jar the knee or pull it back too fast. Beginners can have someone support them, or they can use a wall or chair for balance. Another variation is to practice with a partner, facing each other and touching each other's hands. The challenge of the pose is not to lean forward, but to rise upward. Naṭarājāsana seems like a simple pose, but it can be intense, depending upon the flexibility and strength of the practitioner.

Psychophysiological Benefits

The bow in this standing posture combines the strength of the lower body with the flexibility of the upper body. This bow represents growing balance within all phases and activities of our life. The arm is the bowstring and is taut, giving leverage to the heart center to lift to the heavens while the bottom foot moves deeper into the earth with the gravitational pull, like the weight of Śiva's mighty bow. The arc of the bow bends with the strength and purity of our intent.

The pose strengthens the lower body and gives flexibility as well as strength to the upper body through the tension of two poles. The back of the neck elongates, and as the skin moves down the back, this can be an excellent pose for releasing neck tension. While Naṭarājāsana strengthens the physical body, it also acts on the subtle body through the strengthening of the nervous system, as well as the pranic channels or nāḍīs, the subtle nerve currents. The pineal and pituitary glands are brought into balance, represented by another of the manifestations of Śiva, Ardha Śiva, in which one breast is convex and the other concave, symbolizing an androgynous balance between the feminine (pineal) and masculine (pituitary).

One of Śiva's multitude of forms, Naṭarājāsana—the Supreme Dancer—is a reminder to us of the play of the Universe. His dance is sometimes veiled and other times unveiled for devotees who recognize the Para Atman, the Supreme Soul and ultimate reality, seated within his heart. Śiva's dances tell us to remember the illusion of life and to expand our consciousness to experience life as Līlā, divine play. As the Lord of the Dance, Śiva creates, maintains, and destroys until we realize that all forms come from the same source, and that there is no separation. We are already One with the Universal Source of all creation.

Utthita Trikoṇāsana

Extended Triangle Pose

Ut means to "rise upward," and *hita* (from the root, ri) means to "rise upward again." *Kona* means "angle" and tri means "three." This is commonly known as Triangle Pose.

Philosophical Introduction

Trikoṇāsana forms a beautiful energy field or yantra (geometrical pattern). Yantras are said to be the dwelling place of the deity by whose name it is known. In this pose, the body assumes the form of Sri Yantra, the sacred geometrical force field or vortex within the heart Cakra (Anāhata). Trikoṇāsana is a matrix wherein creation manifests (Shakti or Prakṛti) and returns to its unmanifest form (Śiva or Puruṣa). The diagonal lines of trikoṇa give a dynamic quality to the geometry of the pose. Whenever the body takes the form of a yantra in asana, it becomes an invocation to the invisible energy associated with these particular angles. Thus, Trikoṇāsana is a *pūjā,* an offering, and along with all standing poses, a salute to the gods and goddess of Vishnu's ten-sided Universe.

Triangle Pose honors the sacred number of three. Many things in life manifest in patterns of three, including Brahma, Vishnu, and Śiva; the Father, the Son, and the Holy Ghost; Mother, Father, and Child; and the three guṇas. Tri, the Sanskrit root for three, is found in *trinetri,* the third eye, and in *tripundra,* the sacred mark of Śiva and Trishul. It is seen as the trident carried by Lord Śiva. Traditional Vedic mantras to the deities are performed in multiples of three. In Vedic astrology, where angles rule the major domain of life, *trikoṇa* is where the trinal houses join and is considered to be auspicious.

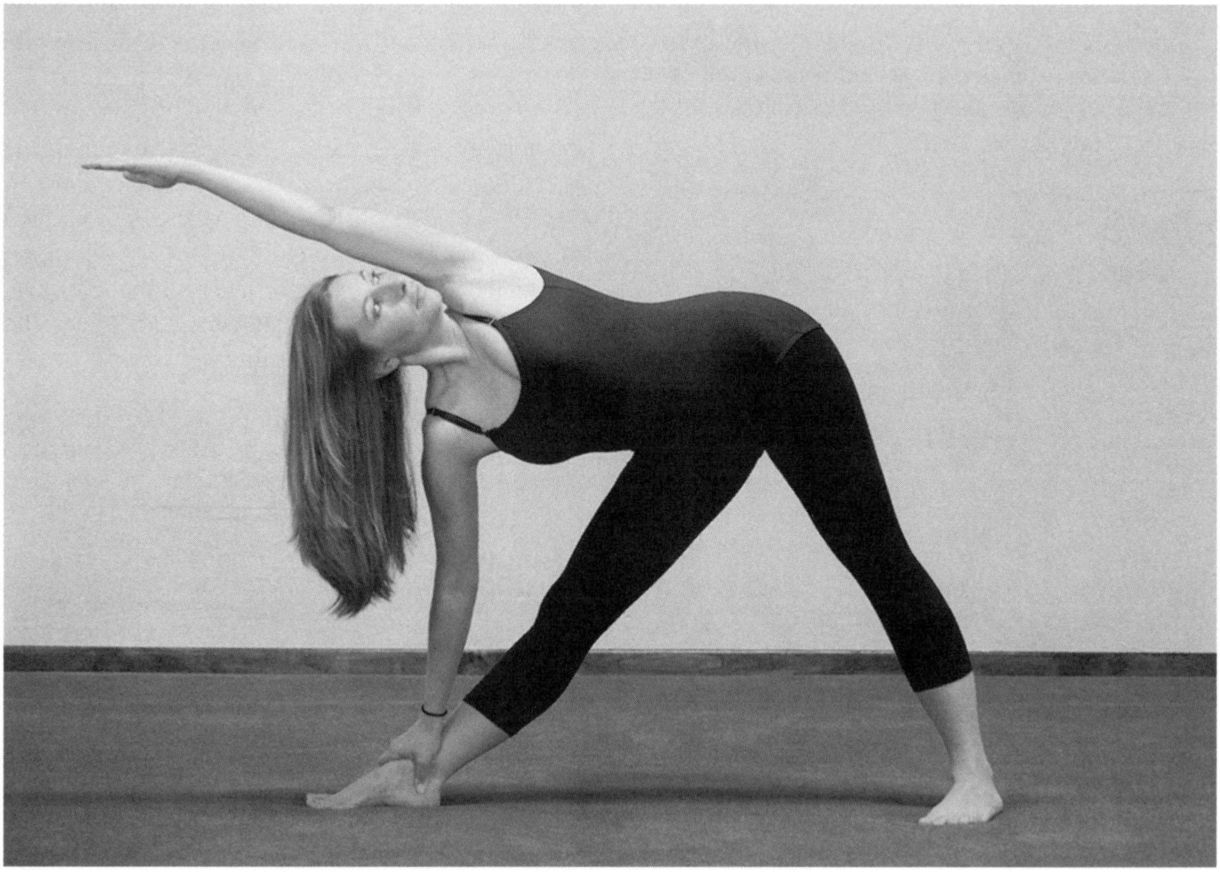

In the full expression of Trikoṇāsana, the upper arm hugs the ear.

The three guṇas—tamas (inertia), rajas (activity), and sattva (dynamic lightness and stillness)—are the constituents that bind the force of all matter and creation. We can see the guṇas operate in our lives. When we feel lethargic, apathetic, or heavy, this may be due to excessive tamas. When we feel restless, agitated or angry, this may be due to an imbalance of rajas. When we are balanced between tamas and rajas and feel lightness, serenity, and contentment, we are in the finest expression of sattva guṇa. The three guṇas can also be applied to asana. When the head is tamasic (inactive), and the spine is rajasic (active), the pose becomes sattvic (dynamically balanced, light, and serene). This exemplifies *Yogaḥ cittavṛtti nirodhaḥ,* the second and most important verse in the Yoga Sūtras, meaning "Yoga is the stilling of the mind waves."

In Sāṁkhya philosophy, the three guṇas are the root of all creation and are considered to be inseparable. They are found within the atom as electrons, protons, and neutrons. They give perception and create the life force within the human body as well as in the world around us. Commentaries on the yoga sūtras say, "The ultimate nature of the guṇas is never visible; what is seen is ephemeral, like an illusion." The guṇas can also be thought of as the waves that oscillate within the mind and all aspects of life. The ultimate goal of yoga is to balance and transcend the guṇas, bringing them into equilibrium with one another so that one is not more of a distraction than the other; this balance allows them to return to their unmanifest state.

The unmanifest state within one's Being is a point (bindu) where all knowledge is in the seed form, from which all things are created and to which all things return. This bindu is considered to be the seed of the entire universe. When the bindu wants to manifest itself, it becomes a triangle. Trikoṇa, the three-sided angle, is created by the effulgent luminosity of bindu.

Bindu, the still point, is Puruṣa or Śiva, immoveable and immortal. Trikoṇa represents Shakti or Prakṛti, the primordial feminine principle that unfolds dynamically, like our limbs in Trikoṇāsana. In this pose, the lower limbs unfurl from the bindu within the procreative plexus in the pelvis, while the upper limbs unfold from the heart center. In his book on Tantra, Harish Johari wrote, "The point inside a central triangle and the center of the yantra is known as Sarva Ananda Cakra, the cakra of total bliss. Śiva is the Bindu and Shakti is Trikoṇa."

Trikoṇāsana depicts the blending and balancing in the mystic union of Śiva and Shakti, the "Being" and the "Doing." The upward-pointing triangle formed by the lower limbs, with the apex at the pubic bone, draws energy upward and away from the world. It represents the element of fire or male energy. This triangle can be seen as Śiva, the upward ascent of consciousness. The downward-pointing triangle is formed by the arm, torso, and leg, with the apex at the point where the hand joins the earth, ankle, or shinbone. This triangle honors the element of water or female energy (Prakṛti or Shakti). The other arm reaches straight up to the heavens, creating a straight line between the hands stretching between the earth and the heavens. This honors both the Puruṣa and Prakṛti, Śiva and Shakti. Prakṛti comes from *pra,* meaning "to bring forth," and *kri* "to do or to act." *Pur* means "to fill," and *uṣa* is "the dawn."

Many years ago, while Mr. B.K.S. Iyengar was demonstrating Utthita Trikoṇāsana at a workshop at Harvard University, he kept asking the two hundred yoga teachers who had gathered to open their armpits. They weren't exactly sure how to do this, so he shouted in frustration, "Open your armpits, I say! You all want to see the light, but your armpits are lying in darkness." As he strode down the aisles, two hundred armpits opened to the light.

In the full expression of Utthita Trikoṇāsana, the upper arm is brought to the side of the head and is drawn upward as the outer edge of the back heel grows deep into the earth. Again, we honor the polarities. Now the head is resting in the apex of the pyramid said to create regeneration. When the arm is brought to the side of the head, it represents neutrality and balance and the joining of the ascending consciousness of Śiva and the descending of Shakti. It seems to say, "Be in the world but not of the world." The two energies of Śiva and Shakti exist in every asana. However, because the triangle is the first yantra to emerge from the bindu, Trikoṇāsana is usually the first standing pose to be taken after Tāḍāsana.

Guidance

1. Begin in Tāḍāsana to establish the breath. Create the base of the triangle by stepping the feet three feet apart or the distance of your leg. Keep the feet parallel to one another. The distance between the feet will depend upon the flexibility of the hips and hamstrings. If there is strain on the knees, it helps to bring the feet closer together.
2. Exhaling, turn the left leg in thirty degrees and the right leg out ninety degrees. Keep the hips parallel to the long edge of the mat. It is important to keep the feet engaged and lifted, as in Tāḍāsana. Lift the inner left ankle, bringing the weight to the outer edges of the foot, and press down with the ball of the right foot as the knee rotates over the median of the ankle. Center the right knee over the midline of the ankle and foot to help realign the hip joint. This equalizes the adductors (inner thighs) and abductors (outer thighs) and equalizes the pressure on the bones of both legs. Keep the toes light and separated.
3. Inhale, breathing into the back body, rounding it slightly and lifting the shoulders with the breath.
4. Exhaling, bring the shoulders down from the ears, lengthen the back of neck, and let the arms fly upward like wings.
5. Inhale and again allow the breath to move into the back. The breath takes consciousness with it. Wherever the breath begins, let it be the teacher to the denser parts, until the entire back body can open and expand with the inhalation.
6. On the exhalation, grow down through the inner left leg, stretching from the left side of the public bone to lift the inner ankle. At the same time, keep the right inner ankle lifted and grow down with the ball of the big toe. The upper right leg and knee rotate externally while the bottom leg rotates slightly internally.
7. Inhaling, spread the breath across the back.
8. Exhaling, allow the spine to move into the front of the body while reaching the tailbone (coccyx) toward the earth, without dropping the heart center. This elongates the lumbar spine.
9. Inhale and allow the breath to fill the back body from hips to shoulders. The arms and hands are the extension of the heart. As long as they are held from the heart center of Sri Yantra, they will not grow tired.

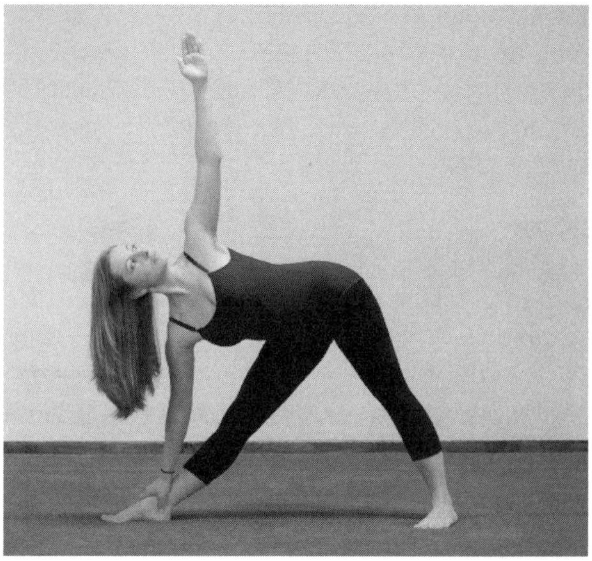

Keep the sides of the torso equally lengthened in Trikoṇāsana.

10. Exhale, externally rotating both thighs, bringing the tailbone down to elongate the lumbar spine, and extending out of the right hip to bring the right hand down to the ankle or shin or to a block. If the hips can stay open and parallel to one another, then bring the fingertips or hand down to the floor in front of the toes. The hand may also be placed on the top of the foot. Keep both sides of the torso equal to one another. Extend the left arm upward.
11. Inhaling, maintain the position and allow the breath to round the back.
12. Exhaling, move the tailbone back and lengthen the lumbar spine, freeing the upper back and allowing the spine to move into the front body like a backbend.
13. Inhale and allow the breath to round the back.
14. Exhaling, lengthen the spine vertebra by vertebra toward the head and into the front body, opening the heart center.
15. Inhale and create space with the breath, rounding the back to open between the right and left sides of the rib cage, the kidneys, and shoulder blades.
16. Exhale and elongate the spine, moving the tailbone in the opposite direction of the head, and bringing the spine in to the front of the body like a backbend. Allow an organic rotation to begin from the base and ripple upward until the heart and the head look toward the light.
17. Inhaling, expand the back laterally with the breath, relaxing the neck.

18. Exhaling, extend the bottom arm toward the earth and the upper arm toward the heavens.
19. Inhale and allow the breath to expand and round the back, bringing the heart center towards the thoracic spine.
20. Exhale, elongating between each vertebra by moving the tailbone back as the spine rotates, turning the heart and face upward to receive the light. This rotation may occur gradually over a period of time.
21. Inhale and do nothing. Make no adjustments, just watch how the breath comes in to the body.
22. Exhaling, draw the spine in and the shoulders down and back as the upper arm moves as close to the side of the head as possible. If the shoulder rises toward the ear, stop at that point and release the top of the shoulder to avoid neck compression. Otherwise, continue extending the arm over the side of the head.
23. When you are ready to complete the pose, inhale, and on an exhalation, bring the upper arm back up to the heavens, letting its heavenly aspirations draw the body upward into the five-pointed star position. Release back to the standing pose, Tāḍāsana.
24. Take the pose to the other side, staying for the same number of breaths.
25. Return to Tāḍāsana and observe the benefits of the pose.

Note: In the beginning phases, it helps to place the outer edge of the back foot against a wall for support and to strengthen the leg. The wall gives something for the foot to press against, activating the adductors and abductors and enabling the hamstrings to lengthen, as well as providing leverage for the spine to elongate.

Years ago, I realized that in Trikoṇāsana and other standing poses, many of us teaching and practicing yoga were extending from the inner knee down to the inner ankle to keep the weight balanced on the outer edge of the foot. Since bones grow along the lines of stress, a few of us were becoming noticeably bow-legged. We were not extending from the inner thighs and psoas muscle. The key to Trikoṇāsana and other standing poses is to extend the inner leg from the side of the pubic bone and even from the skin of the pubis. This not only lengthens and strengthens the psoas muscle but also opens and activates the coccygeal and sacral plexuses.

As the upper torso extends to the side, it is important to lift the tops of both knees gently. By lifting the tops of the kneecaps, we can prevent hyperextended knees. Utthita Trikoṇāsana can also be practiced by placing the bottom hand on the seat of a chair or on a block, rather than trying to reach the hand to the floor.

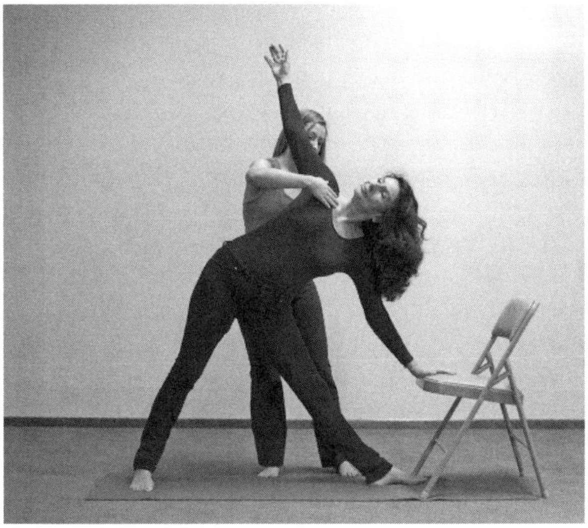

Utthita Trikoṇāsana with chair and partner assist.

When the upper arm extends skyward, the gaze can gently turn toward the hand as the back of the neck elongates. It is important not to turn the head unless the rotation originates from the base of the spine and the upper hip. When the neck tightens, we tighten the lower back, hyperextending the lumbar spine. This can happen when trying to open the chest prematurely, without first establishing openness in the hips. When the rotation of the head and neck comes from a natural evolution in the lower spine, Trikoṇāsana can alleviate, rather than create, neck tension.

Psychophysiological Benefits

Utthita Trikoṇāsana relates to Ardha Candrāsana, Vīrabhadrāsana II, Utthita Pārśvakoṇāsana, and Parivṛtta Jānu Śīrṣāsana. When Utthita Trikoṇāsana is done appropriately, it releases pressure on the lumbar spine and eases neck tension. It can be very beneficial for scoliosis. It works on the respiratory muscles—the outer and inner intercostal muscles of the ribcage and the sternocleidomastoid muscles—as well as on the carotid sinus and the arteries on the sides of the neck. It is excellent for the kidneys, adrenals, and abdominal organs, including the appendix and ascending, descending, and transverse colon. It also benefits the uterine region for women and the prostate region for men.

The full expression of Utthita Trikoṇāsana stretches the oblique muscles and the inner and outer intercostals. Trikoṇāsana firms the thigh and buttock muscles, elongates the hamstrings, and preserves the arches of the feet. When Trikoṇāsana is practiced by extending rather than collapsing the lumbar spine, it stabilizes and strengthens the sacroiliac joints where the sacrum joins with the pelvis. These joints can grow unstable with continued poor posture and the passing of the years. If we rise up out of the hip joints rather than sink into them, our hips can more easily maintain their suppleness and strength.

It is important not to close the hips by going beyond one's svadharma (what is right for the individual) by trying to reach the floor prematurely. This attempt to open the heart center beyond one's current capacity is evidenced by the convex rounding of the upper side of the ribcage. Equally extending the bottom and upper sides of the torso equalizes the prana between the parasympathetic nervous system (the left side of the body) and the sympathetic nervous system (the right side). The spine is equalized when the breath feels equal in the right and left nostrils.

If the feet are not continually brought into alignment, there is a tendency to collapse the adductor (inner thigh) muscles, which puts stress upon the bones of the leg. Some students will try to find the balance by overextending the ankles, others by pressing the medial knee down to the ankle without extending throughout the inner thigh muscles. A complete extension of the thigh of the extended back leg should come from the side of the pubic bone. This will challenge the iliopsoas muscle, one of the largest in the body and one that holds deep emotional memories of the past. As we open and lengthen the psoas on one side the psoas on the other side is lengthened and strengthened and full release is possible.

To find comfort and balance in Trikoṇāsana, it is important to extend the spine first and then allow the rotation of the twist to organically unfold from this extension. If the spine is healthy, when the face rotates upward toward the light, the whole spine rotates all the way from the coccyx. It is the tailbone, or coccyx, that turns the head in Trikoṇāsana, not the neck. This movement begins at the feet, which give leverage for the thighs to rotate externally and open the iliopsoas in the inner groin. This lengthens the lumbar spine. When the upper hip moves back, the coccyx moves toward the front of the pubis, creating the sacral-occipital alignment and activating the parasympathetic nerves. This is the part of the autonomic nervous system that calms, cools, and dilates, creating a sense of growing clarity and relaxation within the action.

Once the foundation is established, and the spine extended and rotated, then the arm can be brought up and over the side of the head. Utthita Trikoṇāsana opens Svādhiṣṭāna (the sacral plexus), and Anāhata, the heart center. In order for energy to reach the heart, it is important to keep the navel passive and relaxed by elongating the lumbar spine. It is the length and suppleness of the lower body that will determine the opening of the upper. Whenever we want to make any adjustments or change in yogāsana, we first start with the foundation. This is a great metaphor for life.

Vīrabhadrāsana II

The Warrior Pose

Vīra in Sanskrit has several meanings: to have unwavering faith and steadiness in any situation, to be steadfast in body and mind, or to be focused and concentrated with unwavering courage. The warrior is one who is balanced in the midst of all life's polarities. A warrior does not fear death but sees beyond the body to the immortality of the soul.

Philosophical Introduction

One of my favorite stories relates the birth of Vīrabhadra, the great warrior who arose from the hair of Śiva. Once, long ago, Dakṣa, a son of Brahma and the father of Satī (the wife of Lord Śiva), held a yagna, a great fire ceremony. The devas and rishis and the lords of heaven all assembled for this auspicious event, but Dakṣa did not invite his son-in-law Śiva, who remained on his snowy abode on Mt. Kailāsa.

When Satī arrived at the ceremony to find Śiva was not invited, she cried out, "Father, only you would belittle such an exalted one. Out of your hatred, your heart has turned from the lord who is loved and honored by the great yogis. What is the use of my keeping this body if it has been born from the one who looks down upon and speaks so ill of the great Lord Śiva?" Satī renounced her father's name and, turning her consciousness inward, she fixed her mind on Śiva and consumed her body in the flames of a self-created fire, giving up her physical form.

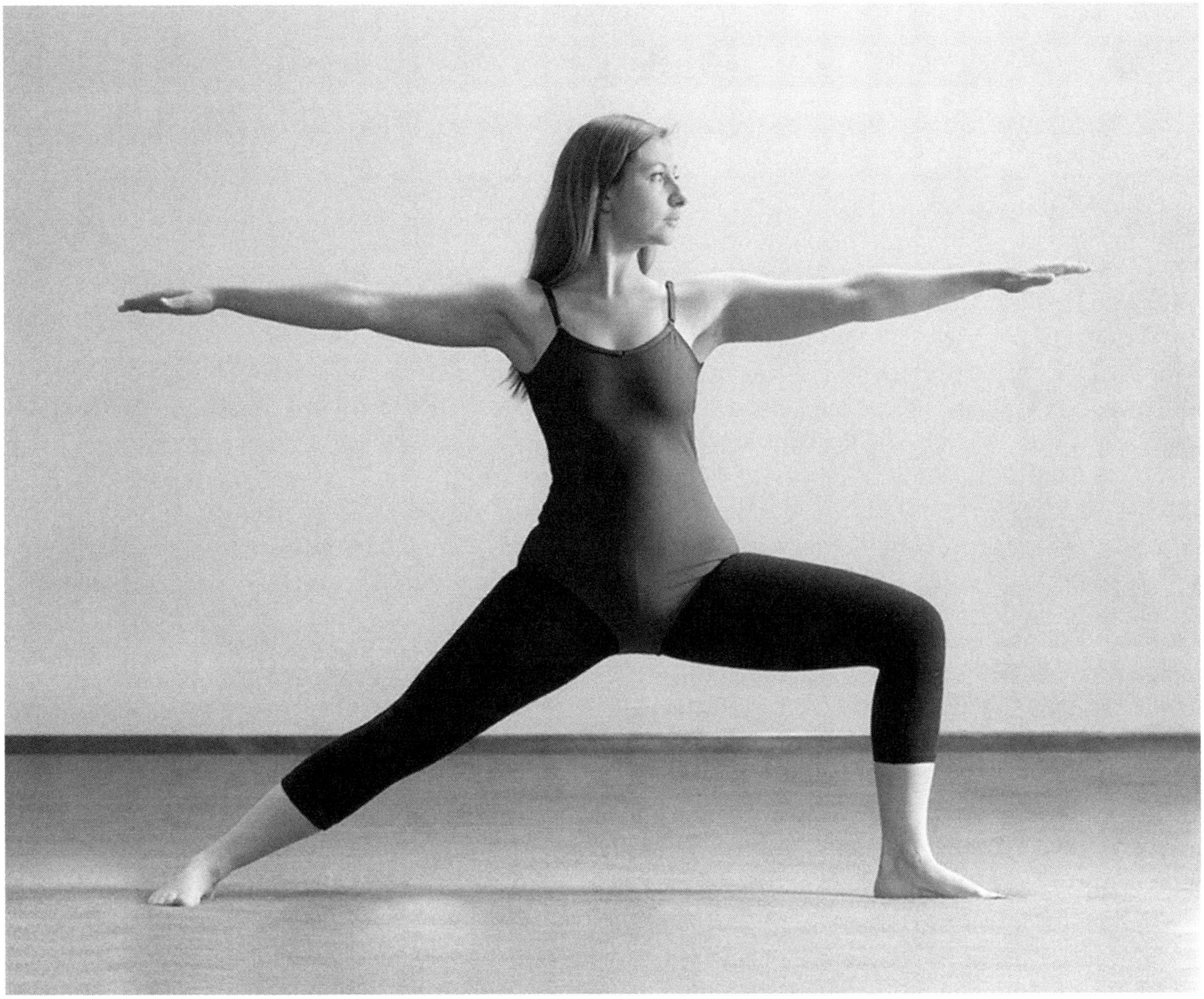

In the full expression of Vīrabhadrāsana II, the gaze extends over the fingertips.

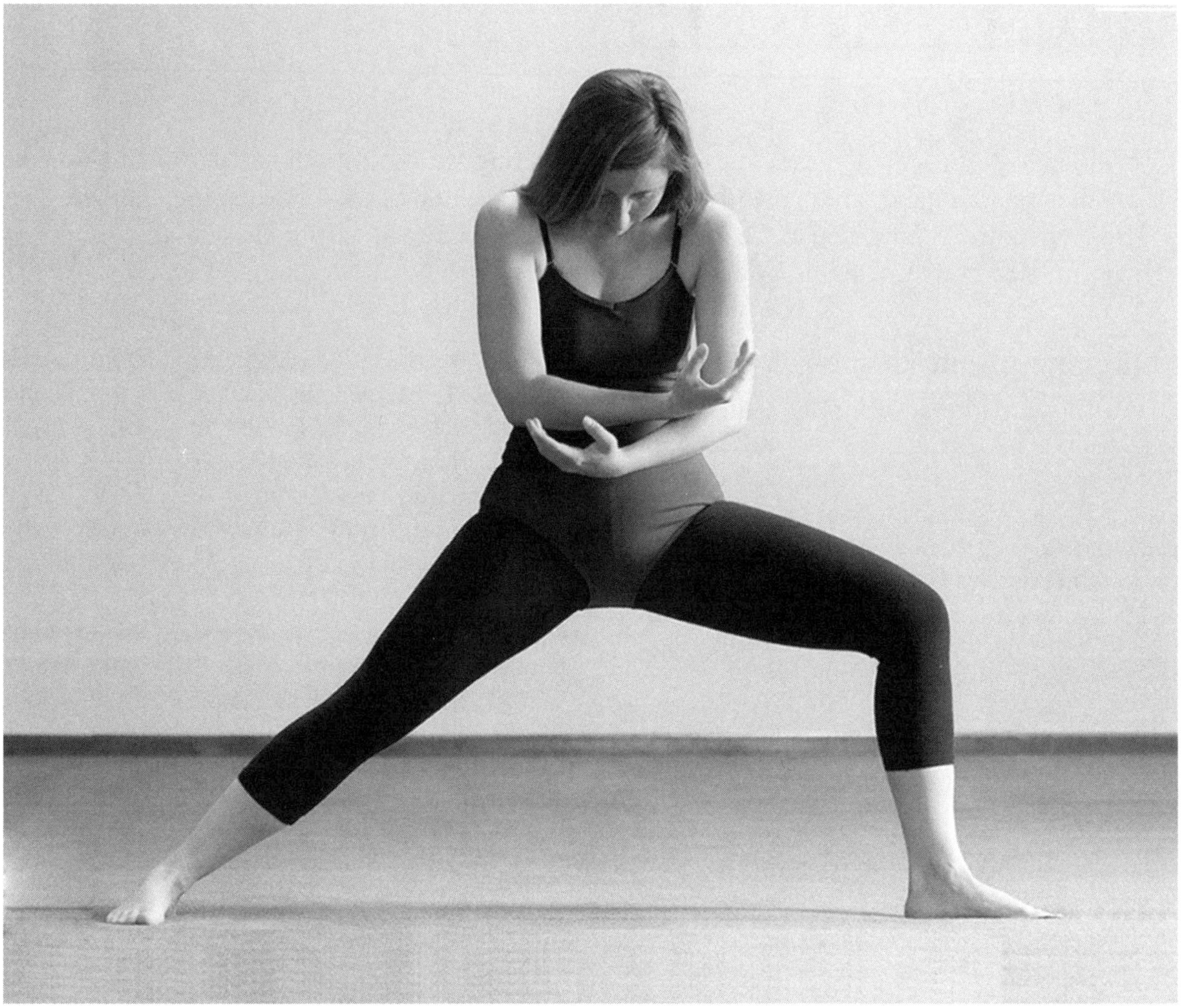

On an inhalation, allow the arms to cross in front of the torso to open the shoulder blades.

The sage Narāda immediately traveled to Kailāsa to inform Śiva of the tragedy. Śiva was so distraught with grief that he tore a lock from his matted hair and cast it to the ground. Out came the mighty and terrifying warrior Vīrabhadra, the manifestation of Śiva's grief and anger. In some versions of the story, Vīrabhadra is joined by Mother Kali, who wears a garland of the skulls around her neck. Kali never shrinks from battle but cuts off the head of the enemy (symbolic of the ego).

Vīrabhadra's power was equal to Kālī's. He was so immense he touched the sky. His thousand arms all wielded weapons that would make him invincible in any battle. Together, these great warriors represent the androgynous balance of the masculine and feminine poles of existence. They asked Śiva how they might serve him, and he commanded them to destroy and desecrate the fire sacrifice.

Vīrabhadra and Kali rallied Śiva's allies and, like a whirlwind, created chaos and havoc at the ceremony. Satī's father Dakṣa was killed by Vīrabhadra's mighty weapons. The reprisal was so devastating that Lord Brahma advised the devas and rishis to go to Śiva's abode on Kailāsa to entreat his forgiveness. They approached with hands in supplication, and Śiva granted a boon: "May all of those who were injured and maimed become healed. May Dakṣa be revived, but with the head of a goat." They returned to continue the ceremony of fire to burn the karmas and bless the world.

Vīrabhadra represents the warrior aspect of Śiva, who is often depicted sitting in contemplation, unmoving and unchanging. However, when it is time to act, the spiritual warrior is powerful, decisive, and immense. Like Vīrabhadra, the warrior has peripheral vision with 360-degree views that stretch into infinity. The warrior transcends self-absorption, rising above his or her own pains that spring from ego or individuated consciousness.

In Vīrabhadrāsana II, even though it looks as if the body is lowering as the knee bends, the upper body is moving up. Polarities exist in everything. As one part moves down, another part moves up. We learned in previous poses, such as Tāḍāsana, to hold equal awareness to both upper and lower polarities. Now, when we practice Vīrabhadrāsana II on the right side and then the left, we also give equal attention to these polarities. In this way, we expand our consciousness gradually to focus on upper and lower, then right and left, and eventually inner and outer. In Vīrabhadrāsana II and the other warrior poses, we use our body as the training ground for expanding peripheral awareness to every part of life.

Guidance

1. Begin in Tāḍāsana by focusing on the breath. Like the wings of an eagle, the breath brushes across the back from the neck to the buttocks, moving horizontally to the right and left of the spinal column.
2. Exhale and bring the feet four and a half or five feet apart, depending on the length of the leg.
3. Inhale and let the breath expand the entire back body.
4. Exhaling, rise up out of the lower body and turn the left leg in 30 degrees and the right leg out 90 degrees. Do not turn the hips with the right leg but keep both hips facing forward as evenly as possible. The heels are aligned. As in all standing poses, remember to relax the toes. Not only are they the nerve reflexes to the brain and sensory organs, clinging with the toes represents abhineveśa, the fifth kleṣa (affliction), which is the clinging to life and the fear of death.
5. Inhale and feel the breath winging across the back.
6. On the exhalation, allow the spine to rise up out of the pelvis, lifting the upper sternum up as the skin slides down the back.
7. Exhaling, release the tops of the shoulders, allowing the arms to fly up effortlessly. Remember that the hands are the extension of the heart. If the arms tire, renew the energy of the heart center with the incoming breath, reaching out to the right and left equally on the exhalations. The arms reach from the sternum, then the armpits, the elbows, the wrists, and last of all, from the knuckles of each finger, with the palms facing the earth. In this pose, we give to the earth as well as receive.
8. Inhale, rounding the back and lifting the back ribs.
9. Exhale and offer the spine into the front body, reaching the tailbone down toward the earth and the heart center toward the light above. Elongate the back of the neck as the upper shoulders release down.
10. Inhale and feel the breath spreading across the back, from shoulders to buttocks, rounding the spine and lifting the shoulders toward the ears.
11. Exhale and roll the shoulders down and back, elongating the back of the neck and offering the spine into the front body like a backbend, lifting the heart center to the light above.
12. Inhaling, bring the breath to the back.
13. Exhaling, allow the breath to rise from the base to the top, lifting the heart center to the light as the skin of the shoulders and back offers into the earth.
14. Inhale, breathing into the back and noticing any areas that the hands of prana have not embraced.
15. Exhale and bend the knee of the forward leg, creating the yantra of the square, a symbol of Gaṇeśa, the remover of obstacles. As the knee bends, lift up out of the basin of the pelvis.
17. Breathe and observe, noticing the balance between right and left, upper and lower, and inner and outer. Find the center.
18. On the next exhalation, maintain the geometrical pattern of the square as you offer the spine and heart upward and extend the back of the neck a little more, releasing the shoulders down.
19. Inhaling, allow the breath to round the back and lift the shoulders.
20. Exhaling, draw the shoulders down, lengthen the back of the neck, and soften and open the throat for the head to turn toward the arm of the bent-knee side, maintaining the strength, balance and steadfastness of the pose.
21. Inhale, breathing into the back.
22. On the exhalation, as the gaze extends over the fingertips, bring the prana or energy of the eyes backward to the base of the skull (the cerebellum) and let the gaze move through the back of the head to "see" the hand and fingers of the opposite arm.

23. Inhale, do nothing.

24. Exhaling, keep the lift of the spine as the knee descends a little further. When the breath becomes shallow or short, it is time to come out of the pose. Simply straighten the bent knee while continuing to lift out of the pelvic base.

24. Inhale and bring the feet parallel to one another.

25. Exhale and return to Tāḍāsana. When you are ready, change sides.

Note: When we feel self-pity or pain there is a tendency to collapse and become self-absorbed. When we are caught in the pit of our own pains, we cannot be there to serve others. Vīrabhadrāsana II teaches us to rise up out of the self and be there for the greater good. Practicing the pose supported by a chair can help students lift up out of the self by opening the hips and lifting the thorax.

Beginning students can sit on the chair, legs relaxed, and focus on lifting out of the pelvis by pressing down on the upper thigh with the hands. Next, they can rotate and extend the back leg to get the feeling of opening and then rotate and bend the front leg, still preserving the lift. Once students have found the openness in a seated Vīrabhadrāsana II, they can simply step away from the chair. Another helpful variation is to brace the back foot against a wall.

Psychophysiological Benefits

The physical benefits of Warrior II are similar to Utthita Trikoṇāsana. Practicing these and other standing poses strengthens the lower limbs, increasing bone density in the legs, pelvis, and spine. Standing poses help to prevent arthritic conditions in the hips and joints of the lower limbs. As we strengthen the legs, thighs, and hips, we gain self-trust, knowing that we have the strength and connection to the earth to rise up out of the pains of the past. Because of the lift up out of the pelvis and the external rotation of the hip, Vīrabhadrāsana II relates to Utthita Pārśvakoṇāsana, Trikoṇāsana, Ardha Candrāsana, and Vṛkṣāsana.

Warrior II brings awareness to the root cakra as well as to the heart and throat cakras. The bent knee forms a right angle or square, invoking the energy of Gaṇeśa and creating foundational support for all life's actions and interactions. As the knee moves down, "we" are going up. This represents lifting beyond old patterns that may have created restrictions and barriers in our lives. Vīrabhadrāsana II helps us to renew faith in our own strength and, like Gaṇeśa, lift the spiritual as well as material obstacles from our path.

The spiritual warrior transcends past pains and hurts, keeping the heart open in the midst of all life's challenges and complexities. The arms extend out from the heart center, and it is said that when we serve from the heart, we never grow tired. If the arms become tired during Vīrabhadrāsana II, bring the awareness to the center of the sternum, breathe in, and on the exhalation let the arms fly out lightly from the heart, forming a straight line.

A straight line, taken into infinity, becomes a circle. The warrior seems to have eyes in the back of his or her head, or 360-degree vision. In yoga, the back body is the intuitive, unseen side. When we bring awareness to this part, we develop our intuitive faculties so that we don't have to turn the head to have a peripheral view of situations. The warrior's circular consciousness or peripheral vision gives her the ability to see all sides of a situation without blaming others or self. The warrior is able to transcend the lower self by lifting up out of the lower body, rising through the spine to stretch the consciousness to the mountaintops. By developing inner strength and expanding consciousness, Vīrabhadrāsana II helps us create a sense of self-empowerment.

Utthita Pārśvakoṇāsana

Extended Side Angle Pose

Ut means "upward," and *hitta* is from *ri,* which means "to rise upward." *Kona* refers to a right angle and *pārśva* refers to the side or flank.

Philosophical Introduction

In this pose, the bent knee forms a right angle. When the arm and hand are in alignment with the lower leg, a square is formed. This is the yantra of the root Cakra, and it is symbolic of Gaṇeśa, the Lord of Thresholds, who protects the spiritual practitioner from any inner or outer obstacles that may arise. As one embarks upon spiritual practices, Gaṇeśa's presence turns stumbling blocks into steppingstones because he brings good luck to those offering invocations. His immense body rides upon the vehicle of a mouse, which reminds us to bear the weight of life's challenges and transcend the downward pull of mind and emotions.

Gaṇeśa is connected with the principal of earth and to the mobility of prana. He is a master of sound and the sacred syllable Om. Gaṇeśa is known to preside over the Mūlādhāra Cakra, the root or support at the base of the spine. This is the area where the goddess Kuṇḍalinī is said to rest in a dormant state, to be awakened by Gaṇeśa. In India, Gaṇeśa is invoked for success at the beginning of important endeavors, and his mantras usually precede any others in a mantra practice.

Gaṇeśa represents change, which appears at every new situation we face in life and in ourselves. He stands as the centurion at the gateway of transformation, representing metamorphosis by letting go of old, rigid, separative beliefs and limited perspectives. His energy is said to bring forth new perceptions, as he opens the gateway of the intuitive mind, allowing for better understanding of our destiny.

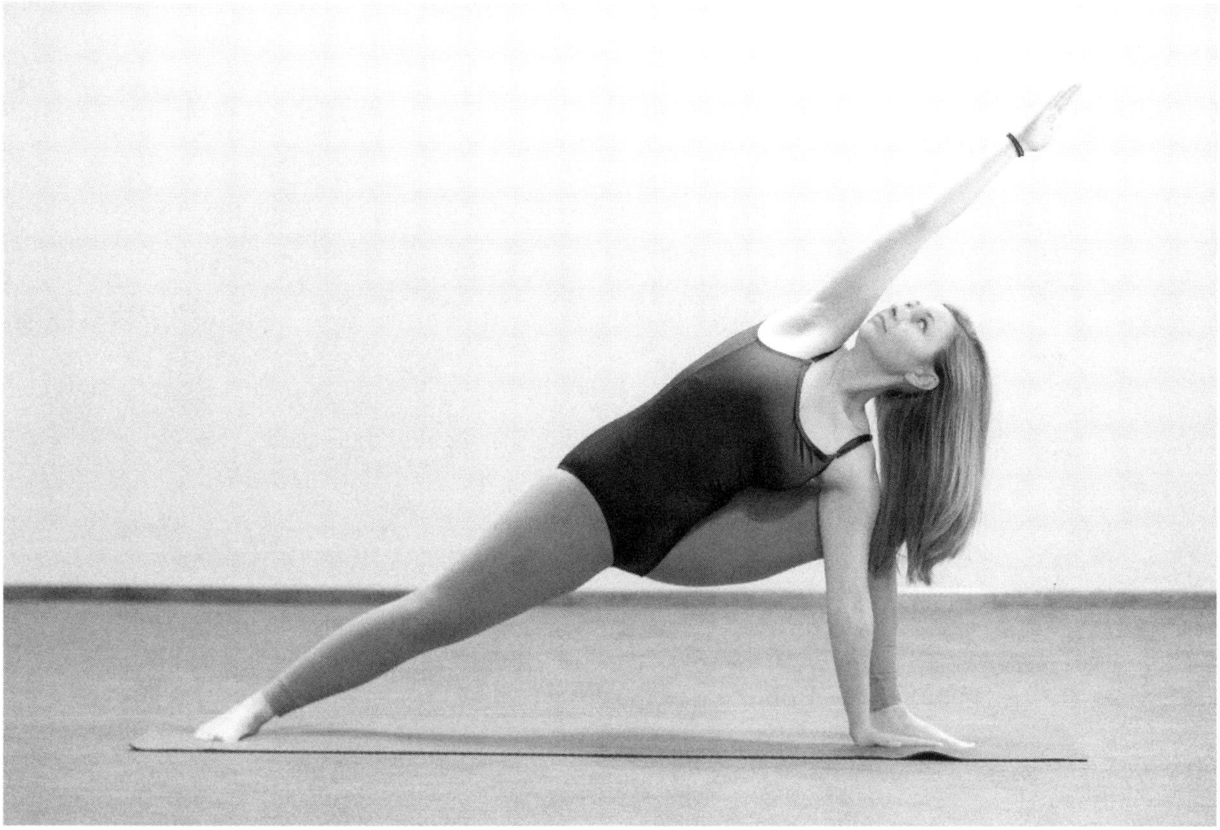

The Pārśva or side flank of this pose forms a diagonal line.

Gaṇeśa has the body of a boy and the head of an elephant, and his pot-bellied form is one of the most loved and easily invoked of all deities. There are several different stories of how Gaṇeśa got his elephant head. A popular story tells that one day, when Śiva was away, his consort Pārvatī was alone. From sandalwood and the dew of her body, she formed a boy to guard her chambers as she bathed. That night, Śiva returned unexpectedly. The boy, never having seen his father, refused entry to the Lord of the Universe. In his anger, Śiva took out his sword and cut off the boy's head. Pārvatī was so distraught that Śiva went out into the night to find a new head. Unfortunately, he could find only an elephant's head, which he placed on the child's body, bringing him back to life. Pārvatī rejoiced and Śiva accepted Gaṇeśa as his son.

Through the loss of his head, Gaṇeśa is a metaphor for transcending the ego, the limited separative consciousness. He is usually depicted holding a bowl of rice or *laddu* (balls of sweetened rice) in one hand while holding the Vedas in the other, showing that we need a balance of physical and spiritual sustenance. His eyes are small, turning into the inner world, while his trunk symbolizes discrimination because it takes a while for the food to reach his mouth, giving time to discern what will be ingested and taken into the system.

The Gaṇeśa yantra of the square formed in Utthita Pārśvakoṇāsana represents solidity and stability. It can also represent stagnancy or static energy. However, when the square is rotated onto its corner, it becomes dynamic. This is seen in the *pārśva* or side flank of the pose, in which the arm and leg form a line diagonal to the earth plane. This prevents the square of the bottom leg from becoming static, and the yantra of the pose becomes a dynamic energy field.

In Utthita Pārśvakoṇāsana, there is equal bilateral extension, honoring the connection to the earth while reaching out toward the heavens. In this, as in all poses, if one part of the body moves in one direction, the other moves equally in the opposite direction. In Utthita Pārśvakoṇāsana, one reaches deeply into the earth through the extended leg, the side of the foot, and the little toe, while the upper flank, torso, arm, and fingers stretch for the heavens. This diagonal yantra equally honors earthly and celestial realms.

The traditional Gaṇeśa yantra has a circle within the container of the square. The circle is dynamic and represents the cyclic force. It is the zero point that contains all forms within itself. (Interestingly, the great pyramid of Egypt was built upon the geometric forms of a square upon a circle.) Within the circle, the Gaṇeśa yantra also includes a triangle. If you practice Utthita Trikoṇāsana, then move into Vīrabhadrāsana II, and then into Utthita Pārśvakoṇāsana, the body forms a triangle, then a square, and then adds a diagonal line from earth to heaven. This creates ever-new forms in our relationship to the magnetic pulls of the earth and the energies of the Universe. In this way, asana can be seen as a living matrix of sacred geometry.

Guidance

Utthita Pārśvakoṇāsana is an extension of Vīrabhadrāsana II. It requires even more concentration (dhāraṇā) to hold all the parts of the body in equal awareness.

1. Begin in Tāḍāsana.
2. Exhale and bring the legs four to five feet apart, depending upon the length of your legs.
3. Inhale into the back.
4. Exhale, bringing the arms up as the tops of the shoulders move down.
5. Inhale and expand out from the inner shoulder blades through arms and fingers, palms facing the earth.
6. Exhaling, turn the left foot in 30 degrees and the right foot out 90 degrees.
7. Inhaling, bring the breath into the back, allowing the breath (not the mind) to round the back.
8. Exhaling, lower the shoulders from the ears and let the arms rise, extending out from the heart center to the tips of the fingers. The arms are dynamic.
9. Inhaling, round the back.
10. Exhale and move the shoulders down, extending the arms from the heart center, and bending the right knee to create right angle to the earth. Be sure the knee doesn't extend over the toes and that both sides of the torso are equal to one another. Bring the right palm or fingertips down to the floor, either in front of the bent leg or behind it. To experience greater extension, you can alternatively place the right elbow on the thigh.
11. Inhale into the back, expanding the breath across the back.
12. Exhaling, bring the spine in like a backbend.

Modified Uthitta Parsvokonasana using the assist of a chair for greater extension.

13. Inhale and breathe into the back.
14. Exhale and elongate the spine, bringing the spine into the front of the body and allowing the spinal rotation to lift the heart. Effortlessly turn the head up to the light, letting this follow the movement of the heart. The rotation of the head and neck comes from the base of the torso, as both thighs are externally rotated, opening the inner groins. This creates an evolutionary spiral of the spine, bringing the bottom side of the torso, the heart center, and the face upward to the light.
15. Inhaling, fill your back with the breath from shoulders to hips.
16. Exhale, bending the left elbow behind the ear and bringing the arm up to the side of the head, behind the ear if possible. Draw the upper shoulder down away from the ear and slowly begin to straighten the arm, but only to the extent that the upper shoulder does not rise to the ear.
17. Stay in the pose only as long as the breath is calm, and then come out of the pose the same way you went in. Change sides, giving equal length to the opposite side.

Note: In Utthita Pārśvakoṇāsana, the further down the arm reaches toward the earth, the harder it is to keep from collapsing the torso or closing the hips. To prevent this, you can use a block or bring the elbow to the knee. Those who haven't developed the strength in the lower body to support Utthita Pārśvakoṇāsana can practice this pose sitting on a chair. This allows them to get the feeling of how to reach down with the lower body, pressing the thigh into the chair. Then they lift up through the torso. After they lift, they can move to the side and create the diagonal line. Practicing on a chair allows them to stretch the pārśva, the side flank, without worrying about the strength of the lower body.

Assist: Working with a partner in this pose will help you lengthen the spine and open the heart center. Your partner will stand behind you and use her thighs to clasp your extended leg. She will gently move the leg and upper hip back toward her as your arm reaches in the opposite direction. Still clasping your thigh between hers, she can use her hands to draw your shoulders toward your hips, moving the skin down the back to prevent neck tension as your arm

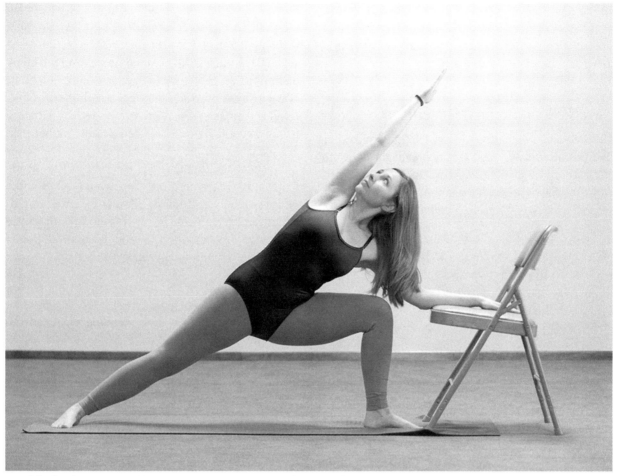

comes to the ear. The coccyx moves back as the head moves forward, which extends the lumbar spine and in turn releases and opens the thoracic spine to bring the heart center closer to the light.

Psychophysiological Benefits

Utthita Pārśvakoṇāsana releases the inner and outer intercostal muscles, freeing the breath through the release in the lungs and diaphragm. The pose also works on the obliques, the rectus abdominus, erector spinae, iliopsoas, trapezius, and all muscles of the upper body.

On a spiritual level, Utthita Pārśvakoṇāsana prepares us to live on the earth plane and in the inner-dimensional states of consciousness at the same time. Practicing this pose, we stretch from the earth to the heavens, from the little toe to the little finger. We welcome the light into our being while connected like the roots of a tree to the darkness of the earth beneath our feet. The light represents the conscious mind, while the darkness represents the subconscious. If we make the decision to release fear and penetrate the unseen depths of the subconscious mind, the leg and lower torso will grow stronger in this process. However, we can only reach as high as we can penetrate the deeper recesses of Being. Make the final reach for the stars without losing the connection to the earth. The reach is like extending beyond old stuck patterns of the past in order to expand consciousness. If we lose the base and overreach with the arm, this reflects a rajasic—restless or competitive—nature trying to get to a goal. This can contract rather than expand consciousness. On the other hand, if one does not make that ultimate reach, this reflects a tendency to get stuck in the comfort zone, which can promote tamas—apathy and inertia. Sometimes we want to stay where we are and don't want to take that little extra step that may be required at strategic points of our life. This, too, contracts rather than expands consciousness.

This pose teaches us to stay balanced in the midst of polarities such as praise and blame, criticism and compliments, success and failure. A square is a neutral foundation that supports and sustains, like Gaṇeśa. It is balanced and strong like the elephant. In the Yoga Sūtras (III:25), Patañjali says, "By practicing saṁyama (concentration, meditation, and samadhi) on the strength of elephants, the power of that strength can be acquired."

Pārśvōttānāsana

Intense Side Stretch Pose

Pārśva means "side" or "flank." Though *tan* is commonly translated as "intensive stretch," it means so much more. In regard to yoga and asana, *tan* implies going beyond self-imposed limitations, the things that have bound us in the past. *Tan* also means "to thin," as in the thinning of the kleśas, life's afflictions. In Pārśvōttānāsana we go beyond constrictions of the side flank of the torso or beyond past limitations.

Philosophical Introduction

Pārśvōttānāsana creates a pole of tension between the base of the spine and the crown of the head. When we transcend self-imposed limitations while in this pose, we can learn how to go beyond the self-imposed limitations in our lives. Our practice becomes a reminder that that no one does anything to us or holds us back, that each of us has the power to make changes and create whatever we wish for ourselves. This brings to mind a contemporary phrase that echoes the ancient yogic concepts of karma and dharma: "There are no victims, only volunteers."

In Pārśvōttānāsana, we offer the upper body to the lower, the torso to the lower limbs. The head humbles itself to the earth. In the fullest expression of the pose, the hands are brought behind the back with the palms together in namaste. The namaste mudrā (gesture) means, "I salute the divinity within you that also is in me." When the mudrā is held behind the back, the hands nudge the back of the heart center, reminding it to hold back no longer but to give and open from its core. The thumbs, which represent the Universal, do not point toward the individual heart; in reverse namaste, they point toward the heavens. This, too, is a pose of bhakti, in which the individual honors the Universal.

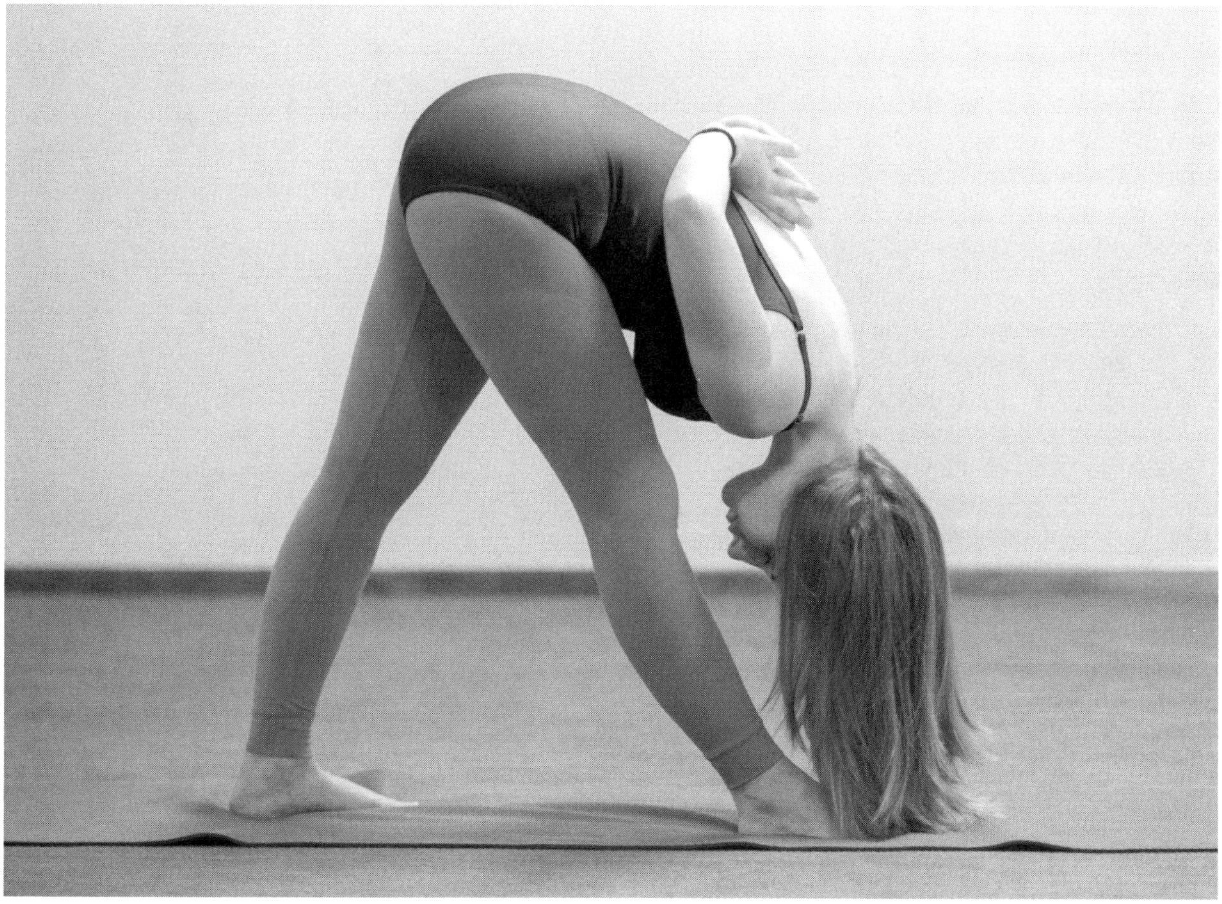

Parsvottanasana, full expression

Pārśvōttānāsana is a wonderful pose to teach us that as much as we move forward into an action, we move back with equal dynamics. In Pārśvōttānāsana, the tailbone moves back as the spine moves forward. Though the tailbone is a small thing, we need to give it even greater attention when most of the body's weight is moving forward. This is like life. When something comes along that takes up all of our attention, time, and energy, we totally disconnect from other things. To maintain a balance in asana and in life, we need to hold two or more polarities simultaneously, giving all parts equal attention.

In particular, Pārśvōttānāsana teaches about past and future. When we find balance in the pose, giving as much attention to what is behind us as to what is in front of us, consciousness is brought into the present moment. It is in the present moment, when there is no pain of remorse over the past and no anxiety about the future, that the mind becomes calm, clear, and balanced.

Practicing Pārśvōttānāsana brings to mind this sūtra (III:52): "Knowledge of the Self and non-self comes from practicing Saṁyama [concentration and meditation] on the moment and its sequence." When a later moment succeeds an earlier one without interruption, it is called a sequence. The moment is defined as "the time taken by an atom in motion leaving one point in space reaching an adjacent point." Commentaries on this sūtra say that in the present moment, the whole Universe experiences change, as past, present, and future exist in that one present moment.

Guidance

1. Begin in Tāḍāsana. Exhale and grow down into the earth through the circumference of the heels, elevating the spine and elongating the back of the neck. The shoulders release away from the ears, and the skin moves down the back.
2. Step the feet two and a half or three feet part, depending upon the length of the legs. Turn the right leg out 90 degrees and the left leg in 60 degrees. Turn the hips and torso with the rotation of the feet.
3. Inhaling, feel the breath spreading across the back in both directions, like wings.
4. Exhale and position the hands (see note) or place the hands on the seat of a chair, shoulder width apart.

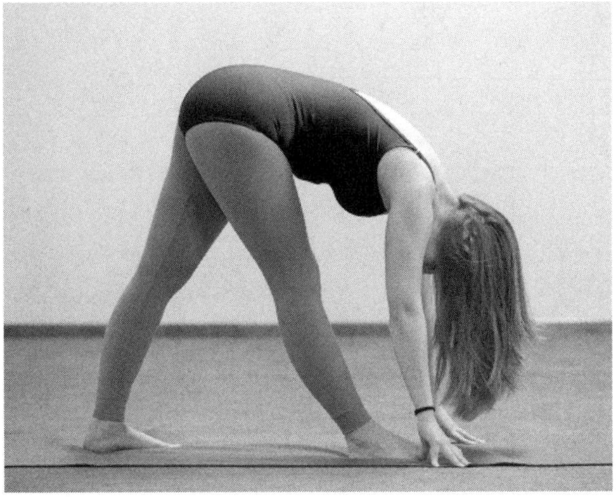

Placing the hands on the floor, or on a chair as a modification, allow the breath to round the back on the inhalation.

5. Inhale, allowing the breath to round the back and lift the back of the ribs.
6. Exhaling, lift the tops of both kneecaps and rise out of the hips, bringing the spine into the front body as though entering a backbend, elongating the back of the neck. Anchor the back heel into the earth, lifting the inner arch and ankle of the back foot, releasing any tension in the toes.
7. Inhale and let the breath round the back.
8. Exhale and elongate the spine, rolling the shoulder skin down the back while bringing the spine into the front of the body and continuing to move the back hip backward. Bring the forward hip back as you roll the front foot toward the ball of the big toe in order to keep the balance of the foot.
9. Inhaling, allow the breath to round the back, bringing it as far down toward the sacrum as possible.
10. Exhaling, release the neck, extending the cervical vertebrae, the base of the skull, and the crown of the head forward. (Do this without lifting the chin, which compresses the back of the neck.) Move the tailbone and both hips back simultaneously to create maximum tension between the two poles of the spine, bringing the mind into the present moment.
11. Inhaling, allow the breath to round the back, lifting the back of the ribcage toward the back of the head and offering the spine to the heavens.

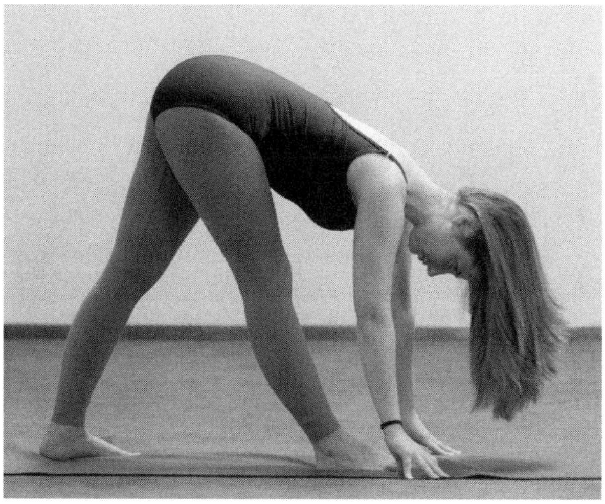

Pārśvōttānāsana, exhalation

12. On the exhalation, keep lifting the back ribs and the floating ribs toward the head as the spine sinks into the front of the body. This elongates the front of the torso and relaxes the navel. Keep the navel passive throughout the pose.
13. Inhale and see if the synovial joints of the ribcage (where the ribs join the spine) can release and create a little more space. Spread the breath in the back, as if spreading it across the earth plane.
14. Exhaling, elongate the spine, bringing it into the front body as though doing a backbend while you enter the forward bend. Lengthen the torso as the weight moves from the tailbone to the back heel. Bring the hips level with one another. If possible, bring the center of the pelvis and the navel toward the legs, and then finally offer the heart and surrender the entire upper body to rest upon the lower.

Note: There is a tendency to lead with the head in Pārśvōttānāsana, bringing the chin up and compressing the neck. This not only blocks the energy between the heart and brain but also reveals our goal-orientation and the tendency to strive in our lives. This striving to get somewhere in the pose takes us out of the moment and usually thrusts the mind and body into the future. In Pārśvōttānāsana, it is important to keep the head neutral and lead with the heart.

In practicing Pārśvōttānāsana, we balance the polarities by balancing the forward momentum of the torso. We do this by bringing attention to the tailbone and extending into the heel bone of the back leg. Both hips move back, and eventually the hips become parallel. The kneecaps lift and act as a springboard for the spine. To create more awareness of the backward movement, place the back heel against the base of a wall for support. The resistance of the wall also serves to strengthen the muscles of the legs and buttocks.

Students with contracted hamstrings can begin Pārśvōttānāsana by placing the hands on a chair. Doing so makes it easier to sense the movement of the spine between the polarities. Eventually, the hands can come to the floor while the forehead rests on the edge of the chair. Supporting the forehead helps the neck release, which in turn releases tension in the lower back.

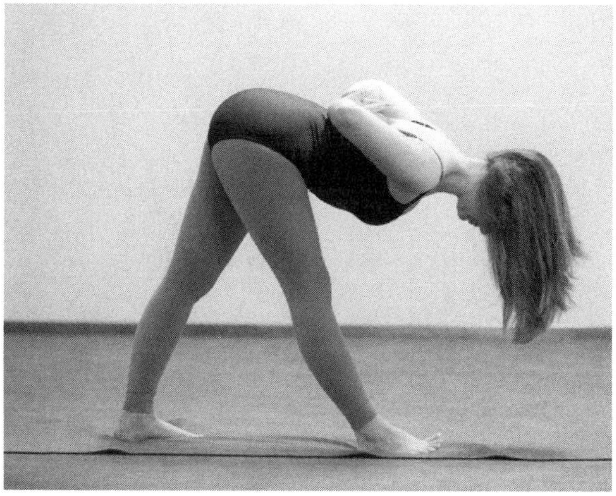

The reverse namaste mudra signifies the balance of the right and left hemispheres of the brain.

The head and heart humble themselves to the earth as the hands offer to the heavens. If the hands are unable to press together in the reverse namaste position, the elbows can be clasped behind the back. Yet another variation is to interlace the fingers and reach the arms up behind the back. When we practice the pose with the hands in reverse namaste, however, the mudrā activates the plexus that innervates the arms and fingers, which relate to each of the five lower cakras (see Lower chakras, page 34). If the hands press together equally, this signifies the balance of right and left hemispheres of the brain. In this way, Pārśvōttānāsana, which moves forward and back, also balances the right and left halves or *pārsva,* the side flanks. Whichever arm variation is taken, it is important to draw the skin of the shoulders down the back as the upper arm rotates externally. This will expand the chest across the clavicle bone and open the heart center.

Psychophysiological Benefits

Because bones grow along the lines of stress, practicing Pārśvōttānāsana and other standing poses increases the bone density of the legs and hips, stimulating circulation within the spine and pelvis. Pārśvōttānāsana, in particular, preserves the flexibility and health of the hip joints and strengthens the musculature of the lower body. It lengthens the hard-to-reach gastrocnemius and soleus muscles of the calf and stretches the Achilles tendon, which relates to intestinal peristaltic flow. Pārśvōttānāsana also lengthens the hamstring muscles in the back of the thighs and strengthens the knees as it opens the minor cakras in the backs of the knees.

Pārśvōttānāsana benefits the procreative organs, kidneys, and adrenals. As we lengthen between the polarities of the spine, Pārśvōttānāsana releases spinal compression and alleviates neck tension. Keeping the neck relaxed aids in the sacral-occipital alignment. There is a direct relationship between the sacrum and the occiput (the base of the skull). Whatever affects one area, affects the other.

When we look at the esoteric anatomy of Pārśvōttānāsana and other asanas, the tailbone moving back represents *tha,* the feminine or lunar aspect of creation. The crown of the head moves forward, representing *ha,* the masculine or solar principle. These two poles *(hatha)* can also be seen as Prakṛti—the feminine principle of creation or Mother Nature—and Puruṣa, the masculine, immutable foundation of Being. As we balance the tension between masculine and feminine poles, light and dark, day and night, this pose exemplifies Hatha Yoga, the union of the polarities.

On emotional and spiritual levels, Pārśvōttānāsana helps us find balance in life as we learn to move in two or more directions at the same time. We also learn to re-center the mind in the present moment and move through life with an open heart.

Uttānāsana

Standing Forward Fold

Ut means to "rise upward" and, as we learned in Pārśvōttānāsana, *tan* refers to going beyond self-imposed limitations. *Tan* relates to the English word "tension" and is found in the names of several asanas, including Jaṭhara Parivartanāsana and Paścimottānāsana. It is commonly translated as "intensive stretch," applying only to the body; however, in asana names, *tan* refers to extensions of not only the physical but also the subtle, mental, and spiritual bodies. These extensions and expansions enable us to process the obstacles known as kleśas, the reasons for our afflictions in life. Once these have been released, we can then quiet the mind.

Philosophical Introduction

The Sanskrit name of a pose reveals the part of the body that is to be engaged and the energy form that will be invoked through the geometrical patterns (yantra) of the body in the pose. Uttānāsana, as its name implies, means "to rise upward and go beyond self-imposed limitations." But how are we to rise upward when the pose appears to be going downward?

Abhyāsa (checking the downward pull) is the first teaching that Patañjali gives for stilling the waves of the mind: *abhyāsa vairāgyābhyāṁ tannirodhaḥ* (I:12). *A* means "to negate," and *bhyāsa* means "outward or downward pull." *Vairāgya* is unattachment. *Tan*—here's that word again—means "going beyond self-imposed limitations," and *nirodhaḥ* is to still the storms or noise of the mind. Thus, the first way to quiet the waves of the mind is by checking the downward pull or reversing the pull of gravity. We can do this emotionally and even spiritually through the upward ascent in the physical body. The concept of *abhyāsa* can be applied to all yoga postures as well as to the postures or positions we take in our life.

In Uttānāsana, we use the downward pull of gravity to transcend gravity by inverting and bringing the head to the earth and the tailbone upward to receive the light. In yoga, the head is a symbol of ego. Wherever our head is going is where we think "we" are going. In this pose, the ego humbles itself. As the crown of the head is offered to the earth, the tailbone—which usually lies in darkness—has the opportunity to rise up and offer itself to the heavens. As the feet grow into the earth, the tops of the kneecaps lift, acting as a springboard for the spine to continue to lift as the upper body descends. Even though the quadriceps muscles of the front thighs are engaged, the hamstrings in the back thigh relax and softly elongate. This creates the appropriate lift of the tailbone, and that in turn allows the downward-moving energy (the apāna flow) to reverse and move upward to the more complex cakras within the crown of the head.

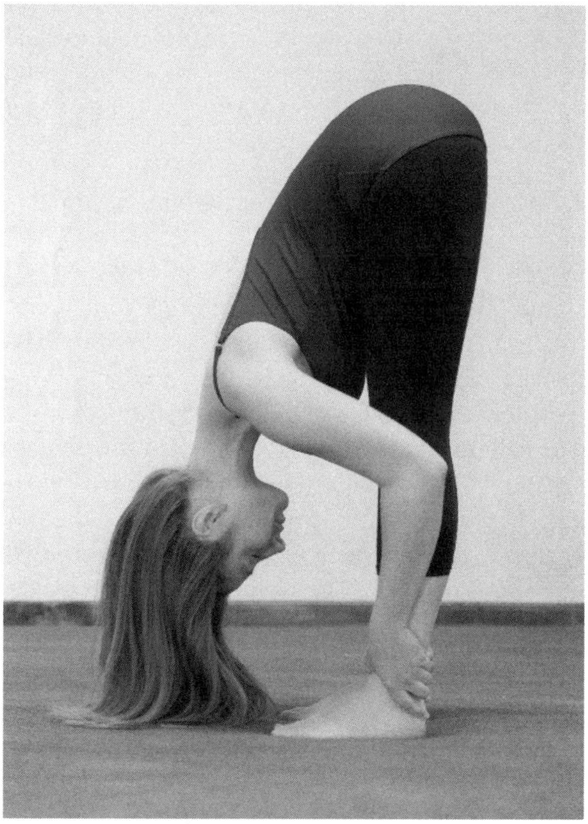

Uttānāsana, full expression.

Yogis say reversing the spinal axis is like recharging the battery of body and mind—bringing the negative emanations from the base of the spine to the positive currents that emanate from the heavens. At the same time, the crown of the head, which has a positive current, comes down toward the negative emanations of the earth. As we reverse the poles of the spine, we gain new perspectives. This effect is similar in other inverted poses, with the exception that our feet do not leave the earth in Uttānāsana.

The feet, according to the Bible and also to the ancient yogis, are symbols of humility and peace. Uttānāsana, which is a forward bend as well as an inversion, humbles the ego as the head is brought down toward the feet. This is a devotional pose that internalizes consciousness while the breath organically brings the upper and lower body together. Uttānāsana becomes an act of Īśvara Praṇidhāna, or surrender to God.

Uttānāsana can also be practiced as dhāraṇā, the sixth limb on the eight-limbed path of Aṣṭāṅga Yoga. Dhāraṇā is concentration, the unwavering steadiness of mind upon its object of contemplation, and it precedes meditation, or dhyana. In Uttānāsana, the upper body is the subject and the lower is the object. It is not necessary to bring the upper and lower together to have a wonderful sense of communion and connection. It is the one-pointed concentration and devotional offering of the breath that brings about this communion.

Uttānāsana stirs up the emotional sediment stored in the pelvis and solar plexus, allowing it to rise with the gravitational pull towards the head, revealing past stored impressions in the psyche. As Swami Jyotir Mayananada said, "When the invisible becomes visible then, and only then, can it be eradicated," or—as we might say in today's world—transformed. In the Yoga Sūtras, Patañjali described what the ancient sages of India had discovered thousands of years ago, that five main impediments (kleśas) hold us back from our true nature. Kleśas comes from *klis,* meaning "to inflict." The kleśas are considered to be the reasons for our pains in life. (For more on the kleśas, refer to page 30.)

These limitations will show up on a physical level in the tightness of our hamstrings and calf muscles, which result in restricted pelvic rotation and back stiffness that prevent us from moving into the full expression of a pose. The pose does not create pain, it simply reveals what is already there. Thus, the *ut* in Uttānāsana is the rising up, not just of the back leg or tailbone, but of the kleśas that are stored in the unseen parts of mind. In yoga, the body is a vehicle to access these hidden parts. When asana practice is centralized around the breath, we can thin the kleshas and go beyond whatever has bound or limited us in the past. Then asana is no longer just a physical exercise that projects outwards, but becomes an "innercise" that brings us deeper into the Self by quieting the mind, which is the essence of yoga: *Yogaḥ cittavṛtti nirodhaḥ* (Yoga Sūtras, I:2).

Guidance

1. Uttānāsana can be practiced with the back resting on a wall and the feet approximately eighteen inches away on the floor, or it can be entered from Tāḍāsana (Mountain Pose), with the feet hip width apart.
2. Inhale into the back, lifting the back ribs and shoulders up toward the ears.
3. Exhaling, keep the lift of the back ribs as you lift the front of the floating ribs and bring the shoulders down, moving the skin of the back toward the buttocks.
4. Inhaling, bring the hands to the upper thighs and press down while repeating the movement of lifting the back ribs and shoulders upward.
5. Exhaling, press the hands against the thighs to give leverage to raise the back, sides, and front of the ribcage off the pelvis and bend from the hips (not the waist). Lift the pelvic rim away from the thighs.
6. Inhaling, stay wherever the pose is at this point while rounding the back with the breath.
7. Exhaling, bring the back spine into the front of the body as if doing a backbend in the forward bend. Roll the shoulders and skin of the back toward the buttocks, giving length to the back of the neck. Allow the head to hang toward the gravitational pull to release any cervical compression.
8. Inhaling, take no movement or adjustments. Allow the breath to spread across the back from shoulders to sacrum.
9. Exhale and lift the kneecaps a little more to activate the quadricep muscles of the front thighs. Soften the hamstrings in the back of the thighs. Do not try to stretch these muscles but allow them to relax and lengthen. Hold an attitude of ease while focusing on the movement of the spine. As the exhalation continues, bring the spine into the front body as if doing a backbend. Keeping the navel passive, lengthen the front of the torso to bring the fingertips to the floor (or to blocks or the seat of a chair), resting the fingertips either above the toes or on the sides of the feet. Do not go too far down prematurely. Feel the back of the spine. If the spinous processes are protruding,

there is anterior compression. Stop at this point: Breathe in and then, on the exhalation, see if the front of the torso can lengthen a little more to bring the vertebra into their natural alignment. If the face and neck are tense or if the navel puffs out, it means the ego is involved in trying to get somewhere in the pose and we have gone beyond what is right for us *(svadharma)*. It is best at this point to continue the pose by bringing the hands down to a chair or blocks. This also helps the navel center to remain passive. When it is passive and the neck extended and relaxed, the mind comes into a quiet and restful state of awareness. If the pose can move from this point, it would be what the Bhagavad Gītā refers to as the inaction within the action.

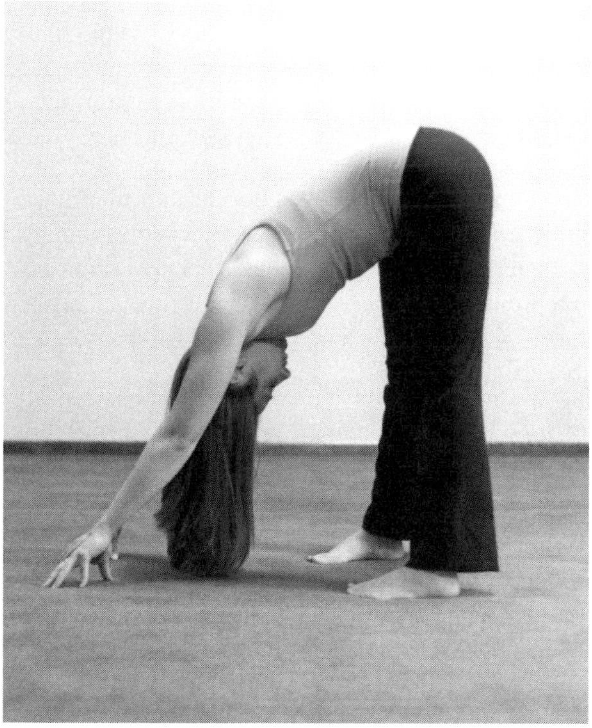

Inhale, reaching through the fingertips as the breath spreads across the back.

10. Inhaling, allow the breath to spread horizontally across the back, lifting the back of the lower ribcage up toward the shoulders.
11. Exhaling, keep lifting the back ribs up as the side and front ribs rise, lifting the upper torso off the pelvis. This gives space to the digestive organs as well as the diaphragm.
12. Inhale, rounding the back and letting the upper arms internally rotate. Lift the shoulders toward the ears as the back ribs lift.
13. Exhaling, roll the upper arms externally to move the shoulders away from the ears and bring the back spine into the front body, opening the heart to the lower legs. (This can be done with the hands on a chair.)

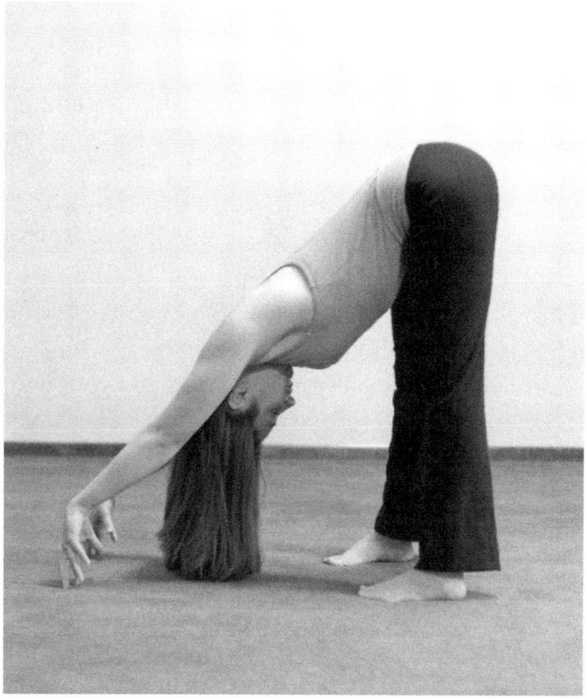

On the exhalations, explore the backbend as the counterpose within the pose.

14. Inhaling, continue to widen the back body with the breath.
15. Exhale and offer the upper to the lower body, bringing the spine toward the front of the body as if doing a backbend in the forward bend. Offer the tailbone (Mūlādhāra cakra) to the heavens as the head (Sahasrāra cakra) humbles itself to the earth. Stay in Uttānāsana as long as the breath will allow. If the breath has stopped or become shallow or arrhythmic, it is time to slowly ease up out of the pose.
16. Inhaling, come up with a rounded back.
17. Exhaling, return to Tāḍāsana—relax the shoulders away from the ears, grow down through the feet, and lift up out of yourself. As the crown of the head lifts to the heavens, the tailbone once more faces the earth, its energy acting like a grounding rod. Caress the earth with your feet as the crown cakra lifts to the heavens and breathe.

Note: Do not *try* to stretch the hamstrings. Focus on the breath and spinal elongation with rotation of the pelvis. Relax and *allow* the hamstrings to lengthen as the tops of the kneecaps and the quadriceps lift upward toward the hips. In all forward bending it is important to keep the navel center passive and relaxed, whether inhaling or exhaling, or moving into or out of the pose. The ego expresses itself in the navel plexus as self-will and competitive striving, trying to reach a goal before the body is ready. It is important to honor where the body is now, as it will reflect any known or unknown resistance within the mind.

When we stay on the edge of our abilities and go only so far as we are able, we practice what is known in Sanskrit as *svadharma. Sva* means "one's own," *dharma* (from *drish*) means "to see," and *ma* is nature. In svadharma, we are "seeing one's own nature." Practicing svadharma in asana means doing that which is right for us personally regardless of how it appears to those around us. In svadharma, we are not overreaching to achieve a goal or to compete with those around us. Doing so could throw the body out of alignment and balance on many levels. (For more about svadharma, see page 31.)

In Uttānāsana and other forward bends, anterior compression of the solar plexus is revealed when the abdomen puffs, preventing the spine from fully lengthening. When this happens, instead of creating more equanimity, the pose can create more restlessness. When practicing svadharma, one does not compete even with oneself. If we can move to our edge, then we can use the breath to take us a little farther (*tan*). As we gently and gradually expand the parameters of the pose we also expand the parameters of our consciousness.

Psychophysiological Benefits

Uttānāsana is central to all standing poses and is the standing equivalent of Śavāsana, which reenergizes the body. In keeping the head and neck passive while moving the thoracic spine toward the front of the torso, the pose becomes a backbend in the forward bend—a counterpose within the pose. This is the model for every asana, keeping the front and back spine—the central axis of creation—balanced and lengthened to prevent any compression of the nerve roots. In Uttānāsana, we use gravity as an ally, extending the spinal vertebrae from the base to the top of the neck. This relieves compression of the skull upon the atlas and axis bones of the neck, preparing the body for twists and all seated forward bends.

Sri Aurobindo Gosh once called yoga "Compressed Evolution." In Yoga, we don't wait lifetimes for the kleśas to manifest; we reach into the cellular structure of our being with the breath and the poses to clear the channels and allow the impressions to reveal themselves. As this happens, there is a lightness that permeates the cellular structure of the body and mind. This *tanu,* or thinning, allows us to go beyond past patterns that have bound and limited us in consciousness. By thinning the midline of the body in Uttānāsana we release emotional barriers. Practicing this way brings the kleśas to the surface where they can be experienced and released.

The Sūtras tell us that when the kleśas are scorched, they can no longer germinate. This brings one into the state of *nirbīja samādhi*—samadhi without seed. According to the scriptures of yoga, this is the highest samadhi because the soul is liberated and not subject to eventual rebirth.

If, however, if we are interested only in stretching the hamstring muscles, Uttānāsana is still an excellent pose to prepare the body for inversions, twists, and forward bends. It teaches us how to maintain equanimity in any position of yoga and life.

Backbend Over Chair

Backbending with a chair teaches us how to surrender the spine into the front of the body in order to open the heart.

Philosophical Introduction

Yogis say that you are only as young as your spine is flexible. The hyperextension of backbends gives a youthful vibrancy and elasticity to the spine and create lightness of spirit. Backbends keep the spine, and the mind as well, supple and flexible.

Just as forward bends are an act of passive surrender, backbends are an active form surrender. They are Īśvara Praṇidhāna, an offering to the Universal or surrender to God or Self. In the Yoga Sūtras, Īśvara Praṇidhāna is the devotional practice that Patañjali mentions more often than other methods for stilling the waves of the mind. He says, *samādhisiddhiḥ Īśvarapraṇidhānāt* (II:45), which one commentator on the sūtras translates thus: "Samādhi comes through the surrender or devotion to Īśvara, the Lord of this world, the teacher of even the most ancients."

When the arms reach back during backbending there is no defense. We open to our own vulnerability, which is where we gain the greatest strength. The eyes and head also reach for the back body, the part we usually cannot see, which relates to the subconscious mind. This may bring up memories and long buried saṁskāras, or past impressions stored within the cellular memory of the psyche.

This backbend begins before ever moving the torso backward. The spine itself, like a crescent moon, moves deeply into the front of the body so that the spinous processes of the vertebrae cannot be felt with the hands upon the back. Thus, this backbend begins in a forward bend. This asana teaches us the art of doing the counterpose within the pose. It opens the back horizontally with the incoming breath and elongates the spine vertically with the outgoing breath. The movement of the backbend reminds me of a cross, symbolizing our horizontal expansion and outreach in service to humanity. On the exhalation, when the spine ascends vertically, I feel it is a personal communion with the Creator.

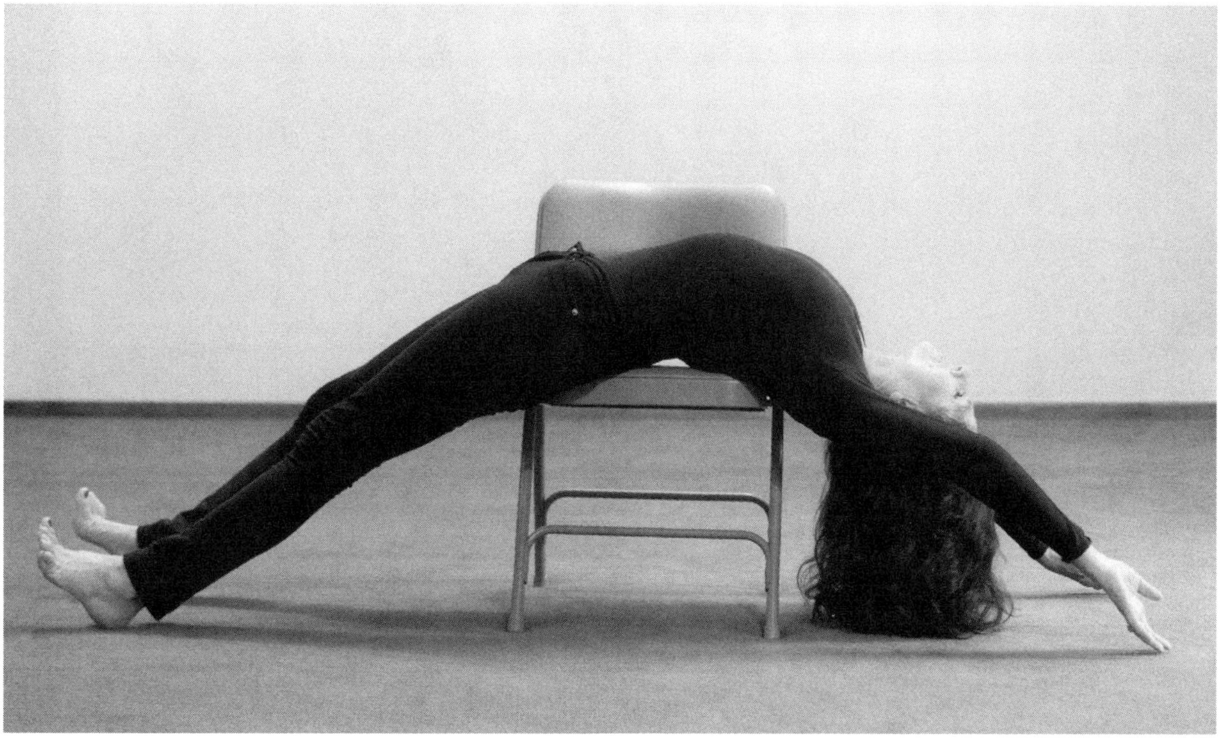

Backbends are an active form of surrender.

If we take this asana or any asana without emphasizing the breath, the mind becomes more active rather than peaceful and calm. It is important in any pose to move only on the exhalation. Remember, it is through the exhalation that the ego unravels itself. In backbends, we move on the exhalation not only to transform the ego but also to release and unravel the body's knots of hypertension and stress.

Guidance

1. Begin by sitting sideways on an armless chair.
2. Spread the legs hip distance apart and press the hands down on the thighs, using traction to lengthen the spine.
3. Inhaling, bring the breath into the back, rounding the back with the breath from shoulders to hips.
4. Exhaling, press down with the hands on the upper thighs, elongating the spine and moving it into the front of the body.
5. Inhaling, widen the back with the breath.
6. Exhale and again press down with the hands on the upper thighs. Move the spine forward as you lift up the front floating ribs, extending the front of the torso and bringing the navel center toward (not to) the inner thighs. Pause when the exhalation ends.
7. Inhale and again allow the breath to round the back, observing the breath to see if it will expand the entire back horizontally from shoulders to buttocks. Let the head relax down.
8. Exhaling, offer the spine into the front body, elongating the torso so that the front and back body are equally lengthened. Bring the navel toward the thighs, keeping the lift and openness of the heart center. This preparation is the backbend in the forward bend.
9. Inhale, staying where you are in the pose as the breath moves horizontally across the back, spreading the right and left sides of the torso out away from the center of the spine. Move the hands down to the top of the knees to give leverage to lengthen the spine on the exhalation.
10. Exhale, keeping the length of the front of the torso as you elongate the back of the neck like a turtle coming out of its shell, extending the neck away from the shoulders as the back skin moves toward the buttocks. (Do not compress the neck by lifting the chin.) Bring the heart center toward the knees as the spine moves into the front of the torso.
11. Inhaling, stay where you are in the pose and round the back with the breath, allowing the shoulders to lift toward ears.
12. Exhaling, elongate the neck even more as the spine comes in like a backbend. Touch the spine to see if all the spinous processes are embedded into the front of the body. If the vertebrae are protruding, don't go down as far. Instead, elongate the spine a little more with each exhalation.
13. Inhale, rounding the back and returning to a sitting position. Sit erect for a moment and enjoy any sensations that may arise and drop away. Sit in the center of your Being.
14. When you are ready to continue, keep the knees bent and slide the hips forward to the side edge of the chair. Supporting yourself with your arms on the seat or back of the chair, lie back so that the shoulders are level with the opposite edge of the chair. Just the head and neck will extend downward.

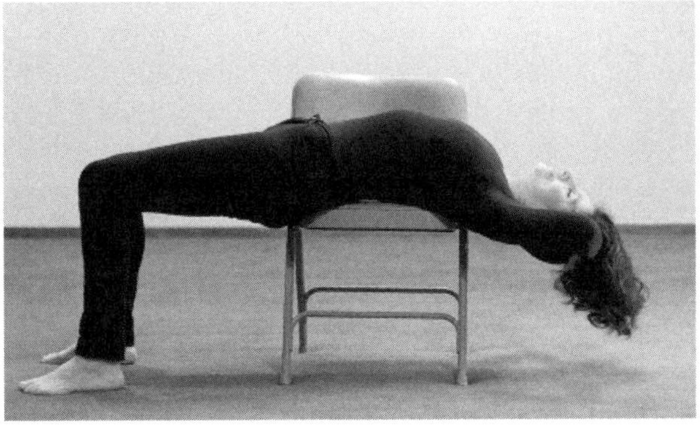

With knees bent and hips at the edge of the chair, inhale and clasp the hands behind the neck.

15. On an inhalation, clasp the hands behind the head, bringing the elbows into the side of the head and lift the head away from the shoulders.
16. Exhaling, with the hands still clasped behind the head to support it, lift the head, lengthen the neck again, and then gently lower the head. (This helps prevent neck compression.)
17. Inhaling, take the breath horizontally across the back.
18. Exhaling, and while extending the neck, come up to the balls of the feet and tuck the buttocks under without dropping the heart center. (This lengthens the lumbar spine and prevents compression.)
19. Inhale and round the back as much as possible, lifting the back ribs.

20. Exhaling, offer up from the base of the pubis to receive the light from above as you simultaneously offer up from your heart center.
21. Inhaling, bring one bent elbow across the chest to open the back of the shoulder blade away from the spine.
22. Exhale and keep the space between the shoulder blade and spine as you reach the arm toward the floor and release the arm toward the earth behind the head.
23. Inhaling, bring the opposite bent elbow across the chest, widening the space between the scapulae even more.

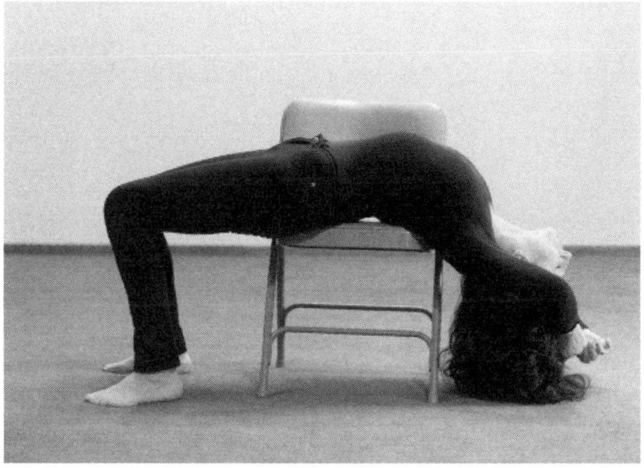

Open the heart center without closing the space between the shoulder.

24. Exhaling, reach that arm above the head, opening the heart center a little more without closing the space between the shoulder blades.
25. Inhale horizontally into the back.
26. Exhaling, stretch the legs out one at a time, keeping the heels on the floor as you extend from the heels and then the balls of the feet without shortening the Achilles tendon. Lift the kneecaps. The knees are the springboard for the spine.
27. Inhale and exhale, staying in the backbend as long as the breath is rhythmic and calm.
28. When you are ready to come out of the pose, exhale and bend the knees, supporting yourself by bringing one arm to the back of the chair and the other to the back of the head. With a straight back, return to the sitting position and prepare for the counterpose.
29. Exhaling, press the hands down on the upper thighs to lengthen the spine and bring it into the front of the body. Continuing to move on the exhalations, lengthen the front of the torso and bend forward from the hips, to complete the backbend in the forward bend.
30. When there is a feeling of completion, exhale and sit up. Close the eyes (if they are not already closed). Turn the palms upward, allowing the hands to rest on the thighs. Enjoy the meditative aftermath or "fragrance of the pose."

Note: The breath helps elongate the spine and the increased length prevents compression. By moving on the exhalation, we create inner space. In doing this, we will be better able to handle stressful situations in life, and won't need as much space around us. A feeling of outer pressure comes when we don't have the inner space to draw upon.

Psychophysiological Benefits

The backbend over a chair is not just for beginners. The chair gives a foundation of support for every level of student to learn to open to the light of the universe, knowing that we are supported and sustained by a power greater than ourselves. It is through this support that we can release habitually contracted muscles to create the inner space that brings about a quietness of mind.

With the support of the chair, we can create equal length to the front and back of the spine and bring circulation to all the vertebrae. This releases tension in the solar plexus and opens the diaphragm for improved breathing. The pose stretches and strengthens the abdominal muscles and the erector spinae muscles, and lengthens the psoas muscle within the groin. It creates space in the digestive organs such as liver, gallbladder, spleen, pancreas, stomach, and intestines. This backbend is wonderful for the kidneys and the adrenals. Due to the support of the chair, backbending does not overtax the adrenals but helps restore and rebuild their reserve in times of stress.

The support of the chair also helps us to lengthen the lumbar spine to prevent compression in other poses. The most mobile part of the spine is between the fourth and fifth lumbar vertebrae. Because this part of the spine is more mobile, there is a tendency to do backbends only from this area. If the entire spine is not engaged and extending equally, the lumbar area is overworked, leading to possible compression and even disk degeneration.

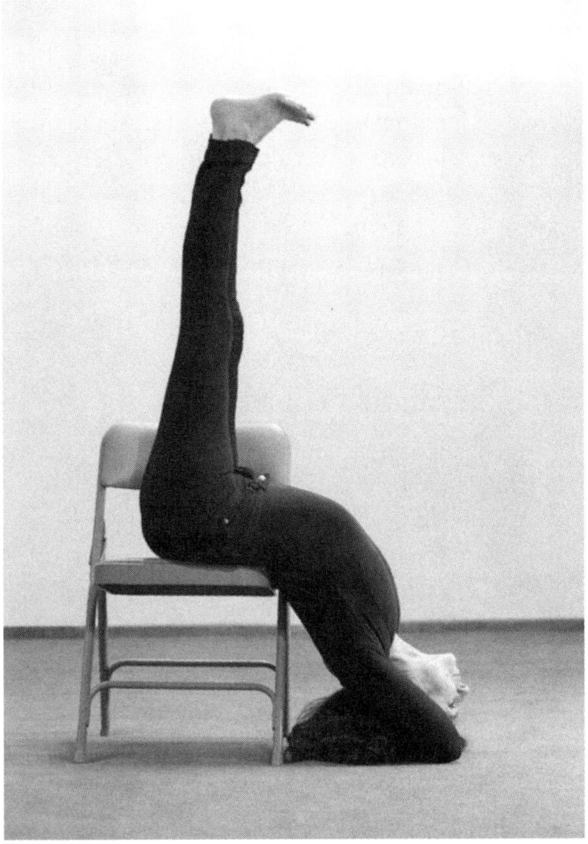

This variation of the backbend over a chair is an excellent preparation for headstand.

Thus, practicing this backbend over a chair is one of the best preparations for forward bends, headstand, and shoulderstand, as well as for Fish Pose and other hyper-extensive asanas. The backbend over a chair helps alleviate neck and shoulder tension and, if aligned appropriately, strengthens the spine and opens a heart that may have been closed for a very long time. It brings us back into the center and reminds us of the vast inner worlds that wait for our exploration. Though it may appear to be a simple pose, this backbend opens us to our own vulnerability, where we gain the greatest strength.

Setu Bandhāsana

Bridge Pose

Bandha means "to bind," and *setu* means "bridge," something that joints two points of separation. In Setu Bandhāsana, we bridge the Ātman to the Brahman, or the individual to the Universal.

Philosophical Introduction

A bridge is meant to bind two opposite sides or shores together. It is a passageway from one place to another, from one body of earth to another. In the Rāmāyana, the great epic of India, Rama builds a bridge to rescue Sītā. After procuring the blessings of Varuna, the God of the Sea, Sri Rāma called for the construction of a bridge made of rocks, earth, and trees to connect southern India with Sri Lanka. This bridge allowed Rama's warriors and Hanumān's legions of monkeys to cross and fight Rāvaṇa, the ten-headed demon who had kidnapped Sītā.

Setu Bandhāsana represents the battle of our primordial instincts, in which we slay the demon of the ego, or the illusion of separative consciousness. As we bridge the gap between our lower and higher nature, we reunite with the light in remembrance of our Eternal Self.

It is interesting to note that earth usually supports and gives form to water, but the bridge, built from earth's elements, signifies water supporting earth. In Setu Bandhāsana, the first cakra of the earth element is prominent over the second cakra, the water element. These elements are offered to the upper body. Prana rises from the primordial centers of our being into the heart center, symbolized by Hanumān, who represents bhakti or intense devotion. Eventually, the prana moves even higher to the throat cakra, ultimately winding upward from the back of the head to the crown cakra, Sahasrāra. The breath, which is the invisible link or bridge between the mind and body, is the prana that flows from the base of the spine upward to the crown of the head, uniting the polarities of bottom and top, Shakti and Śiva, or Sītā and Rāma.

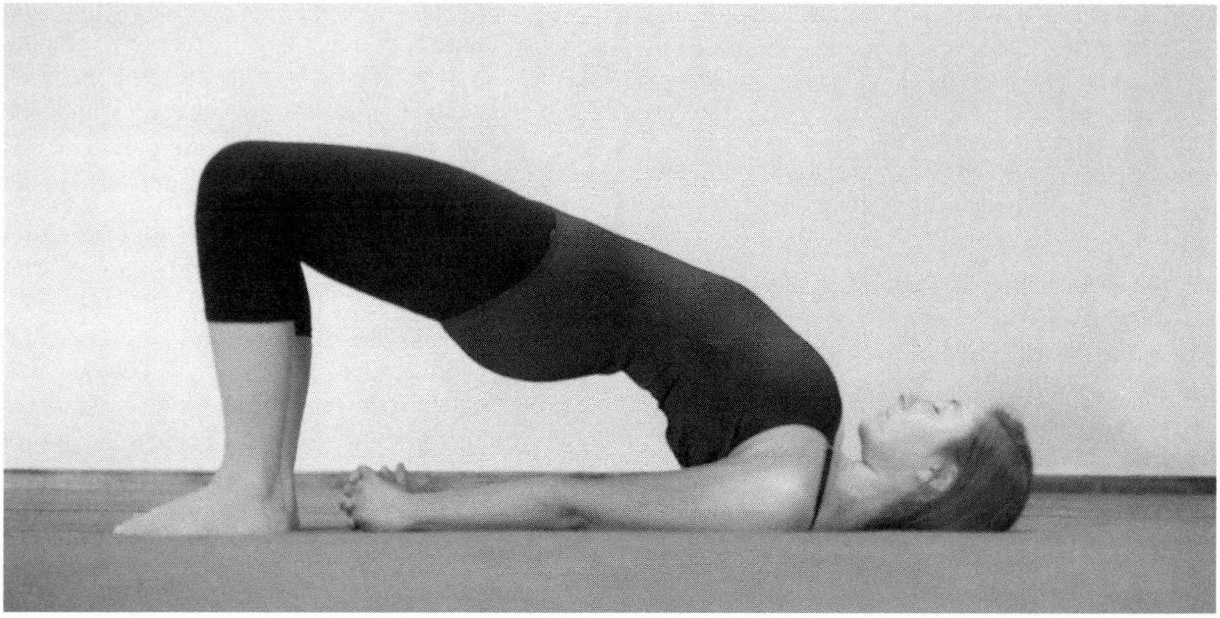

Bridge Pose is a simple but profound preparation of the body and mind for all asanas.

This story is deeply symbolic. The demon represents the many heads of the ego that need to be vanquished or transcended so that Sītā, representing the Shakti that dwells in the darkness at the base of our spine, can be freed to reunite with Rama, the light dwelling in the solar region or crown cakra of the head. In this sense, the bridge links two opposing forces within the self, allowing the practitioner to rise above the alternating currents of conflicting mental and emotional turbulence in order to still the waves of the mind. This is the essence of yoga that Patañjali defines in the second of his sūtras: *yogaḥ cittavṛtti nirodhaḥ.*

Guidance

1. Lie on the back, close the eyes, and breathe abdominally. Bend the knees, bringing the feet to the floor as close to the hips as possible. The feet are parallel to one another and the knees are hip distance apart. This aligns the femur bone in the acetabulum or hip socket. (Bones grow along the line of stress, and we don't want to stress one side of the bone more than the other.) The weight is evenly distributed around the circumference of the heels. Relax the toes: Gripping with the toes indicates contraction of the brain cells.
2. On an exhalation, press down with the heels and lift the hips, offering the heart center toward the head while elongating the lumbar spine down to the tailbone.
3. Inhale, focusing on abdominal breathing, keeping the breath in the lower torso versus the upper chest.
4. Exhaling, relax the head, face, tongue, and lower jaw. Relax the shoulders and arms. Turn the palms to face the light to draw in the energies of the heavens. This also relaxes the shoulders and neck.
5. Inhale, focusing from the back of the sacrum around the sides of the pelvis to the front, comfortably expanding the abdomen with each incoming breath.
6. Exhale and elongate the lumbar even more without dropping the heart center. Keep the upper body and arms relaxed.
7. Inhale and do nothing as the mind observes the breath
8. Exhaling, adjust the weight of the body equally on both feet (keeping the toes relaxed) and both shoulder blades. Relax the buttock muscles. When the buttock muscles are released, the pranic energy can flow freely from the base of the spinal axis—the Mūlādhāra cakra—to the Viśuddhi cakra within the throat center. When the buttock muscles are released, and the weight is distributed equally beneath the feet and shoulder blades, Bridge Pose begins to hold itself. When the body is perfectly balanced, the mind rests, and the pose becomes like Śavāsana. We can even sleep within it.
9. Breathe slowly in and slowly out. Observe the mind getting fidgety and wanting to come out of the pose. Hold beyond this point, releasing the mental effort within the pose. Keep the eyes closed so the brain can rest. Relax every part of the body, the parts that are not "doing the work" and even the parts that are, like the buttock muscles.
10. While slowly and calmly inhaling and exhaling, relax the tongue and let it drop back. Relax the face and head, and then spread that sense of relaxation down to the shoulders and into the arms. When using the lower body, there is a tendency to grip with the upper body. But if we release that grip, we can experience the effortlessness where the asana holds itself. This is a metaphor for life.
11. Inhaling and exhaling, bring the chest to the chin (rather than the chin to the chest). Keep the thoracic region lifted. If this is difficult, place a rolled blanket under the back midsection of the ribs.
12. Inhaling and exhaling, keep the flame within the heart center burning brightly. This feeds the lower procreative centers just as the lower centers feed bhakti, the devotion of the heart center.
13. When you are ready, exhale and slowly come out of the pose the same way you went in. Bring the upper back down first, vertebra by vertebra, elongating the lumbar in the descent, and then let the lumbar rest fully upon the earth. Slide the legs out diagonally to relax the pelvic organs and allow the lumbar area (which relates to the frontal brain) to relax and let go.

Note: Setu Bandhāsana is an excellent preparation for Śavāsana and Sālamba Sarvāṅgāsana. When preparing to do the shoulderstand at a wall, first practice Setu Bandhāsana with the feet on the wall. This lifts the torso in preparation for inverted poses. Setu Bandhāsana with support of a bench or platform is excellent for reversing the apāna flow of prana to prevent excessive bleeding during the moon cycle, and has also been used in India to prevent miscarriage.

Psychophysiological Benefits

Setu Bandhāsana has many therapeutic applications. It is used to relieve lower back pain because it releases anterior compression on the intervertebral disks of the lumbar spine. By drawing the uterus and all pelvic organs back into their natural resting place, it is one of the best poses to prevent uterine prolapse. It is also an excellent posture for preventing hernias. It strengthens the abdominal organs and increases peristaltic activity of the intestinal tract, increases circulation, and stabilizes blood pressure.

Because the body is resting on the flat bones of the shoulder blades, where many of an adult's red blood cells are manufactured, practicing Setu Bandhāsana can increase the production of red corpuscles. The upper back of the shoulders have reflex points that affect the liver, gallbladder, pancreas, spleen, and stomach. Even the breath benefits by the pressure on the shoulder blades, as this activates the lung tissue. Setu Bandhāsana increases circulation at the base of the throat and stimulates the nerve roots at the seventh cervical vertebra, which impacts the thyroid and parathyroid glands, responsible for the body's metabolism and calcium levels. The immune center of the thymus gland is benefited, as are the adrenals. We can relate the major cakras to each of the endocrine glands that benefit from the reverse flow of energy within the torso.

Setu Bandhāsana promotes greater circulation between the spinal cord and the brain. It also benefits the heart, bringing it higher than the head where it does not have to work as hard to pump against the downward pull of gravity. This increases circulation of lymph and cerebral spinal fluid as well as blood. It helps bring circulation into the neck and shoulders, alleviating chronic tension in these areas. For those who have been on their feet or sitting at a computer, Setu Bandhāsana is a wonderful way to start a practice or end the day because it helps release habitually contracted muscles.

Setu Bandhāsana firms the buttock muscles and strengthens the legs. However, unlike typical exercises or calisthenics, which expend energy, Setu Bandhāsana gives energy. Setu Bandhāsana creates an unimpeded causeway of prana, bridging the gap between the polarities of lower and upper, and simultaneously activating the parasympathetic and sympathetic divisions of the autonomic nervous system. The sympathetic nerves come off the thoracic and lumbar areas of the spine, and the parasympathetic nerves stem from the sacrum and the cervical spine. The effect is very different than that of other backbends in which the neck curves in the opposite direction. In Setu Bandhāsana, we bend forward with the head while doing a backbend of the upper torso and the heart center. In other words, we are doing a counter pose within the pose.

When practicing Setu Bandhāsana, we invert the negative pole of the tailbone and the top of the spine, the positive pole, thus recharging the battery of our being. As we practice Setu Bandhāsana, we lift the prana of the Mūlādhāra cakra, or root energy center. If we focus on lengthening the spine in this pose, trapped energy, usually in the solar plexus, can then move freely toward the heart cakra, the throat cakra, and even into the back brain.

The front brain, related to the conscious mind, is active when our eyes are open, but in poses like Setu Bandhāsana or Sālamba Sarvāngāsana, we come to rest upon the cerebellum, the hindbrain at the base of the skull. This is a good preparation for Śavāsana or—for those who suffer from insomnia—for sleep. It is impossible to sleep unless we bring the prana from the cerebrum (the front brain) back into the cerebellum. The pineal gland, also at the back brain, produces melatonin, a natural sleep aid.

When we awaken the subconscious, we may awaken latent saṁskāras, the psychic impressions that are the result of past thoughts and experiences. Commentaries on the Yoga Sūtras tell us that every conscious experience becomes a subconscious impression. When the samskaras emerge and come to the surface for healing and releasing, it is as Swami Jyotir Mayananada has described: The invisible must become visible before it can be eradicated.

Bridge Pose is a simple but profound asana that prepares the body and mind for all asanas. This pose, more than others, reflects the way we often live life: "I am efforting. I am really going to make this happen. I will sustain it no matter what." The beauty of Setu Bandhāsana is that it teaches the art of relaxation within a pose, or as the Bhagavad Gītā says, the inaction within the action" and the "action within the inaction."

Sālamba Sarvāngāsana

Shoulderstand with Support

Sālamba means "with support." *Sarva* means "whole" or "entire," and *ānga* means "part." Sālamba Sarvāngāsana is the pose that affects the whole ("the entire part") of the body and mind.

Philosophical Introduction

Śīrṣāsana, the headstand, is known to be the king of or father of asana for its effect upon the master endocrine glands, the pituitary and hypothalamus. These glands relate to the frontal lobes of the brain and the sympathetic nervous system, the "fight or flight" response activated by the adrenals. In contrast, shoulderstand is known as the queen or mother of all asana. It impacts the lunar subtle nerve channel, *iḍā nāḍī,* which relates to the parasympathetic nervous system. Shoulderstand does this by emphasizing the cervical nerve plexus and, when moving into Halāsana, the Plough, the sacral nerve plexus. This has a dilating and cooling affect upon the system.

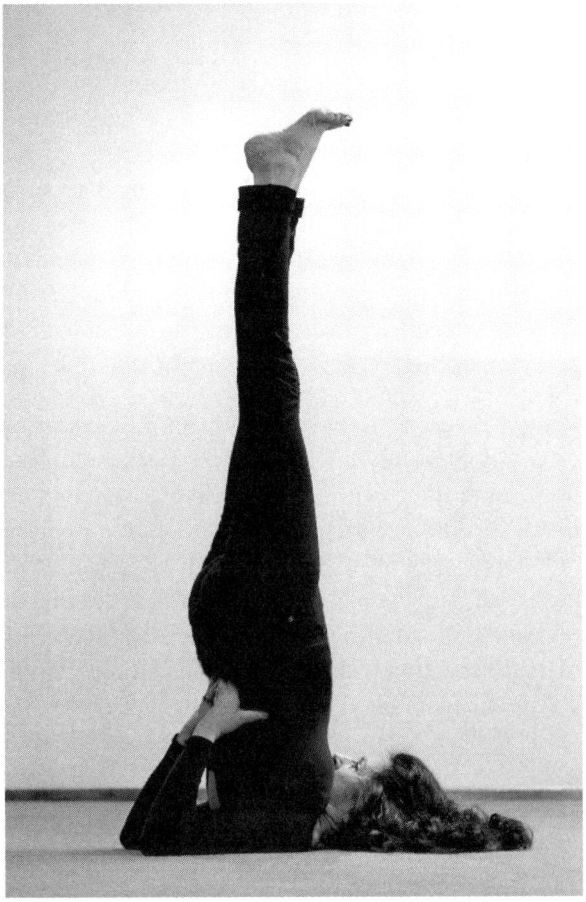

Shoulderstand is known as the queen or mother of all asana

Sarvāngāsana is a beautiful and restful posture that can be practiced as prayer. When moving into the pose with the breath, it may feel as though one is entering a beautiful sacred temple. In this pose, the head rests upon the earth and bows to the altar of the heart, humbling the ego. Whenever the head bows into a prayer position, the senses automatically turn inward in pratyahara, which is a prelude to dhāraṇā, concentration. If the mind is held in concentration for twelve breaths or twelve seconds, it automatically fuses with the object, becoming the practice of dhyana, meditation. In meditation, the subject and object merge like an uninterrupted stream of oil being poured from one vessel into another. And if the state of dhyana is held for twelve breaths or twelve seconds, it fuses into the first stages of samadhi. This sequence (dhāraṇā , dhyana, samadhi), known as Saṁyama Yoga, is described in the third chapter of the yoga sūtras. Sarvāngāsana is a natural *dhyanāsana,* or pose of meditation.

In addition to bowing the head to the heart, this pose has another element of offering or giving that arises out of the fullness of Self, when the legs and the soles of the feet offer up to the light of the heavens. The feet, in turn receive the light and energies from above. The alignment from the base of the skull to the soles of the feet creates a vertical line between the earth and the heavens, symbolic of our relationship to the Divine. It honors the polarities of Atman, the individual soul, and Brahman, the Universal.

The shape of the body in Sarvāngāsana resembles the shape of a candle, and it is sometimes referred to as Candle Pose. When the two legs are brought together in a unifying balance of equal pressure of right and left (as in the prayer or namaste position of the hands), we join the right and left hemispheres of the brain and the mind comes into a focused state of awareness. Sometimes, the flame of a candle may even appear at the forehead center point while practicing shoulderstand. If we practice *trāṭaka,* gazing on the bindu of this point, the pose—and the mind as well—feels steady and unwavering. Sarvāngāsana reminds me of a passage in the Bhagavad Gītā (VI:12): "Let thy mind be like the flame in a windless place."

The shoulderstand has a direct benefit upon the medulla oblongata, which Swami Yogananda called "the seat of the soul." Here the spinal cord meets the brain at the area of the pons, the relay center between the brain and body. When we can eventually reach this area in the pose, the prāṇa of our eyes is pulled backward to the cerebellum, the back brain known as the seat of the subconscious, and the mind and senses are drawn inward into an organic pratyāhāra, a withdrawal or, more accurately, integration of the senses.

The region of the medulla is also known as the cave of Brahman, the creator. It is, I believe, the seat of akāśha, the ether element associated with Viśuddhi cakra, the throat center. The akāśhic records store every imprint of every thought projected into the atmosphere. Edgar Cayce is said to have done his readings and healings from this center.

I have also found that the *saṁskāras,* the cellular memories or latent imprints from the past, are stored mainly in the cerebellum (and other cellular structures), activated by the placement of the head in Sarvāngāsana. Whenever I need an answer, or when I prepare to speak or teach, I practice shoulderstand beforehand. The pose brings me to a place of spatial awareness and holographic information that seems to give clarity and purpose of direction.

Guidance

1. Begin by lying on the floor with knees bent, feet on a wall or the calves on a chair. Bring the hands behind the head, fingers interlaced, and on each exhale, lengthen the neck. Relaxing the neck, gently lift the head so the chin comes closer to the center of the collarbone. Pause on the inhalations. It is important to take time at the beginning of the pose to elongate the neck so that the base of the skull—the medulla—comes in contact with the earth. The placement of the head affects the pons, the relay center where the spinal cord meets the brain. You do not want to put pressure at the back of the skull. That would put pressure on the eyes and sinuses and would do the opposite of what we want to create in Sālamba Sarvāngāsana. We want the energy of the pose to go to the pineal gland, which is at the back of the brain, and not push forward to the pituitary gland, which has a stimulating effect on the frontal lobes.
2. On the inhalation, do nothing.
3. On the exhalation, make adjustments to lengthen the cervical spine. Take a few moments to give space to the carotids, exhaling and extending the back and sides of the neck and even the front of the throat. Pushing the feet against the chair or wall, slide the skin down the back, making space between the upper shoulders and the lobes of the ears.
4. Inhale without moving, and on the next exhalation press the feet into the wall or chair, bringing the hips up into a bridge position.
5. Inhaling, let the breath spread across the back body. Exhaling, move the spine into the front body like a backbend.

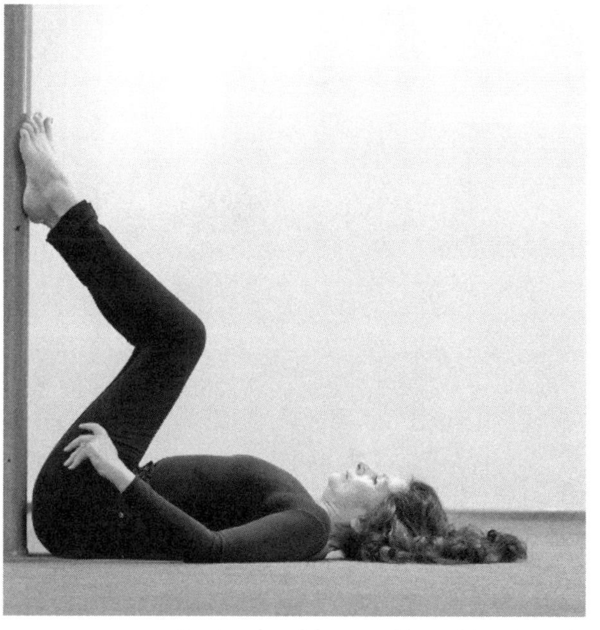

Begin shoulderstand by taking time to elongate the spine while lying on the floor.

6. On the next exhalation, rotate the upper arms, externally anchoring the outer elbows into the earth. Bend the elbows, bringing the palms to the back. Anchor the outer edge of the elbow deep into the earth. This creates a lateral expansion of the clavicle bone, improving lymphatic circulation and lymph drainage. (In Śīrṣāsana, the headstand, we anchor the inner elbow but in the shoulderstand, the outer elbow is the key.)

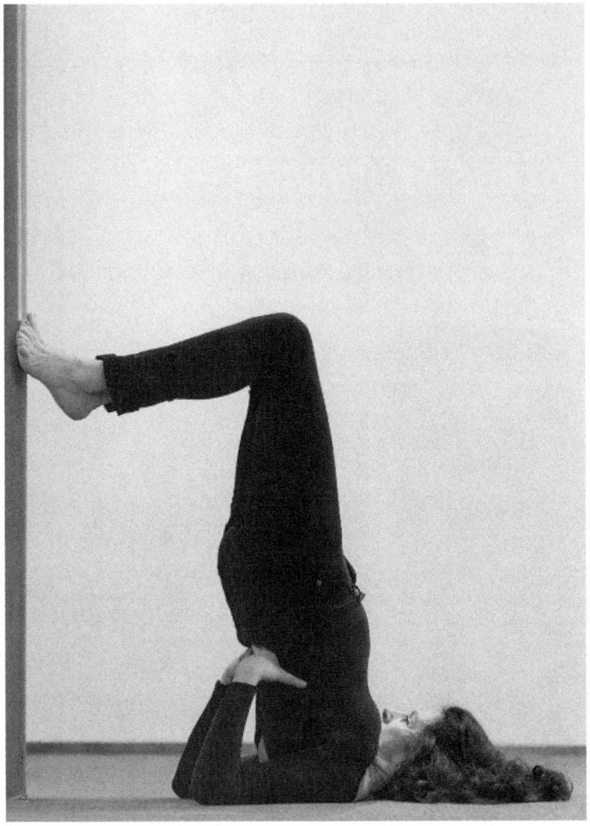

Establish alignment by anchoring the elbows, bringing the palms to the back, and pressing the feet into a wall or chair.

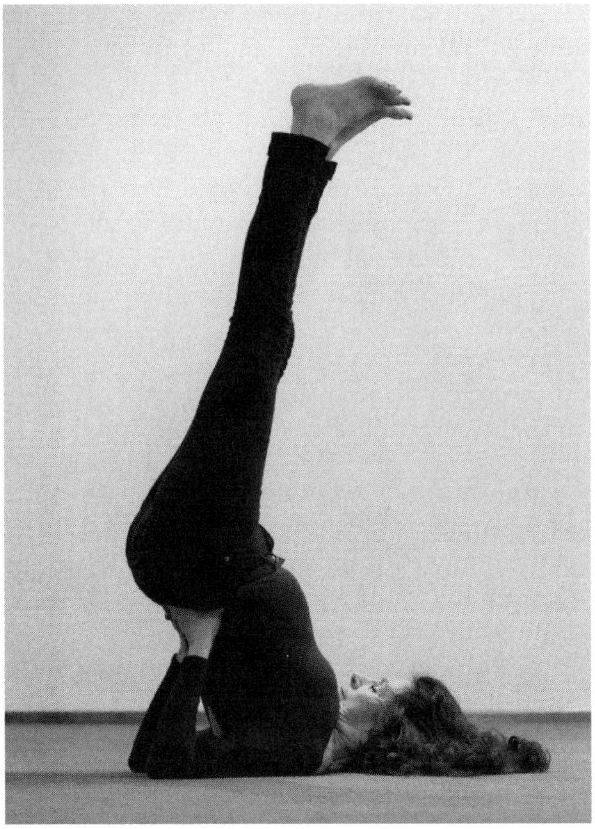

After reaching up through the legs and feet, close the eyes to relax the brain.

8. Inhale and do nothing. Take as much time as needed. Relax the navel to relax the mind. Relax the face continually, as if the head were in Śavāsana. Let the head, brain, mind, and senses go to sleep as the body is enlivened in the pose.

9. When you are ready to move a little more deeply into the pose, exhale, bringing the spine in like the backbend. Bring the hands a little higher on the back to lift the feet one at a time off the wall or off the chair. The perpendicular alignment of the torso, legs, and feet come from moving the spine in like a backbend. Soften and lengthen the neck with each outgoing breath.

10. Moving on the exhalations, extend through the inner legs, from the sides of the pubic bone to the inner ankle, offering up the heel and ball of the big toe to the heavens. This balances the inner leg, which is said to relate to our subtle body, with the outer leg, relating to the physical body. The ideal is to have both big toes in alignment with the inner corner of the eyes. Once aligned, however, it is important to close the eyes to relax the brain and especially benefit the back brain. As the two legs reach up for the light out of the floor of the pelvis, it lightens the pose. Bringing the legs equally together forms the flame of the candle, and extending the legs equally balances the right and left hemispheres of the brain, bringing the flame of the mind to that windless place of one-pointedness, dhāraṇā or concentration.

11. With each exhalation, anchor the upper arm ever more deeply into the earth. This lifts the prominent seventh cervical vertebra from the earth. As Mr. Iyengar used to say, "Sālamba Sarvāngāsana is a shoulderstand, not a neck stand." This attention to the upper arms also elongates the spine and intensifies this pose as an offering of Self.

12. Come out of the pose by reversing the directions.

Note: It is better to advance slowly in this pose using chair or wall for additional support. Traditionally, Sālamba Sarvāngāsana is practiced after Śīrṣāsana, the headstand, if not directly after, then somewhere within the same session. The Shoulderstand and its one-legged variation, Eka Pāda Sālamba Sarvāngāsana, can be sequenced after Setu Bandhāsana and before Halāsana.

Psychophysiological Benefits

The benefits of practicing Sālamba Sarvāngāsana are similar to those of all inversions, particularly Setu Bandhāsana, where energy is also brought to rest in the back brain. Sālamba Sarvāngāsana, as its name suggests, does benefit the whole body. It is especially beneficial for balancing the entire endocrine system. Its emphasis upon the pineal gland, which secretes melatonin, is helpful for insomnia. It balances either a hyper- or hypoactive thyroid due to its direct impact upon the spinal nerve roots of the seventh cervical vertebra, which relates to the heart and thyroid.

Due to the stretch and elongation of the carotids, the shoulderstand is a preventative for heart attacks and strokes. It helps preserve the health of the eyes and ears, and it can even clear the sinus passages. It benefits the cardiovascular system and the respiratory system through its pressure on the back of the lungs. It is excellent for the thymus gland (the true heart cakra), which activates the lymphatic flow and, in turn, the immune center. This pose also prevents abdominal and uterine prolapse and benefits the eliminative organs.

In practicing Sarvāṅgāsana, we are meant eventually to rest on the tops of the shoulders, where acupressure points relating to the digestive organs—such as the liver, gallbladder, pancreas, stomach, and spleen—bring the prana of these organs into balance. If the ligament on the back of the neck has been chronically compressed due to emotional constriction, it will lengthen with practice, alleviating chronic neck tension, eyestrain, and headaches.

Sarvāngāsana, more than any other pose, affects the medulla and the pons, the relay center between the thirty-one pairs of spinal nerve roots and twelve nerve pairs of the brain. This keeps our reflexes responsive and youthful. As we get older, the intervertebral disks begin to disintegrate from poor posture. The disks as well as the bones become increasingly brittle from the lack of circulation and hormonal changes. This is another important reason to take the time to lengthen and make adjustments before going into the pose.

More than any other posture, the shoulderstand impacts the subtle nerve channel known as the *vijñana nāḍī,* "the pathway of shining light." This nāḍī is the main energy channel connecting the heart and the brain, and it correlates physiologically with the carotid sinuses and carotid arteries. With the base of the skull on the earth, these pathways are elongated and are cleared of any plaque buildup that restricts not only the circulatory currents and lymph fluids, but also the subtle pranic currents. When these pathways of light begin to open, we realize the light that has always been. The hard pockets of our heart that have developed through past hurts dissolve, and the pathways of shining light between heart and brain illumine our mind and our Soul.

The way we do asana is the way we do our lives. We can never do the same pose twice; asanas become like life's postures. One day we may have an incredible experience in shoulderstand, a feeling of comfort, quietness of mind, emerging visionary experiences. The next day, we may approach the pose expecting the same results, but this time, the neck is tighter, the mind is restless, and the body is uncomfortable, and we cannot maintain a meditative aspect as we did the day before. Even though we may try to recreate yesterday's experience, the pose asks that we stay in the power of the moment without trying to recreate what was ... so that we can be present to what *is.*

In yoga it is advisable not to compete—not even with oneself. Sālamba Sarvāngāsana is a powerful pose for teaching us how to be noncompetitive, to be in the moment without trying to recreate the past or to project too far ahead in the future. In this pose, there is a perfection of being in the Now. In this moment of Now, we transcend time, space, body, and mind to realize the timeless, infinite consciousness. As Patañjali states in the yoga sūtras (II: 47), "It is through relaxation of effort and meditation upon the infinite that asana is perfected."

Matsyāsana

Fish Pose

Matsya means "fish," and this pose resembles a mermaid or merman, a human torso with a fish tail. This form is symbolic of the evolution of humankind. (For the story about this evolution, see the introduction to Matsyendrāsana, page 195).

Philosophical Introduction

Puranic scriptures refer to Matsya, who was said to be the first of the ten primary avatars or incarnations of Vishnu, the sustainer and preserver of the universe. Matsya is depicted with the tail of a fish and the torso and crowned head of Lord Vishnu. As in much of mythology, there are colorful and varying stories.

In one story, King Manu was performing severe austerities. As he offered his water oblation into the river, a tiny fish became caught in his folded hands. The fish begged the king not to place it back in the water where it would be devoured by bigger fish. Manu complied, placing the little fish in a small clay pot that he carried with him. But the fish instantly grew larger and requested more space. Manu moved the fish from pond to water reservoirs, then transferred it to a lake, which it soon outgrew, and then finally placed the fish in the ocean. Eventually, the king realized that this supernatural fish was Matsya, the first incarnation of Vishnu, and he bowed down as its devoted servant.

Matsya predicted that a great flood would come in seven days and encompass the entire universe. He instructed King Manu to assemble the saptarishi, the seven sages that held the balance of the entire universe in the substratum of their consciousness. Manu was to seek their counsel and gather seeds, animals, and other living creatures, all to be placed on a boat on the day of the great flood. (Similar stories of a great flood are told in many civilizations throughout time, in Sumeria, Greece, and Africa, in New World tribes from the Algonquian to the Mayan, and in the Christian Bible as the tale of Noah and his ark.)

On the day of the deluge, Matsya (who represents evolutionary metamorphosis from its first stages as aquatic life) appeared as a giant horned fish. He used the great serpent Vasuki as a rope to tie the boat to his horns, pulling the boat to safety in the high peaks of the Himalayas. Manu's boat is representative of moksha (salvation), which helps one cross the ocean of samsara. The mountains represent the boundary between earthly existence and salvation in the land beyond.

As Matsya swam through the torrential rain and floods, he gave Manu discourses on the Vedas, Puranas, and Samhitas. After the flood subsided, Manu became the progenitor of the new human race. He is known as the first lawmaker, the author of the Laws of Manu. This allegorical story is also a social commentary, teaching that a good king protects the weak from the mighty, reversing the ancient "law of fishes," which is akin to the law of the jungle.

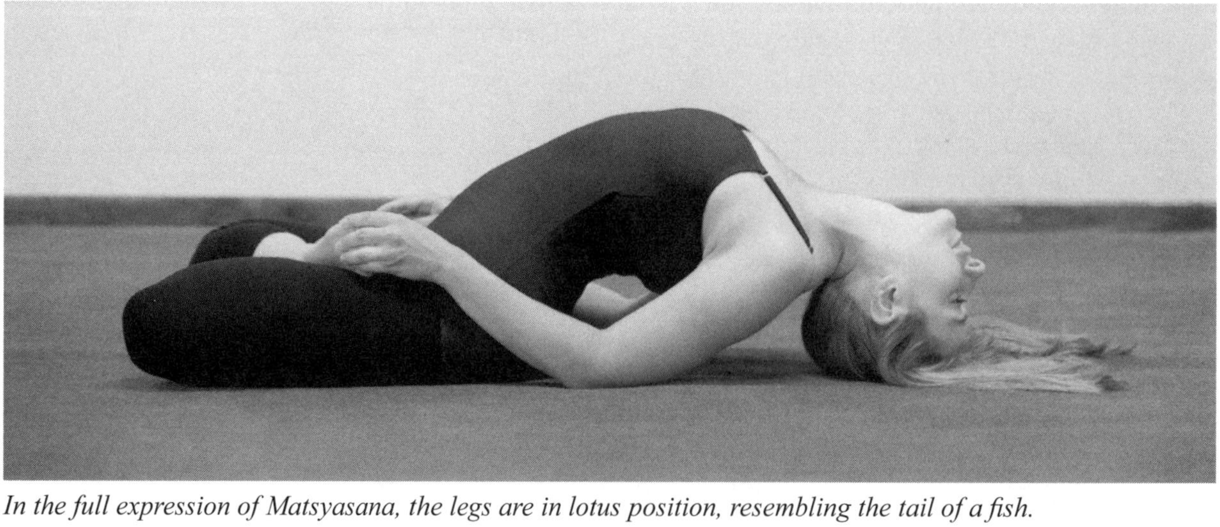

In the full expression of Matsyasana, the legs are in lotus position, resembling the tail of a fish.

In the full expression of Matsyāsana, the legs are folded in the lotus position, resembling the tail of a fish. The upper torso lifts to open the heart center, while the chin points upward and the crown of the head is brought toward the earth. The mouth may be exaggerated by forming vowel sounds, in English or Sanskrit. This stimulates the pituitary gland and other glandular reflexes within the brain.

In ancient times, it was said that whoever listens to the tale of Matsya, remembers him, or invokes him (as we do in Matsyāsana) is absolved of past karmas and is granted success in all endeavors of life.

Guidance

1. Begin in a supine position on the floor. Place a rolled blanket equal to the width of the shoulders underneath the lower ribs. Inhale into the back as much as possible.
2. Exhaling, bend the elbows as close to the hips as possible and push up, elongating the neck.
3. Inhale laterally across the back, bringing the breath into the sacrum and front of the abdomen as much as possible.
4. Exhale and press down with the elbows to lift the heart center. Extend the neck out before bringing the crown of the head down to the block or blanket.
5. Inhale, keeping more pressure on the elbows than on the head, expanding the breath across the entire back if possible.
6. Exhaling, move the spine into the front of the body in a backbend of the upper torso while extending the lumbar area. To make a self-adjustment, use the hands to move the hips down, creating more length. Each time we elongate the lumbar without dropping the chest, we lengthen and release any tension within the neck.
7. Inhale, feel the breath within the back.
8. Exhale, see if the spine will allow you to rise into the pose a little more, being careful not to compress the neck.
9. To come out of the pose, inhale, and on an exhalation, lengthen through the hips and sacrum to elongate the lumbar. Extend the neck out as the chest and upper torso come down to the blanket. Move the blanket to the side and let the spine relax in Śavāsana as you breathe.

Note: In all variations of this pose, it's important to extend the lumbar as the heart center lifts. The beginning version of Matsyāsana is practiced with the legs outstretched. This way, students can focus on the upper body and avoid compression of the lower back. Even so, there will be a bend in the lumbar that corresponds to the natural C-curve of the neck. Matsyāsana is often sequenced after shoulderstand and Plough Pose because it preserves the lumbar and cervical curvatures of the spine. The first stages of the pose can also be practiced as an extension of Setu Bandhāsana (Bridge Pose), using a blanket underneath the back of the ribs to help create the lift of the thoracic region while the lumbar area is lengthened by reaching the tailbone toward the feet.

A teacher or a partner can help the student into Matsyāsana. With two partners, one person can draw the hips and buttocks downward to lengthen the lumbar as the other lifts the upper ribcage. This allows the student to sense how much lift is required to lengthen and relax the neck. The crown of the head is brought to the earth only if the upper back is flexible enough to offer to the heavens so the neck can bend in its natural C curvature without compression. Weakness or stiffness will show as a collapsed thorax. If the heart center is not open enough when we try to touch the head to the floor, we can create rather than relieve neck tension. In this case, it is

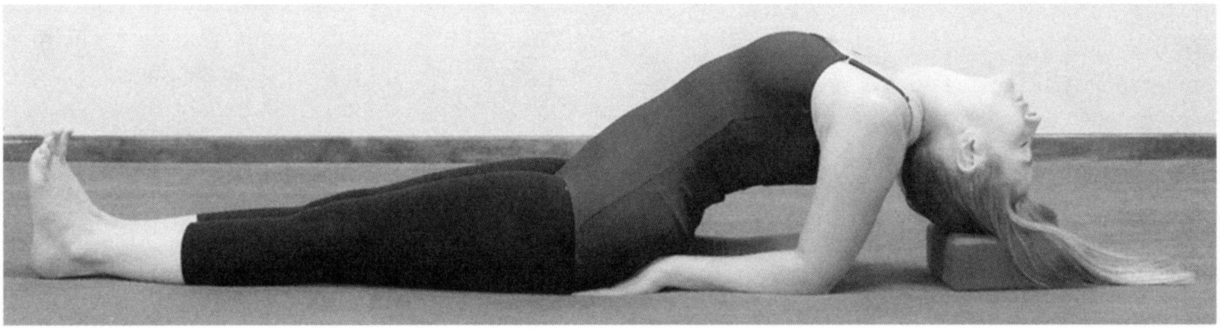

Placing the crown on a block helps prevent neck compression.

advisable to place a block or folded blanket under the head. When the neck is compressed, in any pose of yoga or life, it can restrict circulatory currents from flowing between the spine and the brain.

Another variation of Matsyāsana is to bend the legs underneath, with the hands holding the feet and the elbows on the floor. More adept students can practice Matsyāsana while the legs are in Padmāsana (the full Lotus Pose), the hands holding the ankles, bringing the bent elbows slowly toward the floor. This gives optimum leverage for the heart center to lift.

Fish Pose can also be practiced in the water with the legs folded in Lotus. The body takes the form of the fish and, as the heart lifts and the head tilts back, one can use the hands to flutter like the gills of a fish. The legs, which are the tail of the fish, propel the body through the water.

Psychophysiological Benefits

Matsyāsana helps prepare us for other backbends, gently correcting anterior compression and realigning the sacrum and pelvis as it helps to alleviate back pain. It releases compression in the solar plexus and restores a flattened lumbar curve. It is particularly helpful for opening the chest, preventing kyphosis and preserving the cervical curve. It even helps to correct the reverse curvature of the neck that is sometimes referred to as "military neck."

It is important to take time after Fish Pose (and subsequent backbends) to relax, deliberately slowing the breath and the beat of the heart. When we allow ourselves to rest at the completion of the pose, we create a cascading effect of deep sustained energy that increases as the day goes on. If we practice this pose in such a way that we restore and rebuild the adrenals and kidneys, it can help alleviate fatigue and depression.

Matsyāsana, through the arching of the cervical and lumbar spine, stimulates the prefrontal cortex of the brain and the adrenal glands. It is an excellent stimulation of the thymus gland, which is the physical correlate to Anāhata, the heart cakra. Because of Matsyāsana's stimulating effect on the thyroid and parathyroids, it is one of the best postures for hypothyroidism and the activation of the metabolism of calcium. It has been helpful for hypoglycemia due its beneficial effects on digestive organs such as liver and pancreas.

When we free the neck, we allow the energy to spiral upward, like a fish swimming up from the water element of the second cakra, Svadisthana, a name that means, "Establishing one's own place within the eternal cosmic vibration." As this evolutionary spiral of creation winds upward through the lower centers and flows to the crown, it becomes symbolic of the evolutionary journey, from fish to humankind to godhood.

Fish Pose helps balance the samāna prāṇa (at the navel center), the prāṇa prāṇa (in the region of heart and lungs), and the udāna prāṇa (within the throat center). Those who experience hyperactivity or vata imbalance should not do this pose often. Vāta increases when there is any compression in the neck. Those who have excessive pitta or restlessness in the nervous system should progress in the pose very slowly, using the abdominal breath to help to balance pita.

On a subtle level, Matsyāsana is a powerful pose to awaken Viśuddhi Cakra, which corresponds to the thyroid and parathyroids. Viśuddhi is the center of speech and communication. Where there has been repression or fear of speaking out, Matsyāsana helps to free past saṁskāras and open the channels for words to flow freely. It is said that when the throat cakra is open, Sarasvatī—the goddess of culture, refinement, music, and learning—dances upon one's tongue.

Śalabhāsana

Locust Pose

Śalabha refers to the locust. Śalabhāsana resembles the way a locust or grasshopper lifts its hind legs when it is ready to leap.

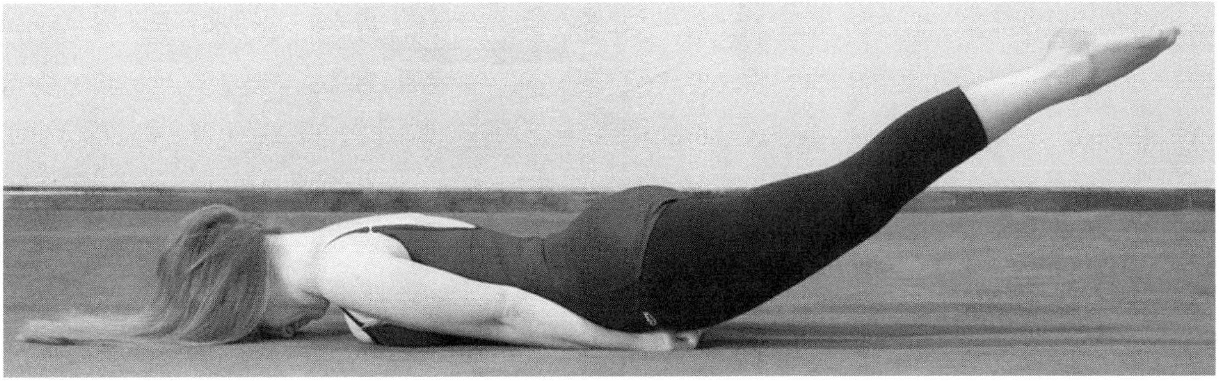

Press the hands into the earth, let the legs leap upward, and maintain an attitude of lightness as you breathe in.

Philosophical Introduction

The grasshopper is the Chinese symbol of good luck and abundance. It represents taking a chance or a leap of faith, to act upon a vision or a thought and jump right in. Those with locust or grasshopper energy do not laboriously take things one step at a time but move quickly, trusting their own inner instincts to guide them before they take that leap. It is interesting to note that grasshoppers only jump forward and never backward.

When a grasshopper leaps into our life, it is believed to be a sign. We are being asked to take a leap of faith, to do something out of the ordinary that may require facing stored-up fears. These fears may be things we have avoided doing, and they are often linked to a change or expanded direction. This could include a relationship, a job, long-held beliefs and concepts, or deep internal changes.

This may be reflected in our yoga practice. What are the poses we have been avoiding? What poses do we most favor? Usually we favor those that are pleasant and comfortable. The ones we want to avoid are those that bring up pain. As we say in yoga, "Yoga does not create pain; it reveals what is already there." Just as we can use the poses as a gauge of our being able to stay balanced in the midst of polarities—such as likes and dislikes or pain and pleasure—the locust and grasshopper remind us to face that which we have been avoiding, going only forward, never going backward.

The locust/grasshopper is also linked to astral travel, meaning to leap into another reality. It is said that the totem of the locust and grasshopper jumps across time and space, traveling from one dimension to another. Like Hanumān, it can leap over any obstacles that may appear within its path. This is a magnificent reminder to honor all life forms as aspects of the Divine, for we never know how and when the Eternal Cosmic Vibration will manifest.

Guidance

1. Begin by lying on the stomach, forehead down and arms alongside the torso.
2. Inhale into the back of the neck, bringing the breath down to the shoulders, widening the distance between the shoulder blades.
3. Exhaling, let the spine descend into the earth, offering it and giving as completely as possible.
4. Inhaling, let the breath ascend, as if offering to the heavens through the upliftment of the back, bringing the breath from the neck, shoulders, and ribcage. With the continuing inhalation, expand all parts of the back horizontally.
5. Exhaling, surrender the spine even more deeply.
6. Inhaling, allow the entire back body to lift with the incoming breath. Use the resistance of the floor (earth) to bring the breath from the shoulders all the way down to the hips.

7. Exhale and surrender the spine even more deeply into the earth, bringing the hands underneath the thighs. Position the hands with palms up or by making fists or placing the palms turned downward next to the thighs. Keep the arms as straight as possible.
8. Inhale, and again let the breath expand into the entire back body
9. Exhaling, press down with the hands. As the hands press into the earth, keep the knees straight, and let the legs leap upward away from the earth. As the legs come up, the muscles of the back body engage, including the soleus, hamstrings, gluteus maximus, and spine extensors. Hold to an attitude of lightness and ease as you continue to breathe in the pose. If the breath stops, it is time to come out of the pose.
10. On an exhalation, lower the legs, turn the head to one side, bring the arms out from the thighs, and rest while observing the breath. Slow the breath to slow down a rapid heartbeat.

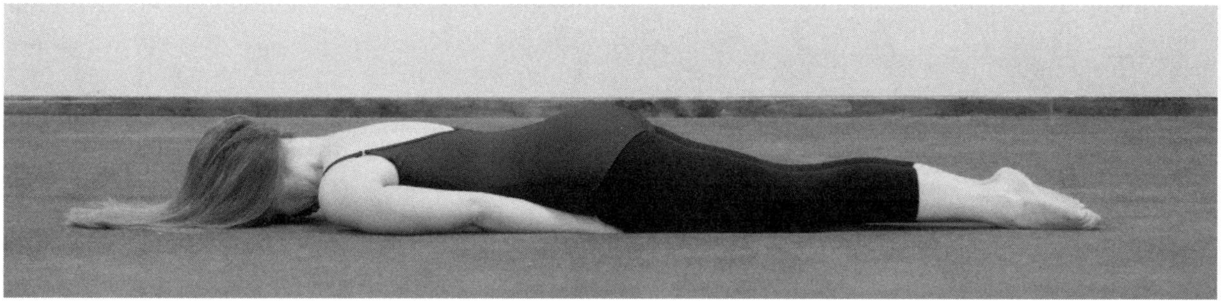

Take time to breathe into the back, surrendering the spine, before bringing the hands underneath the thighs.

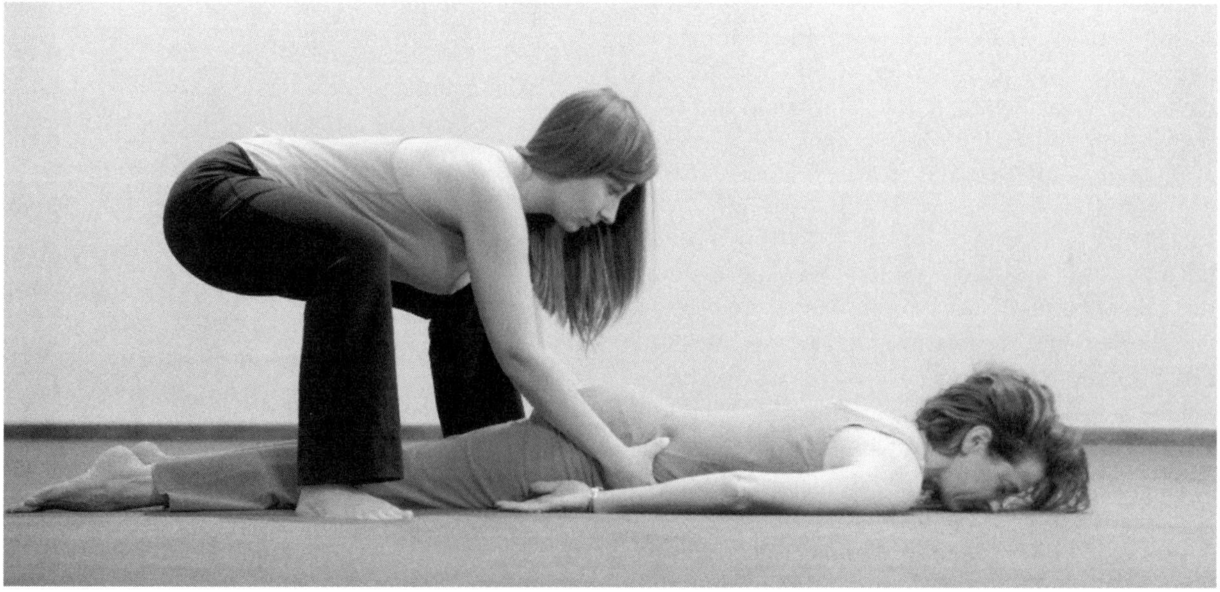

A partner can assist by lengthening the lumbar area to prepare for Śalabhāsana.

Psychophysiological Benefits

Even though this is a difficult pose for some yoga practitioners, it is one of the most effective for re-building the kidneys and adrenals. In the Chinese system of medicine, the kidneys and adrenals are not separate from one another. What affects one affects the other. Śalabhāsana is also excellent for creating an aerobic effect, which strengthens the heart.

It is important to use the breath effectively. The breath and the beat of the heart speed up from the adrenal stimulation, but if we volitionally slow the breath down, the heart rate slows and the adrenals come to rest. This is why Śalabhāsana is considered to be a pose that teaches the system how to deal with stress. As in other āsanas, we create a stressful situation and then steady the breath to steady the mind; thus we raise our threshold of stress. When we learn this skill in āsana, we can take it into the situations in our lives. The things that once caused stress are now perceived differently, and we are able to keep the mind quiet throughout the postures of our life.

It is after the pose that we receive the benefit. Śalabhāsana strengthens the muscles of the lumbar spine, brings circulation to the pelvic organs, relaxes the navel center, and firms the buttock muscles. It is said that we carry energy and power in the gluteus maximus. The pose of Śalabhāsana, taken over a period of time, gives sustained energy that we can take into areas of life.

While strengthening the body, Śalabhāsana also creates spinal flexibility. There is a relationship between physical flexibility and emotional flexibility. Like the grasshopper or locust, we can leap over obstacles when we feel a growing lightness in both body and mind.

Bhujaṅgāsana

Cobra Pose

Bhu refers to the earth plane, and *aṅga* means "part" or "piece." Remember that *āsana* means "pose" and comes from *as,* meaning "to be" or "to breathe," *san* or *sam,* meaning "to sum up" or "become one with," and *na,* the eternal cosmic vibration. In Bhujaṅgāsana, it could be said that one rises up from the earth plane and becomes one with the eternal vibration and essence of all creation.

Philosophical Introduction

In ancient Egypt, the serpent was depicted with a human head, representing our primordial nature. The ancient Egyptians believed that we must escape from the world of matter and leave behind the lower part of nature to focus on higher aspects of the self and reflect the Divine. They viewed the serpent as one that works to prevent the human soul from ascending to the realm or sphere of God, similar to the serpent that tempted Eve to eat the forbidden fruit of knowledge in the Garden of Eden. For Christian Gnostics, however, the serpent represented a positive force of liberating knowledge.

In the yoga tradition, serpents include Takṣaba, the majestic prince of the Nāgas, or serpent race; Vāsuki, who wound himself around Mandara to help the devas recover the elixir of immortality; and Ananta *☒e☒a N☒gas*, the thousand-headed serpent upon which Lord Viṣṇu, the preserver and sustainer of the Universe, reclines and rests. Ananta means infinite, or endless, and this great being known as the serpent of infinity may resemble the figure eight on its side, or a mobius strip.

In Greco-Roman mythology, two serpents form the caduceus, the staff carried by Hermes or Mercury. The caduceus, which became a symbol of medicine and healing, shows the entwined serpents intersecting at six vortices. If we view this as an image of Kuṇḍalinī rising, the two snakes symbolize the parasympathetic and sympathetic aspects of the autonomic nervous system, the ganglia that originate in the base of the spine and end at the top of the nostrils. The third eye center corresponds to the meeting of the heads of the two snakes.

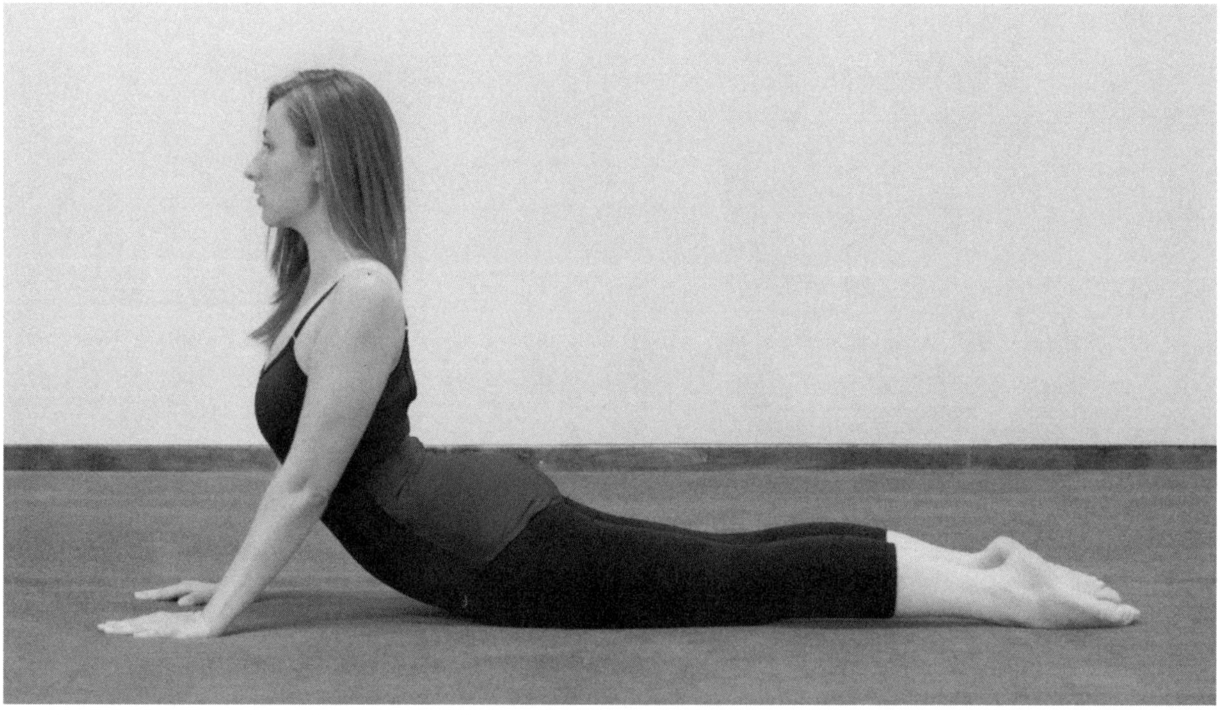

In Bhujaṅgāsana, the heart lifts majestically, emulating a cobra.

The serpent is the symbol of Kuṇḍalinī Śakti, which is the biological and psychological nuclear energy that lies dormant within the human system. It is the procreative power, the primordial energy that dwells on the subtle unseen plane. In the physical body, Kuṇḍalinī is said to lie dormant at the base of the spine between the 5th sacral and 1st coccygeal vertebra. The sacrum, which physically resembles a downward facing serpent, has five vertebrae that fuse at puberty, and the coccyx has four that also fuse at puberty. These bones safeguard and protect the serpent energy of Kuṇḍalinī. The density of this area serves the purpose of keeping us bound to the earth plane. That is, until the goddess Kuṇḍalinī awakens and arises out of her resting place, spiraling upward through the central canal of the spinal cord, piercing through the five lower energy vortices (cakras) on her way to reunite with the masculine pole of Puruṣa in the crown of the head. She is the ultimate primordial energy, the divine Prakṛti, which cannot be seen with the physical eye but can be felt and experienced within the body as well as within the human psyche. Kuṇḍalinī represents unrealized potential and the rise of consciousness from the primordial instincts of one's lower nature toward the evolutionary light of Universal Oneness.

In Bhujaṅgāsana, the heart lifts majestically, emulating the seven-hooded King Cobra. This majestic serpent is symbolic of the seven major cakras or energy vortices within the subtle body, which correspond to the endocrine glands in the physical body. Its seven hoods fan out from the brain stem, which can also resemble the shape of a serpent. The pons in the human brain stem is a relay center between the spinal nerve roots and the sensory nerves that fan out into the brain.

The upper brain or cerebral cortex is associated with inspiration, thinking, and free will. It relates to the sixth and seventh cakras. The cerebellum or reptilian brain—activated in this pose when the back of the neck lifts and lengthens—regulates respiration, biological functions, basic instincts, and genetic coding (DNA). It is associated with the five major cakras from the base of the spine to the throat center.

Even though some philosophers have dismissed the reptilian brain as an unnecessary primordial appendage, it is the cerebellum or lower brain that opens us to the vaults of memory. It brings us into the theta wave state of hypnogogic imagery, where we can access genius-like areas within the collective unconsciousness. This is the place where Edgar Cayce and Albert Einstein were said to access information that transcended dimensional limitations. The reptilian brain holds the secrets or imprints of humankind. It is "the hall of records" where all things are known and all things are stored, the subconscious mind. It is the energy of the lower body and the lower brain that sustains, awakens and energizes the upper regions.

In Bhujaṅgāsana we honor the primordial instinctual nature of our own urges and bring the prāṇa from the base cakra of the spine into the crown cakra. We honor the foundation and potential for evolutionary unfoldment. As the undulating movement of the serpent moves up the spine, the heart and head reach for the evolutionary light of wisdom as if once more climbing the tree of knowledge to find our way back to the Source in the Garden of Eden.

When aligned appropriately the Cobra will internalize rather than externalize consciousness. This is done through the opening of the chest and heart center. When the heart lifts, the head is drawn back, stimulating the cobra brain or posterior brain of the cerebellum. This creates a magnetic pull for the focus *(dṛṣṭi)* of the eyes. Instead of darting outward, the gaze is pulled inward. The focus of the ears, the nose and tongue all seem to follow the alignment of the head. This alignment creates a natural pratyahara, the withdrawal and integration of the senses, where no one sense is more distracting than another. When the senses are integrated into one-pointed awareness, this leads to dharana or concentration, the sixth of the eight limbs of yoga. Instead focusing outward on sensory stimulation that leads to desire and attachment, the prāṇa of the sensory organs turn inward, to the vast realms where nothing is wanted or needed, All Is.

As the back of the neck lengthens more and more, the head is freed on its atlas. When the compression of the skull and the top of the spine is eventually released, something magical can happen. At times, if the alignment is just right, it can feel as if an invisible hood rises up from the brain stem and fans out across the top of the head like a King Cobra. This experience gives a sense of deep internal strength and protection. It feels as if one is dwelling under the cosmic umbrella of the great Śeṣa Nāga that supports Viṣṇu and all creation, like Atlas holding the Earth.

Once I held a rainbow boa constrictor, and this gave me a new understanding of Cobra Pose. When a snake moves, the action begins at its tail, and a peristaltic response ripples up the body to the head. From that day, I began to practice Bhujaṅgāsana from the bottom up, allowing the energy to ripple from the toes to the knees, thighs, pelvis, and navel plexus to raise the heart and head, which then receive the evolutionary light from above. In Bhujaṅgāsana, we emulate the great serpent that provides Viṣṇu's foundation by creating our own foundation for awakening energy from the lower to upper regions of our Being, preparing for liberation and self-realization.

Guidance

Serpents do not have arms, yet in this variation of Bhujaṅgāsana, we use the arms as leverage to extend the spine and prevent compression. In this pose, it is important to lengthen the back of the neck without lifting the chin. This brings the base of the skull off the atlas and axis bones of the neck. At times, it may feel as if the head wants to sway a little from side to side, like the coiled cobra. We do not bring the face and eyes upward: This cobra gazes straight ahead with unwavering, one-pointed intention, as if its two eyes become one.

3. Exhaling, surrender the spine into the front of the body, beginning the backbend before moving the body. At the end of the exhalation, bend the elbows, bringing the palms under the shoulders. Keep the elbows close to the torso.
4. Inhale into the back, expanding the breath to widen as well as lengthen the back ribs. The upper arms may turn in, but keep the Venus mounds of the thumbs and the balls of the index fingers firmly rooted, as if into the earth.
5. On the exhalation, press down with the circumference of the palms, extending from the roots to the tips of the fingers and draw the spine forward as it lifts from the earth. Move in incremental steps with the breath, letting the movement of the lower body ripple upward.
6. Inhaling, pause and allow the breath to round the back.
7. Exhaling, surrender the back of the spine into the front of the torso, preparing the heart to lift to the light above.

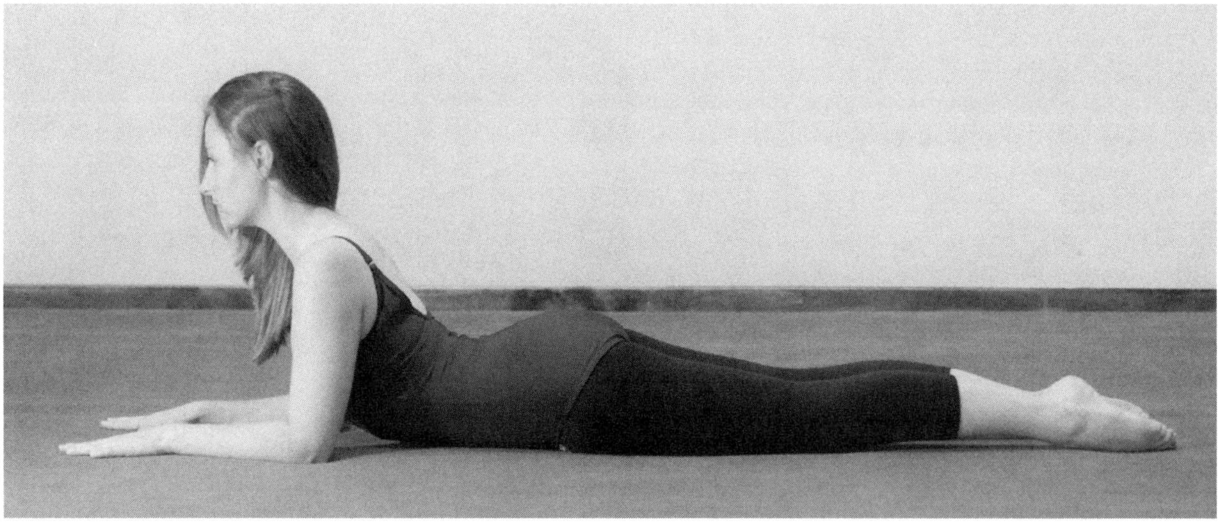

Use the resistance of the floor to expand the breath into the regions of the back, as in this variation of Bhujaṅgāsana known as Sphinx Pose.

1. Lie down on the stomach with the forehead on the earth, the arms outstretched.
2. Inhaling, breath into the back using the resistance of the floor as an ally to bring breath into the back of the neck, shoulders, ribs, lumbar, and sacrum. With each inhalation, see how far the breath can move without strain. Allow the breath to rise effortlessly and consciously but subtly direct it with to the desired areas.
8. Inhaling, pause and allow the breath to fill the back, because when inhaling we activate the cerebrum, the upper brain. This pose should enable us to focus on the exhale when we bring prāṇa into the cerebellum of the reptilian or cobra brain.
9. Exhale, and as the spine offers itself to the front of your chest, lift out of the heart center. Tighten the buttocks to extend the legs out of the hips, moving the heels and toes away from the upper

body. You can move one leg at a time on an exhalation, pausing on the inhalation.

10. Inhaling, press down with the palms and lift the shoulders toward the ears, rounding the back as much as possible.
11. Exhaling, press the palms down, keeping the hands firm as you use the leverage of the arms to draw the shoulders down. Move the skin of the back toward the buttocks to lift the heart center toward the light. The upper arm will roll out slightly as the shoulders are brought down from the base of the ears. The pelvis, legs, and feet are not dragged forward with the upper torso but move backward.
12. Inhaling, keep the back of the neck passive as you press down with the palms to provide leverage to round the back and allow the breath to fill the back of the lungs.
13. Exhaling, relax the buttocks and drag the upper torso forward as if across the earth while leaving the pelvis, legs, and feet behind. This lengthens the lumbar region. Remember not to lift the chin or eyes but to lift from the back of the neck as if a silver thread were pulling the base of the skull off the first vertebra of the neck and opening more space.
14. Inhale and once again allow the breath to round the back, bringing the shoulders towards the ears. The upper arms may rotate internally as the head relaxes forward, the gaze turning toward the earth.
15. Exhaling, see if the spine is ready to lift the heart a little more, remembering always to lengthen the back of the neck, keeping the gaze forward not upward.
16. Inhaling, round the back, allowing the shoulders to soften as before.
17. Exhaling, bring the spine into the front of the torso, lengthening the spine even as you lower out of the pose, using the arms as leverage for greater elongation.
18. Inhale and turn the head to one side, filling the back with the breath.
19. Exhaling, surrender into the earth as if emptying yourself through the breath.
20. Inhaling, turn the head to the other side.
21. Exhale, releasing into the earth while having moved beyond it. Enjoy the benefits of the pose.
22. When ready, press back to Mārjāryāsana (Cat Pose), using the breath to move the spine. Stretch up into Adho Mukha Śvānāsana (the downward-facing dog) or Bālāsana, (Child's Pose). Breathe and elongate the spine.

Note: One of the great errors in Bhujaṅgāsana is to lift the head without offering the heart to the light. When the head is lifted prematurely, this creates posterior compression of the neck and restricts the flow of lymph and of the cerebral spinal fluids that pass from the spinal cord into the brain. A coiled serpent does not throw its head back, but elongates all parts of its being from the base upward, corresponding to the human heart center lifting upward to the light.

Psychophysiological Benefits

Bhujaṅgāsana may be called Cobra Pose because of its direct impact upon the powerful energy hidden within the sacral and coccygeal plexuses. It stabilizes the sacroiliac joint, which is affected by age and postural misalignment, giving strength to the joints where the pelvis and sacrum join. Due to the bend at the lumbar and thoracic regions of the spine, the Cobra pose stimulates the adrenals and, in turn, activates the sympathetic nerves of the spine through the thoracic and lumbar nerve roots.

The pose is excellent for strengthening the lower and mid back and helps to prevent excessive curvature (kyphosis) of the thoracic spine. As the upper body moves forward, the base moves back, creating space between the spinal vertebrae and in the pelvis and abdomen which can help realign the reproductive organs, stomach, intestines, liver, gallbladder, and pancreas.

Bhujaṅgāsana strengthens and firms the gluteus maximus of the buttocks, which is said to hold power as it awakens the Śakti within the procreative centers. The contraction of the buttock muscles also helps protect and strengthen areas of the lumbar spine. However, when a student is more able, the buttocks can be completely relaxed in Bhujaṅgāsana. Relaxing the buttocks allows the upper body to be pulled forward, which creates immense extension and inner space between the pelvic and thoracic areas. This releases compression of the spinal nerve roots that enervate the diaphragmatic muscle. When the breath becomes slow and rhythmic the pose begins to hold itself.

Bhujaṅgāsana can help balance the two nerve currents, sympathetic and parasympathetic, which are referred to in yoga as *piṅgalā* and *iḍā.* When prāṇa is balanced between these two nadis or channels, which run along the right and left sides of the spine, the energy rises and enters into the central canal, the *suṣumnā,* intersecting at the vortices we call cakras. (If we were to superimpose the caduceus symbol upon the body, the serpents would intersect at six points that correspond to the endocrine system on the physical level and the cakras on the subtle level.) Piṅgalā and iḍā meet at the sixth cakra, Ājñā, which awakens with the mystic union of the pituitary gland in the frontal brain and the pineal gland in the back brain.

In the ancient past, the pineal was considered by some to be an actual eye that sunk deeper and deeper into the brain with the evolutionary cycles. When the energies of the pituitary and pineal are in alignment with one another, the hypothalamus (the master endocrine gland) brings balance to the entire endocrine system. With this union, it is as if the mind liberates and expands, taking flight, like the wings of the caduceus, into the inter-dimensional planes of consciousness.

Uṣṭrāsana

Camel pose

Uṣṭra is the camel. Uṣṭrāsana resembles the way a camel bends its knees to rest or to rise from a seated position.

Philosophical Introduction

The camel is an independent animal with a great reservoir of stamina and endurance, known for storing energy and water, which enables it to cross vast deserts without needing anything outside of itself. The camel conquers hunger and thirst, which relates to our own need to fulfill desires, our hunger and thirst after objects that distract us from one-pointed awareness.

At times we may feel as if we are drinking from the oasis of life and tasting the sweet fruits of its fragrant garden. Other times, life's challenges may feel like the crossing of the arid deserts, bringing us to our knees like the camel. Passing through life's desert requires us to look more closely for the beauty that is already there. If we are superficial in our outlook, we will see unrelieved, colorless sand, without basking in the subtle beauty of desert plants, the succulents and cacti that appear to be separate from one another but are connected by a common root system. We may be so caught in the pit of our own pain that we cannot fill our hearts with the sunrise, or bask in the aura of sunsets that spread to vast horizons as far as the eye can see.

Uṣṭrāsana builds an unlimited reservoir of strength, both physical and emotional, to draw upon during the spiritual journey, which may not always be a lush garden oasis. The Camel Pose creates humility and flexibility, as demonstrated by the bend of the knees, the extension of the spine, and the opening of the heart to the bright light of the desert sun, which is always shining.

Guidance

1. Prepare for Uṣṭrāsana by kneeling on a soft blanket or mat, the knees hip distance apart and the toes turned under. Turning the toes under helps to massage the reflexes to the brain and sensory organs. To help elongate the spine and lift the chest, I recommend beginning Uṣṭrāsana by placing the elbows on the seat of a chair.
2. Inhale, expanding the breath into the back.
3. Lengthen the lumbar spine on the exhalations. Bring the hands to the back of the hips, and with every exhalation draw the buttocks down as the chest lifts up. If you are using a chair, press the elbows into the seat of the chair. This gives the leverage to elongate the spine.
4. Inhaling, pause to observe the fullness of the breath.
5. Exhaling, press down with the elbows to elevate the chest, moving the spine in like a backbend and offering the heart center to the heavens. Maintain the perpendicular alignment of the thighs to the earth. The quadriceps (front thigh muscles) are required to relax their grip and elongate.
6. Take as many breaths as you need, using the exhalations to lift the heart center while simultaneously bringing the buttocks down to elongate the lumbar spine. With every exhalation, the shoulder blades and the skin of the back descend, creating space between the tops of the shoulders and the ears.
7. Pause on the inhalations to spread the breath horizontally across the back.

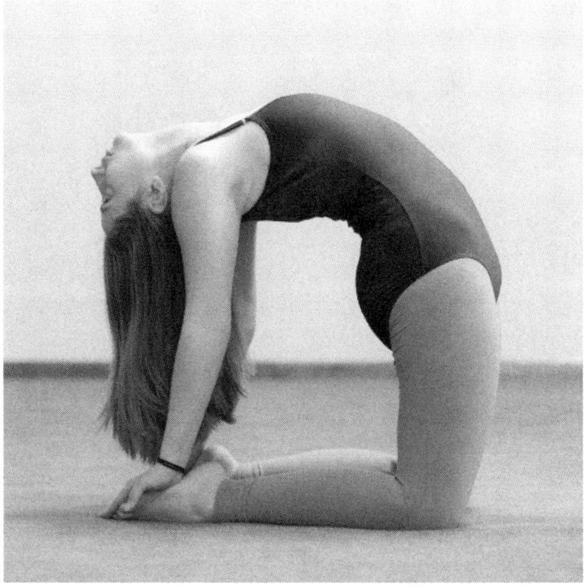

In the fullest expression of Uṣṭrāsana, the hands rest on the heels and the tops of the feet relax to the floor.

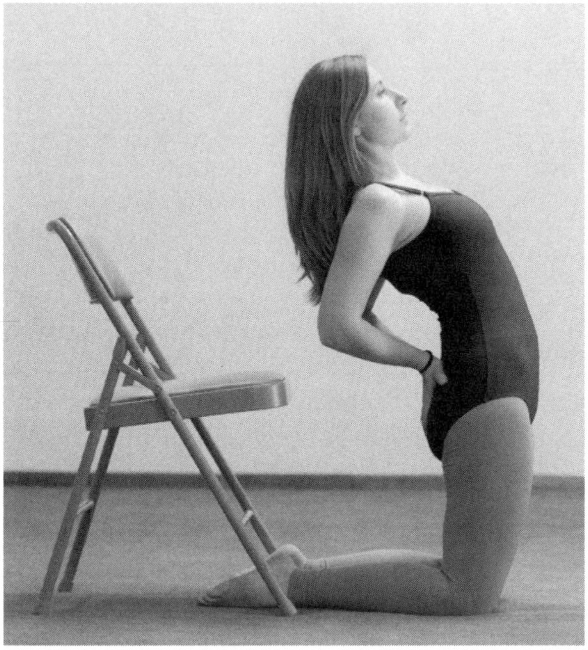

Lengthen the lumbar spine on the exhalations.

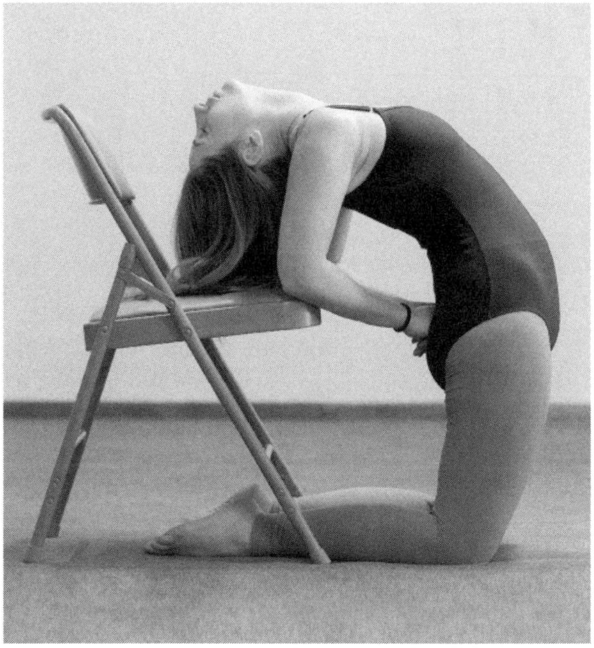

Press down with the elbows to elevate the chest.

8. On an exhalation, deepen the pose by moving the spine like a crescent moon into the front of the body, without compressing the lumbar. Elongate the back of the neck, moving the skin of the back and shoulders down to create even more space between shoulders and the base of the skull.
9. Inhale and do nothing.
10. Exhale, and as the heart lifts, bring the hands one at a time to the heels. Using the leverage of the pressure of the hands on the feet, lift even more on next the exhalation, when the ego unravels itself.
11. If you want a deeper bend of the spine, exhale and relax the tops of the toes to the floor, increasing the amount of extension to the spine. Do this only if there is no lumbar or neck compression.
12. Come out of the pose the same way you went in, using the breath.

Note: A more advanced version of Uṣṭrāsana is to begin by placing the tops of the feet on the floor and then reaching back for the heels. Even more advanced would be to begin in Supta Vīrāsana and rise up from the floor like a camel rising from its resting place in the sand preparing for its journey. Moving between Supta Vīrāsana and Uṣṭrāsana is a wonderful feeling, an undulating movement that echoes the grace of the camel.

Psychophysiological Benefits

Camel Pose gives us strength and flexibility at the same time. It strengthens the knees and the arch of the foot, lengthens the quadriceps and psoas muscles, and releases tension in the pelvis and solar plexus, relieving compression within the abdominal organs, including the spleen, pancreas, stomach, liver, and gallbladder. Like other backbending poses, Uṣṭrāsana helps to balance hypoglycemia and speed up metabolism, stimulating the digestive and pelvic organs, the kidneys, adrenals, and thymus gland, the body's immune center. When the head is extended back, the thyroid is stimulated, making Camel Pose extremely good for hypothyroidism.

When the camel drops into its resting place, the forelegs bend first, and that is reflected in the yantra of a dynamic diagonal line. In the full expression of this pose, where the head is brought to the feet, the circle yantra represents the expansion of consciousness from the bindu, the point within its center.

Practicing Uṣṭrāsana can help us move beyond the fear of the unknown. In Uṣṭrāsana, the head looks back into the unknown parts of one's self that are represented by the back body. To do this without creating compression in the neck requires an immense opening of the heart cakra, which is offered to the light. The lower body remains humble yet strong, while the growing flexibility of the upper body and thoracic spine brings about the increased ability to open the heart, releasing past hurts to the light so that the heart can shine without the shadows of the past.

Like the camel that stores water and food for long journeys, we can take in the food of the spirit, such as the prāṇa from our practice, and store it within us. By increasing our reservoir for prāṇa, we have something to draw upon during those crisis times when we feel that we are crossing the desert. With this stamina comes the ability to adapt to any situation and the insight to help guide us and others through the sandstorms that at times occlude our vision.

Seated Twist With Chair

Even though Matsyendrāsana or Marīcyāsana are the twists most often practiced in yoga classes, the same benefits can be found in the simplest of twisting movements, using a chair for lift.

Philosophical Introduction

Many years ago, the late Ken Keyes, Jr., the author of *Handbook to Higher Consciousness* and *The Hundredth Monkey,* visited my home. A polio survivor, he was permanently wheelchair bound. As we were talking, he suddenly said, "I practice yoga."

I looked at his paralyzed body. "How ...?" I faltered.

He put me at ease. "I'll show you. This is my way of twisting."

He then took a deep and quiet inhalation. As he exhaled, he turned his head to one side and held his breath out. After a while, he inhaled slowly, rotating his head back to center before exhaling. He then repeated the movement on the other side. Afterward, his eyes were like deep shining pools of light. I was accustomed to practicing very complex twists, but when Ken—in his wheelchair with limited use of arms and legs—turned his head with the breath, I finally understood the mystical essence of the twists.

All twists represent the evolutionary spiral of creation. Whenever we twist or revolve around (parivṛtta), I think of turning around the vṛttis, or mind waves, the painful and non-painful oscillations of our thoughts. *Vri* means "to come into existence." My Sanskrit teacher once described vṛttis as electrical impulses that arise in the field of the mind (citta). The waves of the mind are ten-fold and include correct perception, incorrect perception, imagination, sleep, and memory. When the vṛttis are stilled through practice, the mind becomes as still as glass. Then we can see our own reflection. The third yoga sūtra (I:3) describes it thus: "Then the Seer and the Seen become one," or as I prefer to say, then we can realize the Oneness that already is.

In all of the twisting āsanas, the front brain or *manas*—the conscious thinking mind—turns around to look into the shadow side of itself, the hidden depths of the psyche. It looks to the back body, the part that we cannot see with our physical eyes, which is symbolic of *citta*—the subconscious mind—as well as of intuition. In other words, the conscious mind turns to look into the seat of the subconscious. As we bring the conscious to the subconscious (said to reside in the cerebellum), the back brain rotates to the front body, the side that we can see. This evolutionary spiral brings that which is hidden to the light, the side of the rising sun.

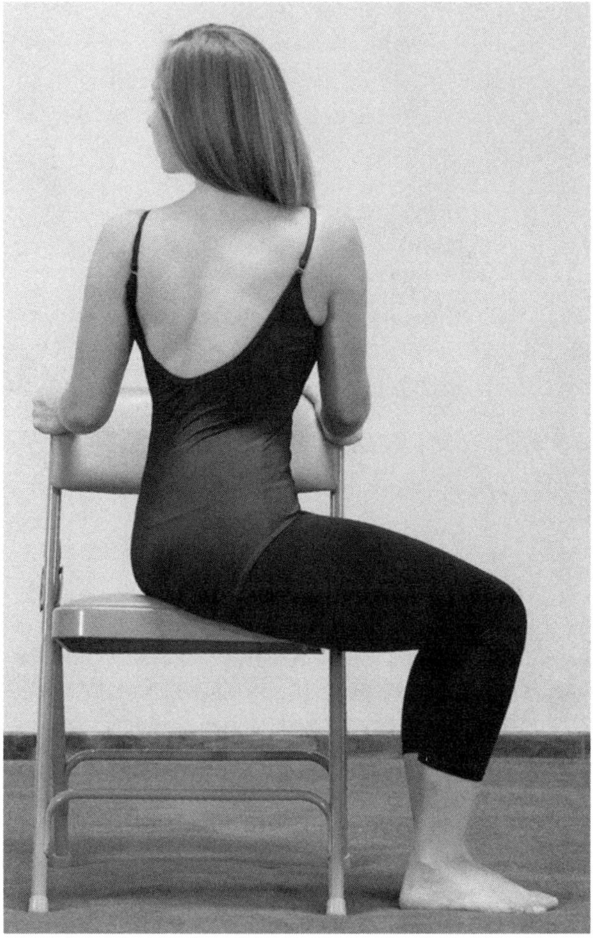

This variation of the seated twist uses a chair to emphasize lifting the torso, symbolic of transcendence.

Twists are poses of transcendence, helping the practitioner lift above self-imposed limitations of body, mind, and emotions. We do this by creating immense space in the midline of the body, which opens neural pathways for cellular memories—saṁskāras or latent impressions—to bubble up to the surface. Here they can be seen and transmuted.

Twists express themselves in a variety of forms. When we vary the twisting movement by sitting, lying down, forward bending, or inverting, we change the internal and structural effects upon the body. When we practice twisting while seated on a chair, the leverage of the arms helps to lift the spine upward, transcending the gravitational pull. This lengthens and strengthens the abdominal and spinal muscles in preparation for more complex twists. Thus, twisting with a chair is an especially good preparation for the seated twists, which have a tendency to collapse the spine.

Guidance

1. Sit sideways on an armless chair, resting both hands on the back of the chair.
2. Inhale, bring the breath into the back, and spread it from the shoulders down to the hips. Allow the breath to flow in, with the mind as the observer rather than a participant.
3. Exhaling, bring the back spine toward the front of the torso as if preparing to do a backbend.
4. With each inhalation, allow the breath to round the back effortlessly.
5. With every exhalation, continue to elongate the spine by lifting each vertebra off the one beneath it, breath by breath. As you elongate the spine more and more, there will be an organic and effortless rotation of the spine toward the back of the chair.
6. On an exhale, press the hands against the back of the chair and pull to give leverage for even more extension and rotation as the shoulders drop down and the skin moves down the back. The back of the neck lengthens without lifting the chin.
7. Continue twisting as long as the spine is comfortable and the breath is continuous and calm.
8. When you are ready to come out, exhale, turning the torso and head back to the center.

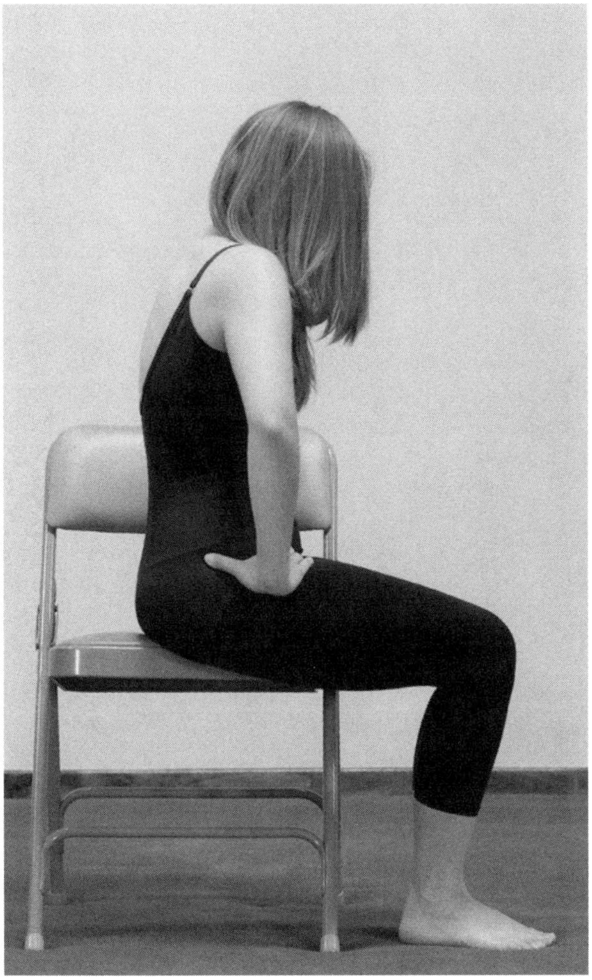

On inhalations, expand the back from shoulders to hips.

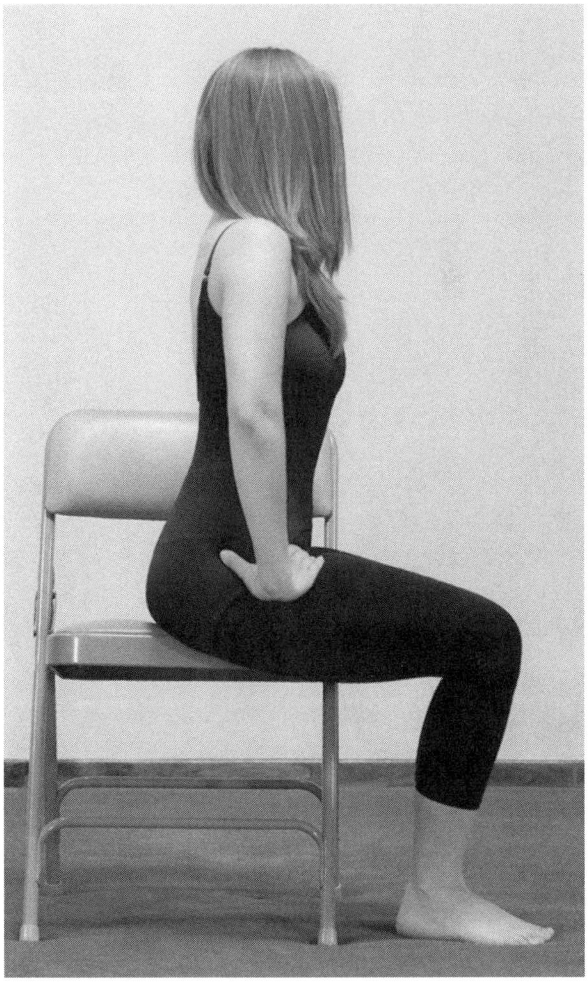

Press hands into the back of the chair or onto the thighs to help elongate the spine on exhalation.

9. Sit quietly, observing the breath, eyes closed. When you are ready, move to the other side of the chair and repeat the twist in the opposite direction.

Psychophysiological Benefits

It is beneficial for all students, beginning or advanced, to practice twisting on a chair in order to learn the art of lengthening and creating internal space. Using the leverage of a chair strengthens the spinal ligaments and surrounding muscles, and teaches us how to transcend the gravitational compression of a sitting twist.

The benefits of twists are numerous. When practiced with spinal elongation, twists help alleviate back conditions, preserving the flexibility and youthfulness of the spine. They help balance functions of the liver, gallbladder, pancreas, spleen, and stomach. They work on the small as well as large intestines, if the spinal rotation can reach down as far to the base of the spine as possible. If the movement of the head follows the rotation of the lower spine, twists can be a wonderful way to alleviate neck tension. In a healthy spine, when the head rotates, the movement should be felt down to the coccyx.

In the twists, as we bring the subconscious to the light of the conscious mind, we may bring up long-buried memories or stimulate dreams. This is because twists activate Maṇipūra cakra, the navel center, which is the center of sight and insight. Twists also balance samāna prāṇa, which is responsible for digestion, adrenal and kidney function, as well as the health of our eyes.

Before taking any rotation, it is important to elongate the entire spine. This action can relieve any spinal compression that restricts circulation to the intervertebral disks. Mr. Iyengar used to say, "I don't know which comes first, compression or depression." As we lift and transcend the compression in our body, it is possible to lift above the compression of the mind and emotions.

Jaṭhara Parivartanāsana

Revolved Abdominal Twist

Jaṭhara refers to the stomach, as well as to all the digestive organs in the midline of the body. *Parivar* is from *parivṛtta,* meaning "to revolve around" and *tan* means "to stretch" or "to go beyond."

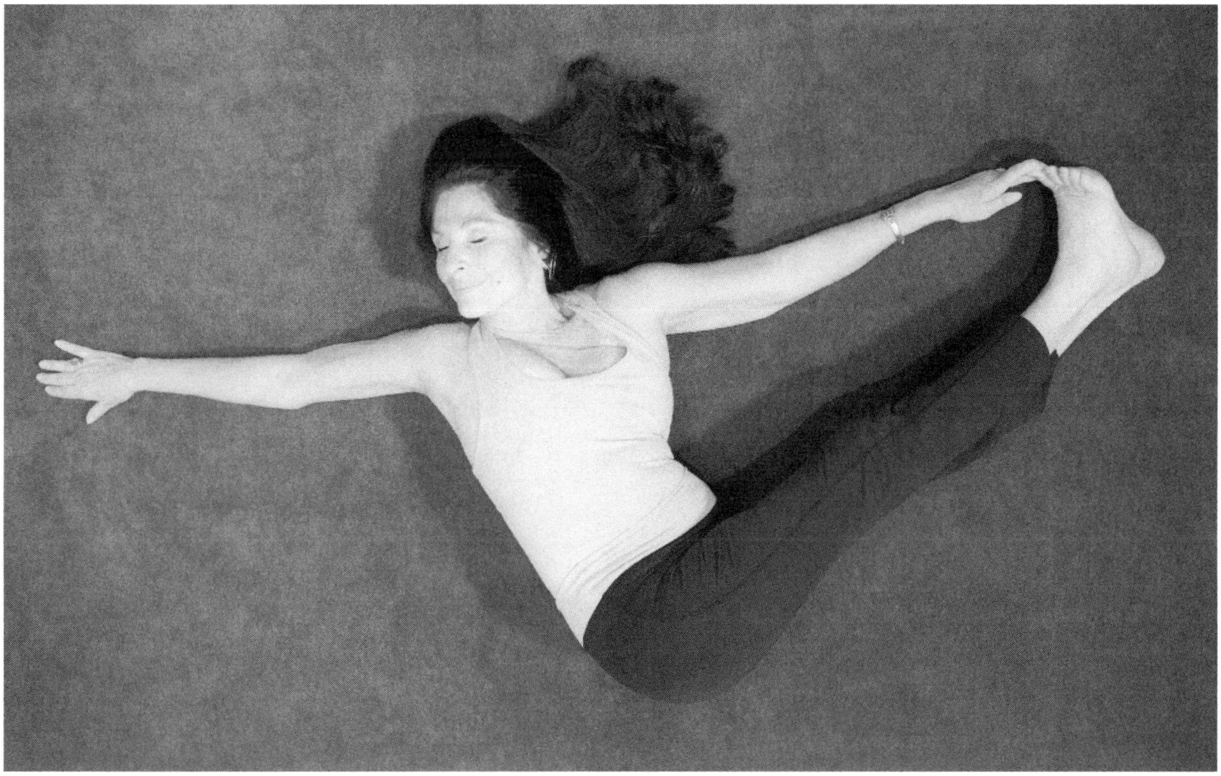

Jathara Parivartanasana, shown here in its classical expression, is known as the Crocodile Twist.

Philosophical Introduction

Jaṭhara Parivartanāsana and its variations are also commonly known as the Crocodile Twist. These variations taken from the supine position are especially beneficial to learn spinal elongation without having to lift against the gravitational pull as in seated twists. The crocodile has the unique ability to twist its body and whip its tail around to catch prey or—as it could be said in relation to the human species—to attain its goal. The crocodile represents sexual prowess and vigor. It moves like a serpant.

The crocodile is the vehicle of Varuṇa, the Vedic god of the seas (and lord of all waters, including ponds, lakes, rivers, and oceans). Lord Rāma invoked Varuṇa to gain permission to build a bridge across the sea in hopes of rescuing Sītā from the abode of the demon Rāvaṇa. The crocodile is also a symbol of the second cakra, associated with the water element.

Brahma, the creator, is said to reside in the first cakra, but what follows creation is that which maintains and stabilizes that creation. Therefore, the second cakra, associated with the sense of taste, is the dwelling place of Lord Viṣṇu, who presides here with his consort Lakṣmī, the post-Vedic queen of the waterways who bestows her devotees with wealth, liberation, enjoyment, and integrity. Viṣṇu is the spiritual power that is in every cell, atom, and molecule of our bodies. It is the energy the pulses through the procreative centers of all species. It is the breath, and the beat and rhythm of the heart. The word *Viṣṇu* means "all-pervasive." It is the prāṇa or life force that maintains the substratum of the Universe.

It is said that Viṣṇu holds the balance between Brahma, the creator at the base of the spine, and Śiva, the transformer energy that dwells in the crown of the head. Viṣṇu represents balanced living and, like his later incarnation of Kṛṣṇa, symbolizes the cosmic *Līlā,* the Divine play of life. The Jaṭhara Parivartanāsana series, like all twists, represents the play of life through the evolutionary spiral of creation.

One unique characteristic of the crocodile is that it swims with only the top of the head and part of the eyes showing. So much more is submerged beneath the water. When we practice Jaṭhara Parivartanāsana, we awaken that which we cannot see on the surface. Twists reach down into the basic primal urges and elements of the Self to bring up the subconscious impressions latent within the psyche. They do this by elongating the spine and rotating from the base of the pelvis and pubis, turning the lower body in one direction and the upper body in another. This awakens the sleeping chambers of old and ancient memories, bringing them to the surface of mind where they can be seen and transformed. Most of these past karmic impressions lie hidden, like the body of the swimming crocodile.

To "shed crocodile tears" means to display false emotions. This happens when we don't come from the depth of our own being, from our authentic self. False façades create a wall of defense or hardness, like the skin of the crocodile, to protect the deeper softer emotional layers of the subtle body. Many years ago, when I was in India studying with B. K. S. Iyengar, our small class followed him around the room like medical interns, viewing different bodies and their corrective alignment. Mr. Iyengar bent down to move one woman's back further into a pose and stopped. "Her kidneys and surrounding muscles are hard," he said. "She is not ready to go further." He stood and moved on, saying, "Hard on the outside, soft on the inside." Then he turned his head and casually threw out another gem. "Hard on the inside, soft on the outside."

This simple profundity stuck with me for years, and I have often observed that when we have a strong inner core, physically and emotionally, we can afford to be soft and open. Conversely, if the inner core of the physical and subtle (emotional) body is weak, the body seems to compensate by armoring itself like the crocodile, with layers of defense mechanisms. This quality of being hard on the outside reflects insecurity, or a lack of confidence or inner strength. When we are not strong at our deepest core, there is a tendency to make up for it by hardening and tensing the muscles and organs, and even the skin and bones, which reflects a need to hold strength in the outer layers.

In the twists, we bring the subconscious to the conscious and the conscious to look into the hidden depths of our psyche. These poses may bring up long buried memories and dreams as they also stimulate the Maṇipūra cakra of the navel center, the center of sight and insight.

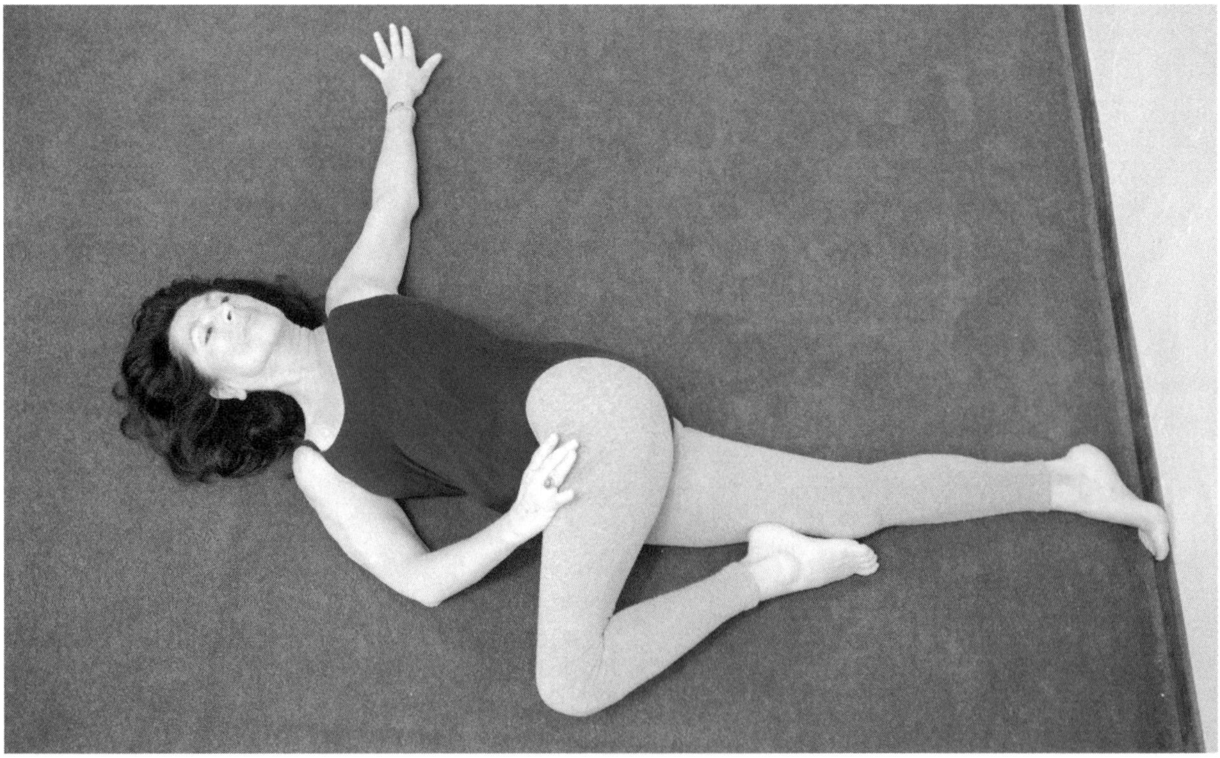

Practicing this twist at a wall helps create greater length through the spine.

Guidance

How we enter this āsana (and all āsanas) is so important. We progress slowly with the breath rather than throwing ourselves into the twist. I recommend synchronizing every movement with the breath, which makes any āsana a powerful conscious and concentrated action.

1. Begin Jaṭhara Parivartanāsana by lying on the floor with the feet against a wall. Inhale and, on the exhale, turn to the right side.
2. Inhale, do nothing, and then exhale, bending the left knee and placing the sole of the foot upon the knee.
3. On the next exhalation, press the bottom foot into the wall and elongate the spine. The emphasis is on moving the thorax away from the pelvis and the pelvis away from the thorax, giving space to the midline.
4. Inhale into the layers of the back from top to bottom. Keep the neck relaxed for the duration of the pose.
5. Exhale while lifting the torso up to lengthen the upper spine toward the head, as the hips move toward the heel.
6. Inhale and spread the breath horizontally across the back.
7. On an exhalation, lift up out of the sacrum and the pelvis as the hip and thigh move toward the foot pressing against the wall. The wall provides leverage to elongate the spine and create space between the lower and upper body with every outgoing breath.
8. Inhale, breathing into the back body, and exhale, moving the spine into the front body like a backbend.
9. On the next exhalation, bend the upper arm and reach out from the spine, creating space between the shoulder blade, ribs, and spine.
10. On the inhalations, do nothing but continue to relax the neck. Create even more space with every exhalation.
11. Exhaling, push the upper thigh away from the upper body with the right (or bottom) arm.
12. Inhale and expand across the back, allowing the breath to lift the left set of ribs up and away from the spine.
13. Keeping this space, exhale and move the spine toward the heart center. As the exhalation continues, bring the outer edge of the scapula (shoulder blade) toward the earth as the inner edge of the scapula moves towards the body but away from the spine creating space at the back of the heart
14. Inhaling, bring the breath into the entire spectrum of the back.
15. Exhaling, straighten the left (or upper) arm away from the spine, using the right (or bottom) hand to elongate the upper thigh, moving the pelvis away from the thorax.
16. Inhale and expand the breath across the back.
17. Exhale and move the spine in like a backbend while leveraging the bottom foot against the wall for extension and elongation of the spine, stretching the spinal muscles and surrounding ligaments.

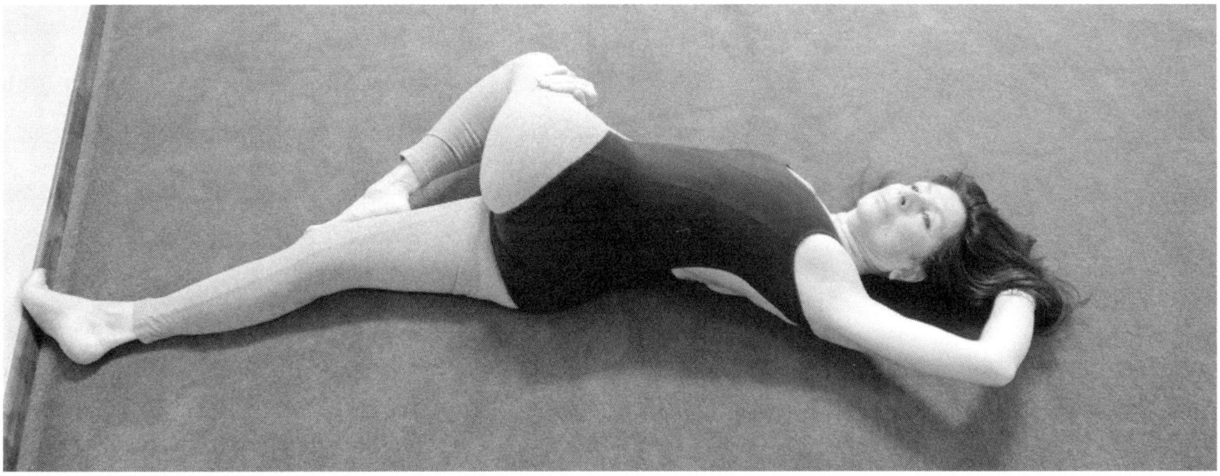

Move the shoulder blade away from the spine on the exhalation and use the hand to lengthen the neck.

18. Inhale, bending the left elbow. On the exhalation, move the scapula a little further from the spine.
19. When you are ready, slowly return to the center while focusing on the breath. Before taking the pose to the other side, take time to allow the energies to neutralize and the mind to re-center. Observe sensations. This is the time when we receive the benefits of the pose.

Note: The intermediate version of this pose would be to straighten the bent knee, bringing the foot as close to the outstretched hand as possible. Continue the pose as if the knee were bent. An advanced version would be to bring both outstretched legs over to one side of the body, toes as close to the hand as possible.

Assist: A partner can stand or sit on the side of the upper crossed-over leg (the left side if the left leg is the upper leg). On the exhalation, use one hand to roll the upper thigh outward and downward away from the upper torso while bringing the other hand to the back to move the spine upward and inward like a backbend. The partner can also stand on the opposite side where the torso and head will turn, having the practitioner hold onto their ankle. The person in the pose can use this as leverage for spiraling the rib cage, deepening the rotation. This helps to release neck tension.

Psychophysiological Benefits

Twists express themselves in a variety of forms—seated, prone, forward bends, inversions—and with each, we change the internal and structural effects. Jaṭhara Parivartanāsana, as all twists, represents the evolutionary spiral of creation. Twisting poses may bring up long-buried memories and dreams as they stimulate Svādhiṣṭhāna (the second cakra) and Maṇipūra (third cakra at the navel center), the center of sight and insight.

Psychologically, when we twist, revolve, or evolve, we are taking the conscious mind and turning it back to look into the seat of the subconscious. I think of it as revolving the *vṛttis,* the mind waves. In all twisting poses, the front brain, the manas, conscious thinking mind, turns around to look into the shadow side of itself. It looks to the back body, which is the part we cannot see with our physical eyes, symbolic of the citta, our subconscious mind as well as our intuition. As we do this, Jaṭhara Parivartanāsana becomes a pose of transcendence, and we can fulfill the *tan*—"to stretch or go beyond"—aspect of the āsana's name by transcending self-imposed limitations in mind, body, and spirit.

We do this by creating immense space in the midline of the body. Jaṭhara Parivartanāsana and its variations are especially beneficial for learning to elongate the spine without having to lift against the gravitational pull, as we do in seated twists. Increased space brings increased blood flow to digestive organs that may be habitually compressed, such as the stomach, liver, gallbladder, pancreas, spleen, kidneys, and adrenals. This twist releases diaphragmatic compression and can even correct breathing difficulties. It relieves neck tension and is especially beneficial when practiced after the shoulderstand and the Plough Pose. It neutralizes the sympathetic stimulation of backbends and the calming, dilating effects of forward bends.

It is believed in yoga that we cannot make changes at a conscious level until first the subconscious is shifted. The twists bring about a shift at a very deep subconscious level, transforming the primordial reptilian nature that reverts to instinct and strikes out when its egoic self-survival is threatened. When we stretch and thin the midline of the body and stimulate the pelvic plexus, we activate the water element of the second cakra. Like the churning of the ocean of milk, twisting the spine stirs the waters, bringing up cellular memory and saṁskāras—deep psychic impressions—from the vaults of the subconscious.

Daṇḍāsana

Staff pose

Daṇḍa means "staff." This refers to the spine, which is also known as the Meru Daṇḍa, the central axis of creation.

Philosophical Introduction

Mt. Meru is the celestial mountain around which everything revolves. This relates to the axis of the spine, where the nerve roots originate and spread out to peripheral areas of the body. Yoga, like chiropractics, is based upon the health of the spinal nerve roots. If they are restricted, nerve impulses and the subtle nerve currents (*prāṇa*) are impeded in their flow to corresponding organs.

A Daṇḍāsana spine is like the scepter held by kings and queens and wise elders throughout the ages. In India, the Śhaṅkarācāryas carry a staff that symbolizes spiritual realization and exalted station, not just in life but in consciousness. In ancient Egypt, the pharaohs held two curved staffs crossed over at their heart center.

In Hindu mythology, Hanumān carries a huge mace, symbolizing the power handed down to him from Rāma, who was an incarnation of Viṣṇu. There is magic in the staff, as demonstrated by Moses who cast down his staff in front of the Pharisees, transforming it into a serpent. In many cultures and religions, wise men have walked vast stretches of the earth with staffs, reflecting a long journey from darkness into light. To this day, kings and queens hold a scepter, a symbol of power and their high station and authority.

Meru also refers to the crowning jewel. Originally, the Divine Right of kings may have been so named because the royal heads were once those whose crown cakras were open. Kings and queens obeyed the descending command of Divine Grace for the welfare of the people. The jewels within the crowns attracted and invited the lords of the heavens into one's being.

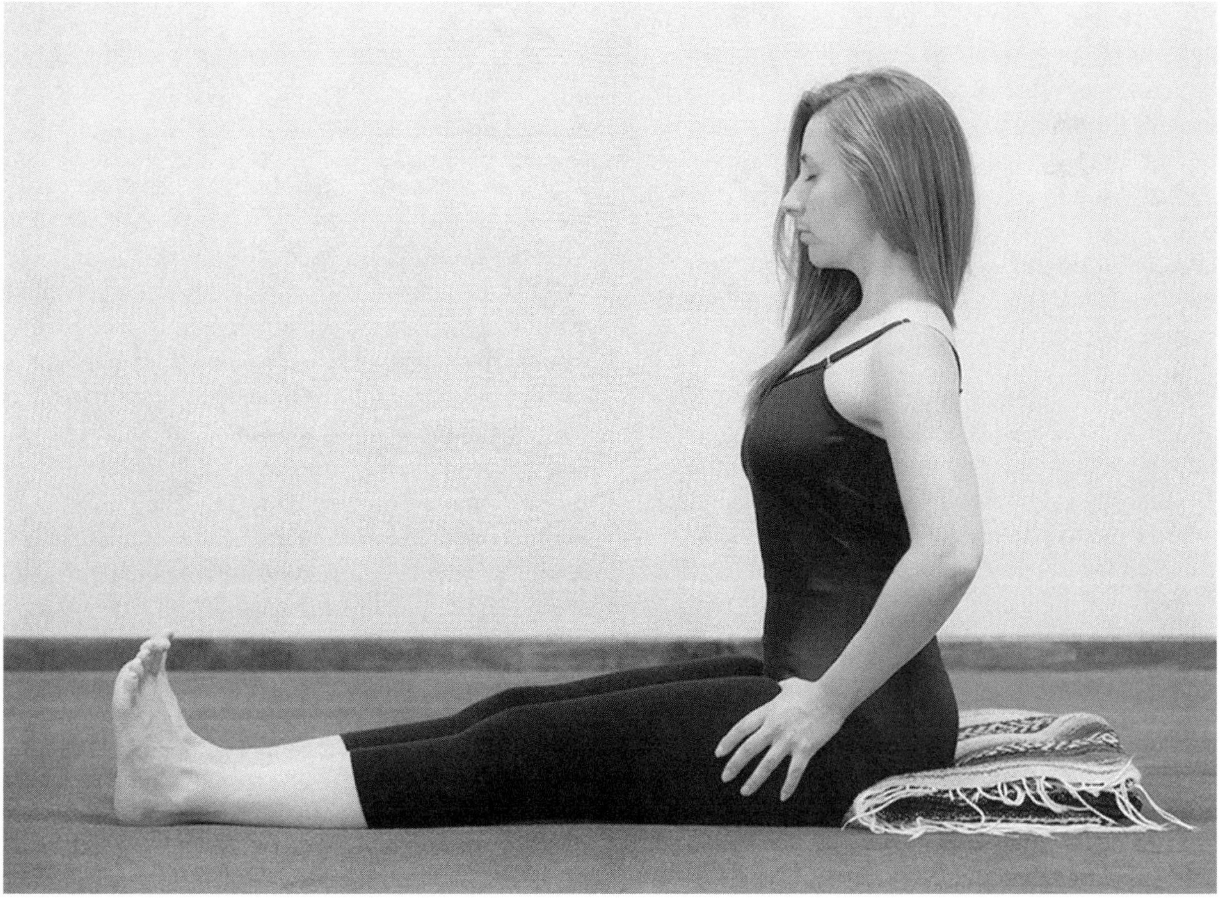

The yantra of Daṇḍāsana forms a right angle or square.

When divine energy descends, it spirals around the head like a crown, into the center of *Sahasrāra* (the crown cakra), and then spirals down into the lower inter-dimensional vortices of the body. This invisible force was not bound by the third-dimensional world and could offer the sight, wisdom, clarity, and compassion needed to carry out "right" actions for the future good of the people. The royal ruler's connection to the heavens was supposed to keep the balance of nature, promoting fertility of the crops and prosperity for all.

Over the ages, the original purpose of the staff has been forgotten. The staff or scepter was a grounding rod for the electrical impulses that manifested from the divine through the brain into the spinal cord. When universal energy spirals down through the crown cakra, the physical and subtle nerves, if not adequately strong and resilient, may be overtaxed by too much voltage. You could say the staff grounds the currents of enlightenment that descend into the *suṣumnā,* the central nāḍī that relates to the physical spinal cord. As Sri Aurobindo Gosh would teach in Integral Yoga, "in meditation the Ascent (of the individual Kuṇḍalinī energy) is followed by the Descent (Divine grace)."

When Divine grace pours into its chosen vehicle, the descent of energy awakens the sleeping Kundala, the coiled serpent that rests in the sacrum and coccyx with its head turned downward. As the power of the Divine force descends into the spine, it dilates the nadis or subtle channels, so the awakened bio- or psycho-nuclear energy can rise like the flow of warm lava or like cooling waters, and not as a burning fire that would dry and weaken rather than replenish the nervous system.

The yantra of Daṇḍāsana forms a right angle or square. The square invokes the divine energies of Lord Gaṇeśa, who is propitiated before any important endeavor. A story told by Harish Johari reminds me of the essence of Daṇḍāsana:

Śiva, the father of Gaṇeśa, was the guardian of the gaṇas—a mixture of gods, sub-gods, humans, demons, spirits, and other beings. Since Śiva was in meditation most of the time, the gaṇas found it difficult to communicate with him. Lord Viṣṇu persuaded Śiva to appoint a new leader and, to find out who was worthy, the gods and sub-gods decided to hold a contest between Śiva's two sons, Gaṇeśa and Kartikeya. Everyone gathered to witness the contest. Viṣṇu was appointed judge, and Śiva and Pārvatī sat in the center. The contest required the two brothers to circle the universe and return as quickly as possible. The fastest would be heralded as the Lord of the Gaṇas.

Kartikeya immediately jumped on his vehicle, a peacock, and flew off into space. Gaṇeśa remained seated on his vehicle, the mouse, and didn't move. Lord Viṣṇu urged him to hurry and catch up. But instead of rushing after his brother, Gaṇeśa rode around his parents, Śiva (who represents Puruṣa, the eternal essence of being) and Pārvatī (who represents Prakṛti, the primordial cause of all existing phenomena).

When Gaṇeśa returned to the starting point, he announced, "I have completed my task."

The witnessing gods and sub-gods were astounded. "It's not true!" they cried.

Gaṇeśa bowed before Lord Viṣṇu (who understood what he had done), and explained his action to the other witnesses: "The phenomenal world of name and form is but an expression and manifestation of the Divine Mother and Divine Father. They are the source and essence of all that exists. Everything else is illusion."

The gods and goddess applauded his wisdom, accepting him as Lord of the Gaṇas, which is why Gaṇeśa is also known as Gaṇapati.

Like this story of Gaṇeśa, Daṇḍāsana reflects both the macrocosm and microcosm. As we aspire upward from the spine, it is like the microcosm of lifting our body, mind, and soul to aspire to the macrocosm of the Universal. As we open our heart and crown cakra, the macrocosm reveals itself, showering grace upon and through our spine, the pillar of light, to unite with the microcosm. Gaṇeśa is that macrocosmic energy, and the little mouse symbolizes the microcosm. Each time we make a micro step to lift to the essence of the Universe, the Divine takes one hundred steps toward us. The centrifugal center of the spine, the Meru Daṇḍa ("mountainous staff"), is what Gaṇeśa circled around. It is symbolic of Śiva/Puruṣa and Śakti/Prakṛti. As Gaṇeśa did this, he triggered the descent of consciousness (the macrocosm), which is followed by the individual ascent (the microcosm).

When one invokes Gaṇeśa by forming his yantra of right angles, it is believed that the spiritual as well as material obstacles will be lifted from the unfolding path of spiritual awakening.

Guidance

1. To begin Daṇḍāsana, sit with the legs outstretched. Settle just in front of the inner points of the ischial tuberosities (buttock bones). Above the apex of these bones is the sciatic notch, where the largest nerve of the body passes through. It is best to position the pelvis just in front of these bones for the sciatic nerve to receive maximum flow.
2. Exhaling, draw the flesh of the buttocks back diagonally, placing the back of the thighs on the earth.
3. Pause to inhale into the back body.
4. On the next exhalation, press down with the fingertips, moving forward into the back thigh, extending the backs of the knees and the heels. Then, without shortening the Achilles tendon, extend through the ball of the big toe.

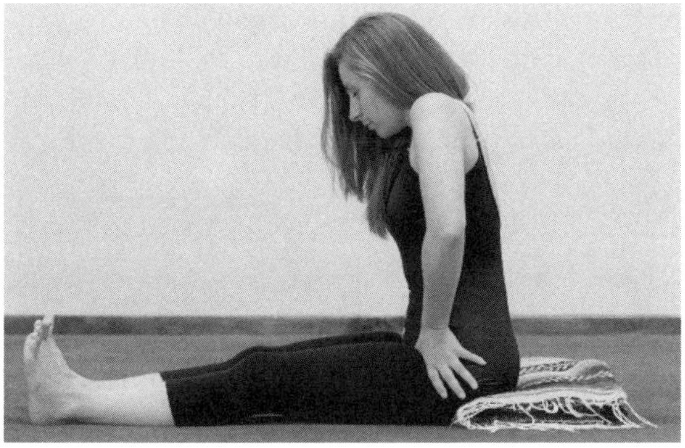

With hands in the thigh crease,
inhale into the back and turn upper arms inward.

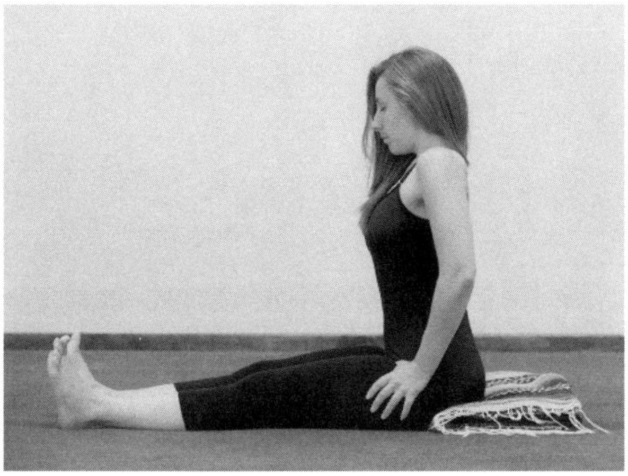

Press down into the thighs and lift,
lengthening the spine with each exhalation.

5. Inhale, rounding the back and turning the upper arms inward. Let the head hang forward.
6. Exhale, press the fingertips beside the hips and elongate the spine. Move it like a backbend into the front body. With each exhalation you are lifting, lifting, and lifting while moving the spine in like a backbend.
7. With each inhalation, gently round the back, spreading the skin out from the spinal vertebrae from shoulders to buttocks. The upper arms will automatically rotate in as the back rounds.
8. On an exhalation, lengthen the inner legs (symbolic of the subtle body) from the side of the pubic bone to the inner ankles. It is important to lengthen the inner legs and outer legs (symbolic of the physical body) equally.
9. Inhale, turning the arms in and rounding the back, letting the breath spread across the back from shoulders to buttocks.
10. Exhale, and without moving the hands, roll the upper arms externally, bringing the spine upward and then into the front of the torso as the skin moves down the back to give length to the back of the neck. (Do not compress the neck by lifting the chin.)
11. Inhale, again rolling the arms internally and rounding the back, spreading the breath out from the spine horizontally to expand the ribcage.
12. Exhaling without moving the fingers, roll the upper arm externally, lifting the spine to offer it to the heart center. Lift, lift, lift each vertebra on the exhalation and create space between the descending back skin and the base of the skull. Keep extending out from the inner groin to the inner ankle.
13. Continue in Daṇḍāsana as long as the breath is deep and rhythmic.

Note: Daṇḍāsana is significant in that it brings us closer to the earth than when we are seated in a cross-legged position. If short hamstrings prevent sitting slightly in front of the buttock bones, then elevate the hips by sitting on a blanket high enough so that there is no undue anterior compression of the lumbar spine. This allows you to relax the lumbar spine and elongate the rectus abdominus muscle.

Psychophysiological Benefits

Daṇḍāsana is the base or preliminary pose for all seated poses, particularly Jānu Śīrṣāsana and Paścimottānāsana. As well as being central to all sitting poses, Daṇḍāsana is a place to rest and re-center between seated poses. Daṇḍāsana gently elongates the hamstring muscles in the back of the thighs and the soleus and gastrocnemius muscles of the calf, while strengthening the quadriceps muscles of the upper thigh.

Daṇḍāsana gives the student a relaxed opportunity to learn how to equalize the stretch of the inner and outer leg, which represent the subtle and physical body respectively. It also is an opportunity to learn how to extend the Achilles tendon and, preserving this stretch, move the ball of the big toe forward to give greater strength to the arch. This movement relaxes the reflex to the spine, an important preliminary for taking any seated forward bends.

Daṇḍāsana strengthens the spinal nerve sheaths subtly as well as physically, so the practitioner can receive a higher frequency of illumination. Ideally, the spine in Daṇḍāsana is aligned as it is for meditation. For this to happen, the heart center needs to lift, bringing the head back so that the crown aligns with the base of the spine. Then the mind can be in a thoughtless state of awareness.

In cross-legged sitting poses, the outgoing energies that move through the feet are recycled back up into the spine and upper cakras. Outstretching the legs in Daṇḍāsana transmits energy downward and outward. As the thigh skin moves to the buttocks and the calf skin to the heels, the sub cakra energy center at the back of the knee is given space to open. Daṇḍāsana is an excellent pose to balance excessive vāta energy, which flows upward above the diaphragm, allowing it to be diffused and balanced through the feet. Some yogis say we store deep saṁskāras or cellular memory at the base of the pelvis. In Daṇḍāsana, we allow these memories to surface and be released through the channels to the soles of the feet and out into the universe.

Psychologically, Daṇḍāsana teaches us independence. When the back can hold itself, we are independent of the need for support. We become less dependent on others for our own emotional needs. Practicing the pose leads to deep inner strength indicated by the square yantra that represents Gaṇeśa. In this yantra, we are grounded in the microcosm but in communion with the macrocosm of the divine.

Paripūrṇa Nāvāsana

(The Full Boat)

Ardha Nāvāsana

(The Half Boat)

The English word "navy" grew out of the ancient Sanskrit word *nāva*. The Boat Pose has two parts, one with oars and the other without oars. *Paripūrṇa* means "fullness," and Paripūrṇa Nāvāsana is Full Boat Pose, or the boat with oars. *Ardha* means "half," and Ardha Nāvāsana is Half Boat Pose, or the boat without oars. Ardha Nāvāsana is a more challenging variation of Boat Pose, requiring greater balance and abdominal strength.

Philosophical Introduction

Many times, I have thought "Oh God! Thy sea is so great and my boat is so small." At those times when life seems overwhelming, I think of Herman Hesse's novel *Siddhartha*, about an ascetic who through solitude and meditation found peace and contentment. During his wanderings, this monk found his way to the court of a king. The king asked him what he did, and the monk replied, "I wait, I watch, and I fast."

The king was impressed with the monk's answer and by his serene countenance. He invited him to stay in his court as a spiritual advisor. A few years passed, and gradually the ascetic became tempted by palace comforts such as rich foods and wine, and he entered into a tryst with a beautiful courtesan. Over time, he lost his serenity and peace of mind and became gross and slovenly. His undisciplined life and insolent behavior forced the king to banish him from the court. After many trials and tribulations he found work as a river boatman. Every day he ferried travelers back and forth across the river from one shore to the next. Slowly once more he began to feel the peace and serenity he had lost over the years. He guided travelers to their spiritual as well as earthly destinations, and his reputation spread far and wide as others found solace in his gentle presence and wise words. His revelations came from the movement of floating and the sound of the oars dipping effortlessly into the water. The boatman had at last found truth in the water's currents and ripples, always changing within their constancy. He saw his reflection in the still waters and realized that the seer and seen were One.

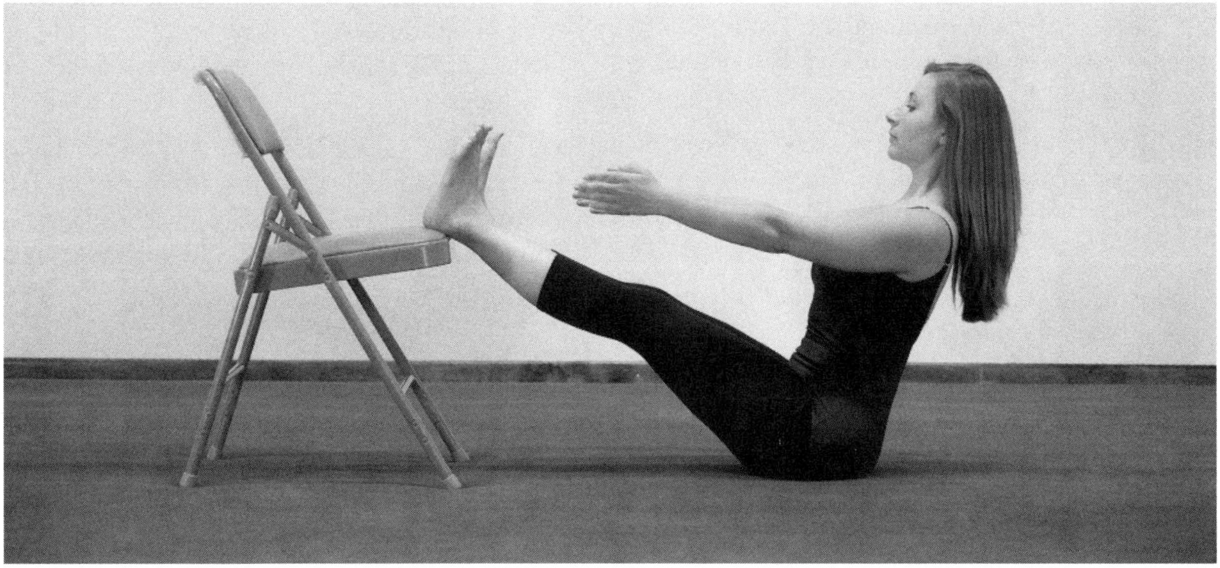

In Nāvāsana the fingertips are extended to emulate the oars of the boat.

Nāvāsana is a challenging pose because it can reveal the difficulties in staying balanced and centered as we ride upon the waves of life. Whether on a turbulent sea or a gentle brook, navigating with the assistance of oars is easier than without. In Paripūrṇa Nāvāsana, with the arms outstretched, it is easier to balance than when withdrawing the oars of the arms and placing the hands behind the head, as in Ardha Nāvāsana. The essence of either variation of Nāvāsana is to find the place of alignment in the midst of the waters where one's own reflection reveals itself.

In Paripūrṇa or Ardha Nāvāsana, the body takes the form of a descending triangle. The downward-facing Trikon is a yantra of the Divine Śakti. Thus Nāvāsana can be seen as the invocation of Śakti energy, particularly of Goddess Sarasvatī, who in ancient Vedic times was depicted near a flowing river, which may relate to her early history as a river goddess. Adorned in white, she rides upon a swan. The swan is a symbol of discrimination because it was said to have the ability to separate water from milk and take only the cream. Sarasvatī is also depicted as floating upon the waterways in the center of a white lotus, a symbol of lightness and purity that grows out of the darkness of the mud beneath the waters. In post-Vedic times, Sarasvatī became associated with literature, arts, and music, representing intelligence, Divine knowledge, creativity, education, and eloquence. She floats upon the universal waterways reminding us to do the same.

Guidance

1. To practice Paripūrṇa Nāvāsana, begin in Daṇḍāsana. Inhale into the back, spreading the breath from the shoulders to the hips.
2. Exhaling, keep the spine uplifted and the heart open, and bend the knees into the chest with feet on the floor.
3. Inhale and do nothing except allow the breath to spread across the back
4. Exhale and take hold of the neck of the big toe with the thumb and forefinger or, depending on the length of the hamstrings, hold the sides of the feet, the ankles, or even the calves.

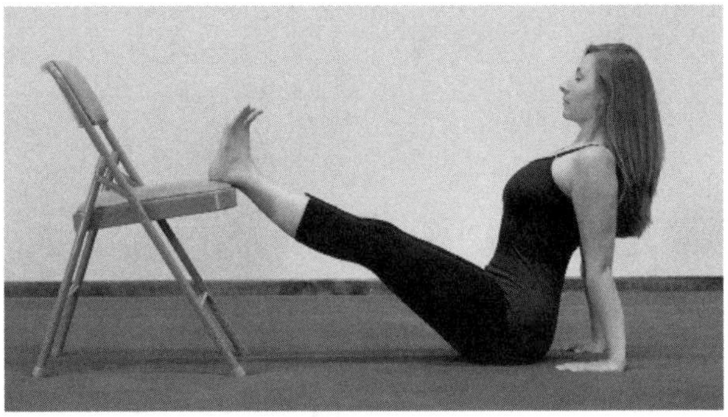

Press the hands into the floor to help extend the spine.

5. Inhale, and then on an exhalation, bring the spine into the front of the body—like a backbend—and raise the legs. If possible, bring the apex of the downward-facing triangle just in front of the buttock bones. The legs may not lift up as high, but the spine will grow stronger.
6. Inhale into the back, rounding it with the incoming breath.
7. Exhale, lifting the top of the kneecaps gently but firmly toward the thighs, bringing the spine in like a backbend. Elongate the back of the neck and keep the gaze steady.
8. Inhale, and then exhaling, move the spine up and into the front of the body like a backbend, bringing the front of the torso toward the thighs as the legs move toward the torso.
9. Inhaling, keep the gaze and the mind steady.
10. When you feel ready, exhale and release the legs, extending through the fingertips to emulate the boat with oars, Paripūrṇa Nāvāsana.
11. If you choose, you may enter the half boat, Ardha Nāvāsana, from the full boat pose. On an exhalation, bend the elbows and clasp the hands behind the neck or head.
12. Even though Ardha Nāvāsana is the boat without oars, you can still "row the boat" by moving the elbows forward and back with the breath. Begin by inhaling, rounding the back. Keep the hands clasped behind the head as the elbows come forward on the inhalation.

13. Exhaling, move the back spine into the front body as you draw the bent elbows back.
14. Inhale, rounding the back and bringing the elbows forward.
15. Exhale and draw the elbows back. Continue rowing the boat this way as long as the breath allows; this opens and strengthens the upper back.
16. When you are ready, come out of the pose the same way you came into it.

Note: Supporting the hips with a folded blanket or firm cushion will help lift the thorax. Adjust the blanket or cushion so that you are balanced just in front of the ischial tuberosities or buttock bones. It is better to bend the knees in order to keep the back straight than to straighten the legs and have the back round. Round the back only on the inhalations; elongate the spine and bring it in like a backbend on every exhalation.

You can use the aid of a chair or a wall for Nāvāsana, which offers two ways of elongating and lifting the spine. You can lean the shoulders against the wall for support, or you can turn around and put the feet up on the wall, pressing the hands on the floor beside the hips to create more lift. The idea is to relieve compression, not create more. Students who have chronic anterior compression should first focus on spinal elongation in the standing poses before practicing Nāvāsana.

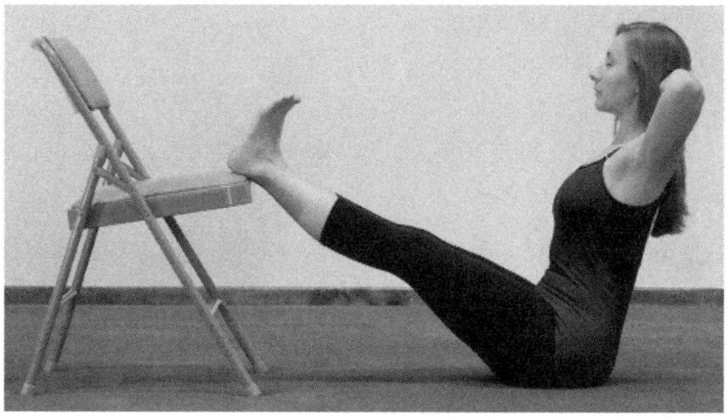

Ardha Navasana, the boat without oars, is especially effective for strengthening the abdominal muscles.

Psychophysiological Benefits

Nāvāsana is a good preparation for Sarvāṅgāsana, the shoulderstand, because it strengthens the muscles used to lift the legs into the posture. Both variations of Nāvāsana strengthen the abdominal muscles, especially Ardha Nāvāsana, the boat without oars. The boat pose also strengthens the lumbar and sacral spine, bringing circulation to both areas. It lengthens the hamstrings (back thigh muscles) and strengthens the quadriceps (front thigh muscles).

Balancing creates emotional as well as physical stability. Nāvāsana teaches us how to flow with life's ebbs and flows. It is also an excellent pose for learning ekāgratā (one-pointedness of mind) or practicing trātaka, one-pointed gazing. Focusing the gaze helps balance the body and strengthens the "muscle of the mind." Finding the center of stillness within Nāvāsana helps us lift above the tsunamis of emotions that at times threaten to engulf us. We learn to rise up and masterfully ride the illusory waves of separative consciousness.

The nursery rhyme we learned as children was profound: "Row, row, row your boat gently down the stream. Merrily, merrily, merrily, merrily—life is but a dream." When we remember our oneness with the Divine, we realize that life *is* but a dream.

Jānu Śīrṣāsana

Head-to-Knee Pose

Jānu means "knee" and *śīrṣ,* "head." Since bringing the head to the knee would cause us to round the spine too much, it helps to think of Jānu Śīrṣāsana as a forehead-to-shinbone pose.

Philosophical Introduction

Far more significant than its name implies, Jānu Śīrṣāsana is a devoted offering, as described by the fourth niyama (observance) of Aṣṭāṅga Yoga, *svādhyāya.* This niyama has been loosely interpreted as the study of scriptures, but what the sūtra (II:44) actually says is this: *svādhyāyāt iṣṭadevatā saṁprayogaḥ,* meaning, "One's own meditation on that which one wishes to shine like [a role model] brings forth the oneness and union of yoga." This is a statement of Bhakti Yoga, the path where emotion is transformed into devotion. I practice Jānu Śīrṣāsana as a devoted offering of the upper body to the lower body. The upper body represents the individuated self and the lower, the altar that is a palpable reminder of a power greater than the self.

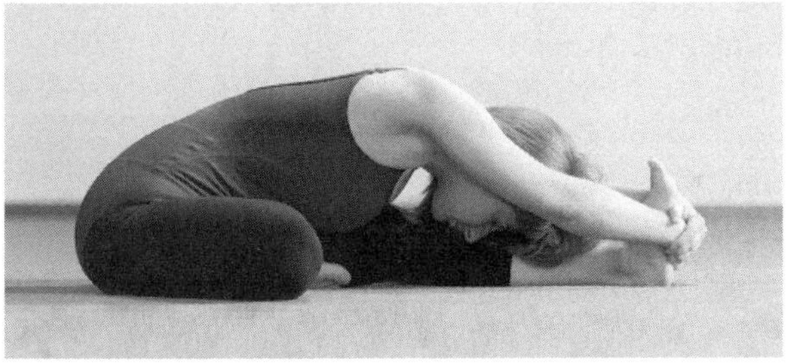

In Jānu Śīrṣāsana, the upper body is an offering to the lower body.

Many years ago, my Bhakti teacher, Sant Keshavadas, told a simple story of the moth and nightingale to help illustrate the difference between the paths of Bhakti and Jñana Yoga. The story of the moth and nightingale also emphasizes the differences between dharana (concentration) and dhyana (meditation), and it gave me a deeper understanding to practicing āsana. The tale begins on one of those perfect summer nights, when the sky was the color of a blue lotus and the full moon shimmered its radiance upon the earth. A moth fluttered into a perfumed garden, where the air was scented with night-blooming jasmine. The aroma of the garden filled the moth's senses with an intoxicating, unearthly fragrance.

The moth became entranced as a melodious song wafted through the garden. He flew in toward the sound and discovered a delicate nightingale warbling its heartfelt song as it was shedding a river of tears. "Oh nightingale," the moth asked, "Why are you crying?"

"Can you not see?" the nightingale answered. "I am serenading my beloved, the rose. These are tears of joy that stream from the outer corridors of my eyes and tears of sorrow that stream from the inner corridors of my eyes. I cry with the ecstasy of love for my beloved and, at the same time, the agony of being separate from my beloved. This is my way of showing my love for the Infinite through one of its many forms, the rose."

The moth pondered this for a moment. "Hrumph. Come, Nightingale. I will show you love." The moth flew to the light within the garden, circling its flame and spiraling in closer and closer. The nightingale watched with wonderment and shock as the moth reached the center and consumed himself in the flame, becoming one with the light. Then, after a few moments, feeling once more the pangs of separation from its beloved, the nightingale returned to its corner of the garden to serenade the rose.

This story is a beautiful metaphor for the differences between individuals in their approaches to yoga. Do we approach our practice like the Bhakti, the nightingale? Or like the Jñani, the moth who becomes one with the flame? Which is greater, the all-consuming approach of the moth, or the separative offerings of the nightingale? If we approach the practice of āsana as a bhaktin, we perceive one part of the body as separate from another. We enter into the pose as a devoted self-offering, in which one part of the body offers itself to the altar of the other. We offer our breath to the altar of our limbs, moving from the base and heart of our being.

Or do we feel the two parts fusing together in a sense of Oneness, like the moth consumed in the eternal flame and light of spirit? The Jñani is like a sugar man who walks into the ocean to measure and analyze its depth. As he goes deeper, he melts into and becomes one with the sea. There is no longer anything to measure. There is no standard of measurement.

There is no separation between the sugar man and the sea; they are one.

This is a metaphor that I have carried into āsana practice throughout the decades. Jānu Śīrṣāsana and Paścimottānāsana, in particular, are poses that can awaken the Bhakti of offering the upper body to the lower, like the nightingale with its beloved the rose. At a certain point, whether or not the upper and lower bodies touch, you may feel as though the parts of your being merge and become one with the Source.

Guidance

The first point of emphasis in practicing Jānu Śīrṣāsana is maintaining the Daṇḍāsana spine, in which all of the spinal processes of the vertebrae are moving anteriorly. As the spine lifts, it is moving upward and into the center of the body so there is no anterior or posterior compression of the intervertebral disks. This compression can be felt with the hand during the pose. If the spinal processes protrude, this means you need to elongate the spine a bit more: Stop, breathe, and lengthen before proceeding further in the pose.

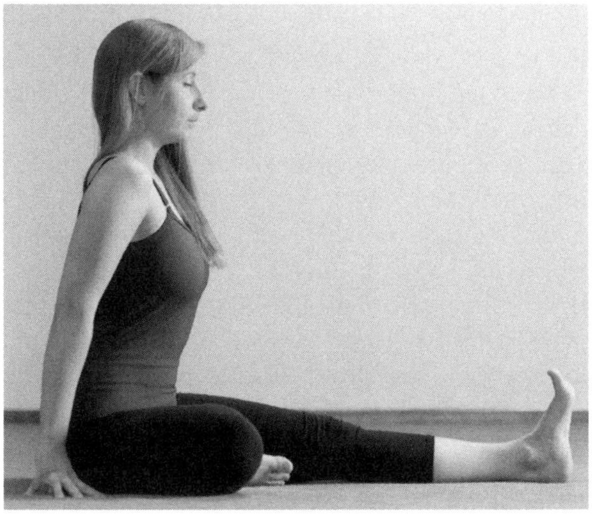

Jānu Śīrṣāsana, starting position.

1. Begin in Daṇḍāsana, establishing the breath.
2. Exhaling, bend the left knee, bringing the foot to the inner thigh of the extended leg. If the openness of the hips allow, bring the heel of the bent knee to the center or even the left side of the pubic bone. Anchor the hip of the bent knee downward and backward so that the thigh rotates externally. Place the fingertips on the floor to each side of the hips.

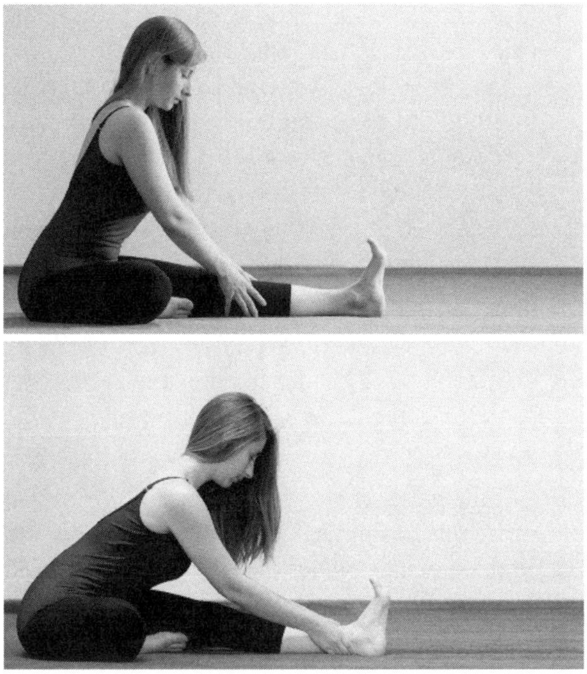

Shift the position of the hands as you progress through the pose, moving the spine like a backbend on the exhalations.

3. Inhale, do nothing but breathe. Bring the breath into the back, from the shoulders upward toward the neck.
4. Exhale and press the fingertips downward, extending the neck up as the shoulders move down toward the buttocks, creating space between the earlobes and the tops of the shoulders.
5. Inhale into the back, rotating the upper arms internally and relaxing the head and neck as you expand the breath from shoulders to hips.
6. Exhale, pressing the fingertips down and rotating the upper arms externally as the shoulders descend downward.
7. Inhale, and again let the breath round the back, doing nothing.
8. Exhaling, press down with the fingertips and turn the navel toward the extended leg. Bring the torso toward the thigh, drawing the kneecap up gently as the torso descends more with each exhalation. The hands at the sides of the hips give leverage to extend the spine. On the exhalations, move the spine anteriorly, like a backbend, to the front of the torso.
9. Inhaling, bring the breath into the back, expanding it as far as possible across the spectrum from shoulders to buttock.

10. Continue focusing on the breath, elongating the spine on the exhalations. If pain arises in the backs of the legs, stop and back off your edge a little. Find the calmness of the breath before proceeding, moving only on the exhalation. If you feel a sensation of pain, imagine inhaling into that area and, on the exhalation, release the tension that surrounds and protects the painful nucleus. To stay within your *svadharma*—what is right for you—stay on your edge without overreaching.
11. Breathe and let go into the devotional offering of the nightingale. When you are ready, change sides.

Note: If the upper rim of the pelvis or hip is pulled backward due to short hamstrings, it is important to use a folded blanket under the buttocks to help with the lift. If the bent knee doesn't reach the floor, it too can be supported with blankets. Support is usually used for students who are heavier or less flexible. If there is neck tension when in the pose, it is helpful to add a blanket between abdomen and thigh, as well as a blanket under the forehead. When the neck is elongated and relaxed, the lower back and sacrum start to release.

Psychophysiological Benefits

Jānu Śīrṣāsana is introduced before Paścimottānāsana, the full forward bend, because it is easier to extend the spine toward one leg. Stiffness isn't due only to the hamstrings but also to fluid buildup in the sacrum and pelvis. The lymph system in the pelvic area can become coagulated from sitting too much. Also, for women, if the circulation is sluggish, stagnant blood can build up in the pelvic or uterine area. In Jānu Śīrṣāsana, there is an internal rotation of the thighs that opens the back of the sacrum. This stimulates the parasympathetic nerve flow from the sacrum, which then releases the cervical spine, bringing about a sacral-occipital alignment. When you can find a comfortable way to "hang out" in this pose, relaxing the neck, then the pelvic region starts to open and release.

Jānu Śīrṣāsana releases neck tension if the pose is entered into with the breath. It lengthens the hamstring muscles. The spine is stretched, increasing intervertebral circulatory flow, which can possibly help rebuild degenerative disks over time. Besides releasing lymph buildup in the sacrum and pelvis, this pose aids elimination by stimulating the parasympathetic nervous system and massaging the abdominal organs. By influencing the parasympathetic nervous system, Jānu Śīrṣāsana and other forward bends help relieve stress on the adrenals and kidneys. In the ayurvedic sense, forward bends balance vāta and pitta, calming and slowing any mental hyperactivity. These poses balance prāṇa in the ascending, descending, and transverse colon, as well as in the procreative and reproductive organs, including the ovaries and prostate gland.

In this pose, we don't just bring the head to the knee, as this could cause anterior compression of the spine. Instead, on each exhalation we reach, lengthen, and soften the neck, while drawing the spine forward to lay it upon the altar of the shinbone. It sometimes feels as if the prāṇa that flows in the torso is uniting with the prāṇa of the extended leg. When we practice Jānu Śīrṣāsana in this manner, we become the Pūjari, the one who conducts the ceremonial rites of Pūja.

Forward bends, like Jānu Śīrṣāsana, close the gap between the Atman and the Brahman, the individual and the Universal. When we offer the head toward the knee, the head is the symbol of ego and the bent knee is a symbol of humility. When our knees are unable to bend, it indicates that somewhere in our psyche we are holding something back. In Jānu Śīrṣāsana, if we learn to offer the total Self without the conflict of resistance, we learn to trust again. This newfound trust can spill over from our yoga postures into the postures of our lives. This is *svādhyāya,* our own meditation upon that which we wish to shine like.

Jānu Śīrṣāsana is a beautiful pose of Bhakti, in which we offer our Being in one part of our body to the Divinity in the other. As we hold the field of love for ourselves and others when we are in the pose, the gap between the upper and lower body, Atman and Brahman, the individual and Universal, can close and merge like the moth who became one with the light of universal love.

Marīcyāsana I

Seated Twist and Forward Bend

This pose is named for Mārīca, a magician and an uncle of the demon king Rāvaṇa.

Philosophical Introduction

Mārīca was a shapeshifter who used his magical prowess to change forms from human to animal, from birds to insects. Driven by lust and desire, Rāvaṇa urged Mārīca to change into a deer so beautiful that it would tempt Sītā to ask Rāma to bring it to her. The plot was to lure Rāma deep into the forest, leaving his beloved unprotected so that the demon could steal her away. When Mārīca refused, Rāvaṇa threatened him: "If you do not do this, you will die by my hand."

Mārīca chose to become a deer, preferring to die by the arrow of Rāma rather than at the hand of his demon nephew. He shifted his shape into a magnificent creature with horns sparkling like sapphires, hooves of precious gems, and golden flanks with spots that gleamed like silver. Sītā's desire caused Rāma to follow the deer further into the dark forest, and thus she was captured by Rāvaṇa, representing the powerful energy of our instinctual nature and the separative consciousness of ego.

In the evolutionary aspects of creation, the soul assumes innumerable forms. Mārīca assumed a magnificent form only to be killed by Rāma's arrow. But in choosing to die by the hand of God, Mārīca transformed. Marīcyāsana I and its variations honor that part of our nature that can shift shapes, rising out of the egocentric self to that of our Divine Nature.

When we practice these twists, prāṇa from the base of the spine spirals up like the evolutionary force of creation through the awakening of the Kuṇḍalinī Śakti, bio- or psycho-energetic transformation. Like Mārīca, we too can make a choice either to sink into our lower instinctual patterns, which lure us deeper into the dark forest of our primordial self, or to rise and evolve out of that nature to the mountain peaks of transcendent consciousness.

Guidance

Marīcyāsana I is both a twist and forward bend. It cannot be emphasized enough how important it is to keep the head and neck relaxed throughout all movements of the pose. The essence of all yoga is to still the waves of the mind. Every pose then becomes *dhyanāsana,* a pose of meditation, in which the head and neck are relaxed and receptive.

1. Begin in Daṇḍāsana. To align the spine, you may need to use a chair or place the buttocks on a folded blanket. (See note.)
2. Exhaling, bend the right knee, bringing the heel as close to the perineum as possible. Place hands beside the hips to give leverage to lift the spine with each out breath.

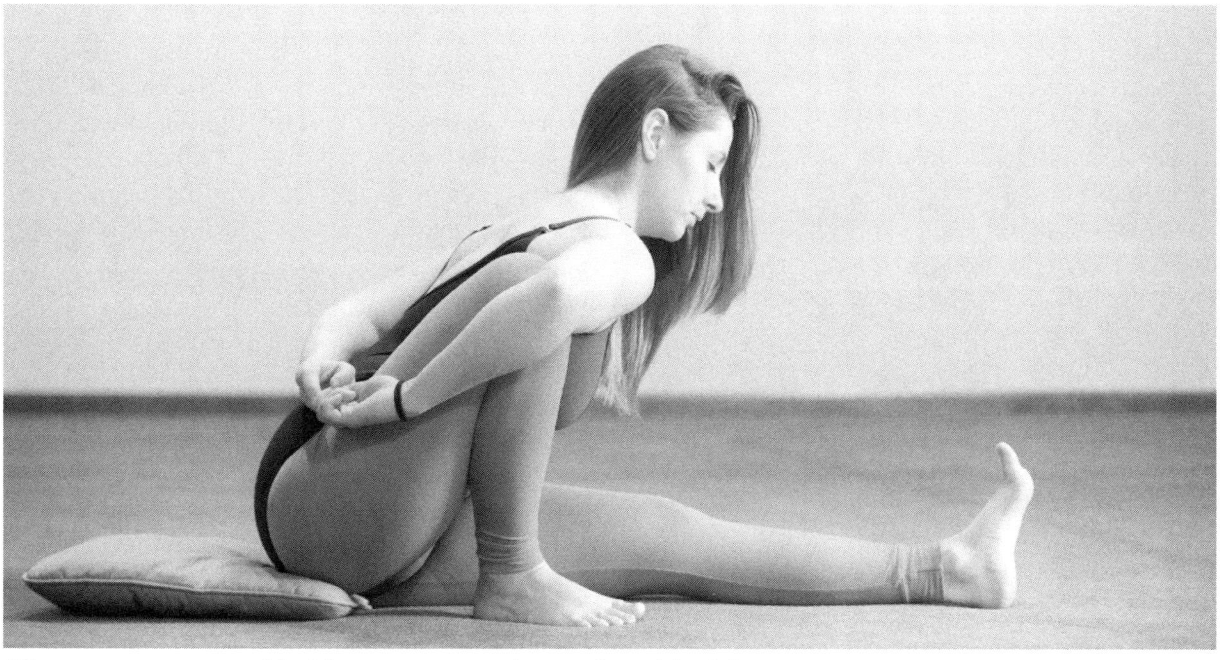

When practicing twists like Marīcyāsana, emphasize the uplift of the spine.

3. Inhale and allow the breath to spread across the back. The inhalation offers an opportunity to take the breath down into those regions that have been compressed and contracted. See if the breath can move from the lateral muscles of the back all the way down to the base of the hips.

4. Exhaling, press down with the hands (or fingertips) and lift the spine, bringing the spine into the front of the body like a backbend. As the back of the neck extends upward, allow the skin of the back to move downwards. Relax the neck.

5. Inhale, allowing the breath to fill the back as before.

6. Exhale and again press down with the hands to elongate the spine and bring it in as though beginning a backbend. Extend out of the inner groin of left leg, all the way to the inner ankle. Extend the heel, stretching the Achilles tendon, and without losing that length, extend to the ball of the big toe. This action strengthens the arch of the foot and softens the spinal reflex within the arch.

7. Inhaling, keep the extension of the left leg and foot while you round the back with the incoming breath.

8. Exhale, pressing down with the left hand to lift the spine. Bring the right arm toward the extended leg, coming forward as in Jānu Śīrṣāsana. Bring the back of the right armpit to the shinbone. Press the arm against the shinbone and rotate the upper arm internally as the lower arm wraps around the back of the waist. There is a tendency to let the bent leg collapse to the side. To correct this tendency, press the inner thigh toward the arm as the arm resists the inner thigh. Keeping the leg aligned creates greater strength in the adductors, the inner thigh muscles.

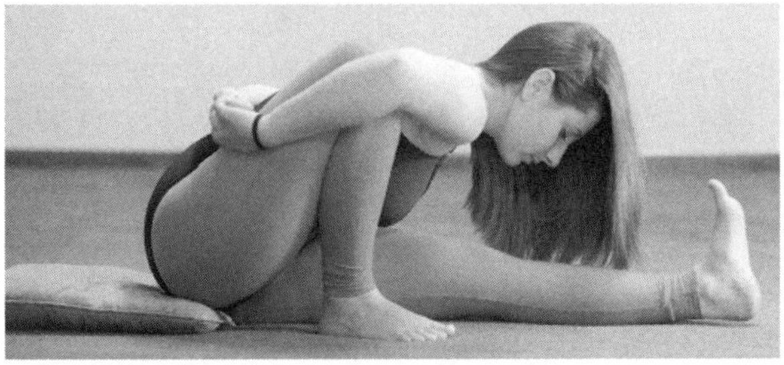

Keeping the leg aligned strengthens the inner thigh muscles.

9. Inhaling, stay where you are in the pose. Take no adjustments as the breath expands across the back from shoulder to the base of the hips.

10. Exhale, lifting the spine and bringing it into the front body as if attempting to do a backbend. Moving the hip and leg back helps to bring the spine forward. Bring the left hand around the back of the waist to clasp the right hand. If this is difficult, you may use a strap.

11. Inhale and let the breath round the back without unclasping the hands.

12. Exhale and press down with the right heel to lift and elongate the spine. Moving the skin of the inner left leg from the pubis to the inner ankle, bring the navel toward the earth in a forward bend. Bend from the hips, not from the waist. The objective is to offer the pelvis to the earth, and then the navel, and finally, the head.

13. Remember, throughout both inhalations and exhalations, to keep the neck and throat passive and relaxed so that the mid and lower back can release.

14. If the torso leans to one side, exhale and extend out of the compressed side to make the lungs equal to one another. Balancing the lungs balances the breath in the right and left nostrils, and in turn, balances the twin hemispheres of the brain.

15. With every exhalation, allow the spine to offer itself toward the head and into the heart.

16. To complete the pose on this side, return to Daṇḍāsana. Breathe and extend the spine before taking the pose to the opposite side.

Note: For many, shortened hamstrings pull the pelvis back and cause compression of the anterior spine. Using a chair helps to create the lift needed for this pose, allowing the spine to rise up out of its past compression. Beginners can sit on the chair with one leg bent toward the torso and the other leg hanging down from the chair, relaxing the hamstrings and making it possible to feel the elongation of the spine as each vertebra is lifted from the next. Even seasoned students will find it helpful to place a folded blanket under the buttocks to elevate the spine for maximum extension. When the heel and buttock on the side of the bent leg can press down at the same time, the spine is lifting. This creates extension and a wonderful sense of lightness and relaxation within the pose.

Psychophysiological Benefits

The bilateral movements of twists equally benefit the sympathetic and parasympathetic divisions of the nervous system. All twists have similar beneficial effects upon the organs of digestion, the stomach, liver, gallbladder, pancreas, and spleen. Marīcyāsana, in particular, activates energy down to the root of the spine and procreative centers, benefiting the adrenals, kidneys, bladder, and the prostate or ovarian regions for men or women. The placement of the legs stimulates the small intestine and the ascending, transverse, and descending colon. Marīcyāsana neutralizes the energies of backbends as it strengthens the hips, knees, and ankles.

In Marīcyāsana, we rise up out of the basic instinctual nature of the first and second cakras. As the spine elongates on every exhalation, the heart offers itself to the light of higher consciousness without denying the base. It is the base cakras that free the upper cakras. We don't deny or repress their energy but, like the transformation of Mārīca, we convert them, bringing them with us into the upper realms. Marīcyāsana, like Matsyāsana (Fish Pose), represents the evolutionary spiral of creation and reminds us that we are all in varying states of spiritual evolution. This pose displays a revolutionary transformation of our darker urges, which are brought up to the light of Being for healing. Like Mārīca, we can all create the magic of revealing and healing any saṁskāras that remain hidden in the deeper recesses of our cellular psyche.

Practicing Marīcyāsana I can bring up feelings of confinement or past disempowerment—any experience that may have resulted in claustrophobic feelings of being closed in. This is especially true if we reach around with the arms before emphasizing the uplift of the spine. Without the spinal elongation, we compress the lungs as well as the diaphragmatic muscle. When the breathing is constricted, it may activate feelings of confinement. Conversely, when Marīcyāsana is practiced appropriately, we may be able to alleviate feelings of confinement either physically or emotionally.

It is not easy to lift in Marīcyāsana. It is so easy to sink into one's self. When we lift the spine, we aspire to something greater than our microcosmic self, an ascent to the macrocosm of the Divine. As we ascend with the central axis of creation represented by the spine, we invite the descending grace of consciousness to enter into the newly created spaces. This awakens the dormant creative impulses at the base of the spine so that they can rise up and meet the descending energies. We then experience Divine Union, where the universal and individual are one.

Paścimottānāsana

Full Forward Bend

Paścima means "west," the side of the setting sun. When the sun sets it grows dark, and we cannot see with our physical eyes. The verb *tan,* some say, means "intensive stretch," but it suggests much more. *Tan* also means going beyond our past self-imposed limitations—not limitations that others have imposed upon us, but the restrictions we have consciously or subconsciously created for ourselves. Thus, Paścimottānāsana is an intense stretch of the west or back side of the body, which takes us beyond past boundaries. This is a pose that awakens the posterior nerves of the spine and the hindbrain, the cerebellum, which is said to be the seat of *citta* or the subconscious mind.

Philosophical Introduction

In Tantra Yoga there are ten directions. East, West, North, South, and their variations are said to have presiding gods and goddess. In this pose, we honor the energy of the Lord of the West, and at times, we may even feel the gentle warmth of the setting sun streaming through the nerve roots of the spine.

Many years ago I studied with Mr. Iyengar in India. It was a cold January morning as I sat in Daṇḍāsana, wearing shorts on the hard marble, while Mr. Iyengar called out detailed instructions of how to move into Paścimottānāsana. As I struggled to seek comfort in a most uncomfortable position, a fleeting thought entered my mind: "Why have I traveled fifteen thousand miles, leaving my children and my husband at a great expense, in order to sit on a hard marble floor on a cold morning and be in pain?"

In this moment of suffering, I also remembered the words of Sant Keshavadas, my Bhakti Yoga teacher, who said, "In pain, one remembers God. In pleasure, one forgets God. One who remembers God in both pain and pleasure equally attains immortality."

It was in this time of great agony, as my head bent toward my shinbone in Paścimottānāsana, that I came face to face with a deep primordial, instinctual fear of death. My deepest fear at that moment was that if I surrendered fully into the pose, the ego would dissolve into itself.

"So this," I thought, "is *abhineveśa,*" one of the greatest obstacles in our spiritual path, what the yoga sūtras call the clinging to life and the fear of death. My body tensed with fear. What if this thing called "I" would drop into a cavern of the unknown? This fear caused my body to tighten even more. The mind was holding back, creating resistance while the body was trying to move forward into the pose. This internal conflict set up even greater resistance.

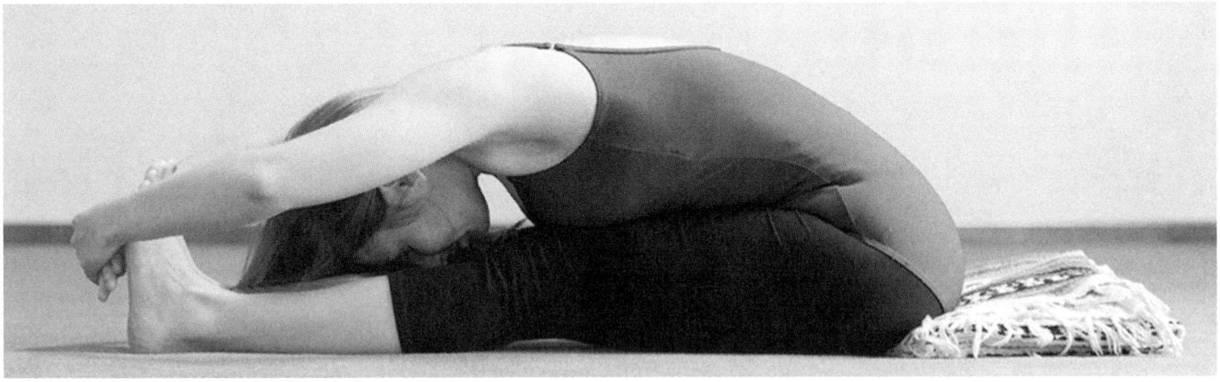

Pascimottanasana symbolizes the coming together of the individual and Universal.

As soon as I asked myself that question, another arose: "Am I working out future pains or future karmas?" I remembered the sūtra that says we cannot avoid the pains of the past because they have already occurred. Nor can we avoid the pains of the moment because they are in the process of occurring. As Patanjali noted in the yoga sūtras (II:16), *heyaṁ duḥkham anāgatam:* "The only pain that can be avoided is the pain yet to come."

I saw Mr. Iyengar's feet approach my side. "Do you see the distance between your upper and lower body?" He fluttered his hand between the vast space that separated my torso and legs.

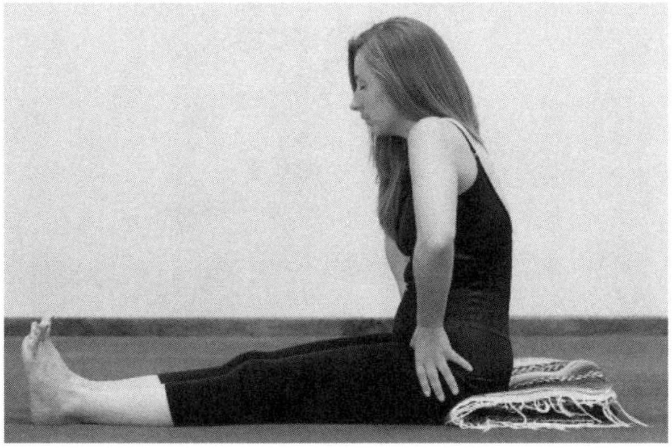

Expand across the back on the inhalation.

"Yes." My voice quivered with even more fear.

"This is the distance between you and God!"

He then stepped on my back, and suddenly the upper and lower body became one. There was no pain or pleasure, no this or that, no front or back body, no subject and object, no here or there. The little me disappeared into an infinite sea of effulgent light. There was no pain, only bliss and an indescribable peace.

Through this pose, I better understood the story of the moth and the nightingale (see page 126) and how much courage it took for the moth to fly into the center and become one with the flame. It did not hold itself back but gave and offered its all from the depth of its being, beyond all resistance physically and emotionally. Only then, I realized, can we have a glimpse of becoming one with the Source.

Seated forward bends bring us into very deep communion with the Divine. Like Jānu Śīrṣāsana, Paścimottānāsana symbolizes the coming together of the individual and Universal, closing the gap of separation or the realization of the Oneness of Atman and Brahman. Forward bends such as Paścimottānāsana are a form of passive surrender. They are the practice of Īśvara Praṇidhāna: *samādhisiddhiḥ Īśvarapraṇidhānāt.* This describes the fifth niyama of Aṣṭāṅga Yoga, outlined in the yoga sūtras (II: 45): "Samādhi comes to those who surrender to Self or God."

This particular forward bend is a devotional practice. As long as there is a sense of separation of upper and lower bodies, we are the nightingale. When we feel the upper and lower merging into one another, we become the moth entering into and becoming One with the light of the Universal flame.

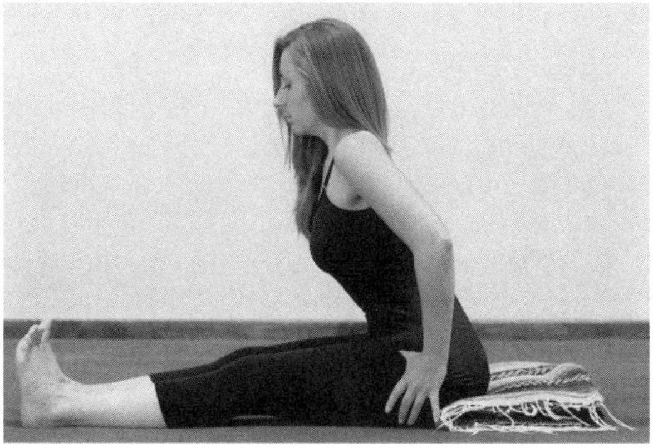

Exhale, initiating forward bend at the hips.

Paścimottānāsana represents exploration of the unknown uncharted waters of Self. It truly is an act of surrender. If we practice this pose as a bhakti, offering the upper body to the lower body, it is not necessary to close the gap physically, even if there appears to be a space between the upper and lower bodies, or between one's self and God. Like the nightingale, we can close the gaps in our souls when we remember that these two parts of ourselves are already One.

Guidance

1. Begin in Daṇḍāsana. Place a blanket or support under the buttocks to get the lift and forward tilt of the pelvis. Extend the inner and outer legs equally. (Remember, the physical body relates to the abductor muscles of the outer leg, and the subtle body relates to the adductors of the inner legs.) Draw the flesh of the thighs back as you extend the heels forward, keeping the length of the Achilles tendon. Notice the slight internal rotation of the thighs that opens the back of the sacrum. Press the fingertips or palms on the floor beside the hips.
2. Inhale and do nothing. Simply feel the wings of the breath spreading across the back. Inhale from the shoulders down to the hips.
3. Exhale, and let the breath draw the spine upward and forward as you bend at the hips, not at the waist.
4. Inhale while keeping the mind still; feel the breath expanding and widening the back from shoulders to hips.
5. Exhaling, elongate the spine upward and bring it in, like a backbend, pressing the hands on the earth to lift the pelvic rim up over the flesh of the thighs. Still exhaling, come forward, bringing the navel plexus (not the head) closer to the thighs.

6. Inhale, pausing to bring the breath into the back ribs, lifting the bottom ribs.
7. As you exhale, keep lifting the back ribs, and at the same time, raise the front ribs to bring the lower torso toward the thighs. The torso doesn't go down as much as it elongates. A useful image is to feel a golden thread pulling the crown of the head toward the feet.
8. With each outgoing breath, offer your entire being upon the altar of life. When the breath becomes erratic or shallow, come out of the pose slowly and lie back in Savāsana.

Psychophysiological Benefits

Poses related to the full forward bend include Jānu Śīrṣāsana, Ūrdhva Mukha Paścimottānāsana, Ardha Nāvāsana, Paripūrṇa Nāvāsana, Halāsana, Uttānāsana, Pādānguṣṭhāsana, Pādahastāsana, and Triang Mukhaikapāda Paścimottānāsana. Like many of these, Paścimottānāsana lengthens the hamstrings and the gastrocnemius and soleus muscles of the calf. If we have harbored anger in this region, when we elongate and create space we have an opportunity to transmute any negativity toward self and others. Paścimottānāsana also preserves the contours and flexibility of the hips. It massages all of the abdominal organs and the procreative glands and also can release the diaphragmatic muscle, freeing the breath.

Because of its impact upon the cervical and sacral nerve roots of the spine, Paścimottānāsana activates the parasympathetic nervous system. This makes it a good pose for insomnia and high blood pressure. It increases the digestive juices and dilates blood vessels, which has a cooling affect upon the body and a calming effect on the mind. Even people with high blood pressure can practice inverted poses if they first practice Paścimottānāsana to dilate the blood vessels.

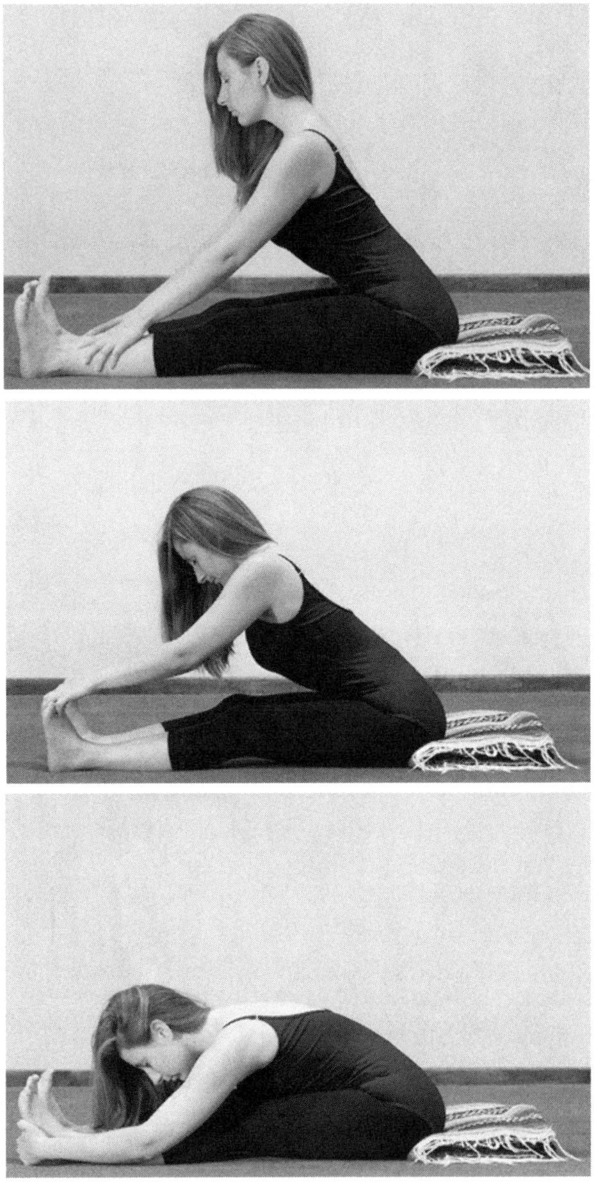

Focus on elongating the torso as you progress through the pose, moving the spine in like a backbend on the exhalations.

On an energetic level, Paścimottānāsana stimulates the apāna prāṇa, the downward flow of energy that governs the eliminative centers of the body. Once we can extend and lower the torso far enough, the buttocks will lift so that the backs of the thighs, rather than the pelvis, will be on the floor, and then the pose creates a natural mūla bandha.

To allow the energy to flow from the base cakra upward, it is important to keep the navel passive. If the solar plexus becomes engaged and pushes forward this stimulates the frontal brain, and that is opposite of what wants to be created here. As the elongation into the pose deepens, a natural uḍḍiyāna bandha occurs, bringing the prāṇa to the heart and eventually to the crown of the head. The energy then recycles through the feet and forms a loop or a cycle of pranic currents that create the yantra of the circle, which symbolizes the expansion of awareness from the inside.

By activating the posterior spinal nerve roots, Paścimottānāsana influences the back brain, the pons, the medulla, and the cerebellum. These are the intuitive parts of our being, which we associate with the feminine aspect of the universe. Paścima, the side of the setting sun, is closely related to the subconscious mind, the part of our mind that is not as accessible as the conscious or the preconscious parts of mind. The conscious mind is easily accessible and is represented by Pūrva, the side of the rising sun. When the sun rises, we can see. As we look down the front of the body, we can see it, unlike the back of our being.

In reference to Paścimottānāsana, Mr. Iyengar once asked, "How do you know you have a back body?" No one could answer. He continued, "The back body is like God. You cannot see it; therefore, you must retire within yourself and there you will feel it."

An Introduction to Seated Poses

Finding the perfection of asana in seated poses helps us reach the state of meditation. But we may be reluctant to call sitting poses "meditation" because we do not know if we will enter the state of meditation or even if we will be able to concentrate when we "sit." Because most practitioners do not know the art of alignment in the sitting poses, they may spend needless hours trying to quiet their thoughts—something that can be done almost instantly by aligning the body with the gravitational field of the earth.

In seated poses, and in all asana, alignment grows out of the center of the breath. We inhale without intentional movement, only awareness of how the breath spreads across the back from the shoulders to the buttocks, moving equilaterally from the spine. On the exhalation, the back body—which represents the subconscious mind, the part we cannot see—is offered in toward the front body, and the spine lifts vertebra by vertebra, offering the heart center to the light above. This movement taken on the exhalation brings the head back and aligns the crown with the tailbone. As the back of the neck lengthens without dropping the chin, the prana of the sensory organs, which usually darts outward to take in the world, now turns inward. This becomes an automatic pratyahara, the withdrawal and integration of the senses.

With each outgoing breath, we check the downward gravitational pull (abhyasa) by offering the spine upward like the trunk of a tree that grows toward the light. The bottom of the thighs and the front of the tailbone are like the roots of the tree, keeping their energetic connection to the earth. The brain cells become like the leaves of the tree, sensitive to the tiniest breeze, while the trunk of the tree—the spine—is strong, unmoving, and stable. This alignment brings us effortlessly into the meditative seat … and perhaps into Dhyanasana, the pose of meditation.

One day, while I was seated in Padmasana, Lotus Pose, Mr. Iyengar came over and gently moved the side of his knee into my back, lifting the heart center. I noticed that my head moved backward to a place where thoughts no longer seemed to take form. He said, "When the heart becomes the extrovert, the mind becomes the introvert." As my heart lifted, my head was no longer moving forward and stimulating the prefrontal cortex of the conscious thinking mind. As my head and neck moved back, I felt more grounded, with a quiet energy in the cerebellum at the base of the skull, an area yogis refer to as the seat of the subconscious mind.

As the heart lifts and the neck lengthens, energy moves up the back of the head to the crown and then down the front of the face, relaxing the skin of the forehead from the hairline to the brows. This draws the prana of the eyes inward. As the energy of the eyes draws back, prana moves slightly up and back toward the pineal gland. This is a blissful joining point for maithuna, the mystic marriage of the pituitary (the projective masculine energy) with the pineal (the receptive feminine energy). Through this intercourse, Ajna, the forehead chakra, has the potential to reveal the wisdom of the teacher within. Eventually, prana leads to the opening gateway of Sahasrara, the thousand-petaled lotus of the crown chakra. This is where experiential knowledge opens, the infinite unfoldment of the brain cells, just as the lotus opens with the light of the rising sun.

There is a special point at the crown of the head. When this point is balanced over the tip of the tailbone, thoughts cannot take form, and we won't need to wrestle with our thoughts to quiet the mind. The mind comes automatically into a thoughtless state of awareness, allowing what is already within us to reveal itself.

Dharana

Dharana, or concentration, precedes meditation. During dharana the subject focuses the mind on a single object. This object can be a symbol of inspiration, for example, a yantra, a sunset, a beautiful flower, an uplifting piece of art, the picture of a guru or teacher or role model who has qualities to aspire to. We can focus on the breath or on a mantra. We may choose to focus on a deity representing any of the world's religions or, if agnostic or atheist, on an ideal, such as the innocence of a child. We all seem to have faith in something greater than ourselves.

Throughout the years, I was taught that if dharana is held for twelve seconds or twelve breaths it would automatically stream into dhyana, or meditation, when subject and object fuse as one.

Dhyana

Meditation (dhyana) has been described as oil being poured in an uninterrupted stream from one vessel to another. During dhyana, there is no space or interruption of the flow between subject and object.

From the time he was an infant, Prince Siddhartha was sheltered within the palace walls. He lived a life surrounded by luxury, beauty, and youth. One day, when he ventured out beyond the palace walls for the first time, he was shocked to find that in his father's kingdom, there was hunger, sickness, old age, and death. In his dismay, he left the palace and his family on a quest for truth and the meaning of life. He became a wandering mendicant, begging food from door to door, living under the sun and stars. He sought teachers who taught him austerities. He fasted and continued the severity of his practices, and still he could not find the meaning and purpose of life.

After many years, his disciplines took their toll on his body and mind but to no avail. In his anguish to find truth, he came to a tree (later named the Bodhi Tree) and sat on the earth beneath it, saying to himself, "I will not move from here until truth reveals itself."

As soon as he took this vow, all the forces of Mara, the temptress of evil, tried to move him from the earth and sway him from his resolve. "Get off my earth!" she cried.

The prince replied, "Who is to say that this is your earth?"

Mara then brought forth all the forces of temptation. All the storms that arise from the turbulence of the subconscious mind, the citta, whirled around the prince as Mara's armies of dark forces and demonic primordial forms testified that this was her earth. "Now, who will testify on your behalf?" she asked.

Frail from his austerities, the prince said, "I call upon Mother Earth herself to testify that I have a right to be here." He then opened his palms to the sky and pointed his fingers toward the earth, joining the index finger, the symbol of the Atman (the individual soul) to the thumb, symbolic of Brahman (the Universal Soul). Mara and her legions of dark forces became powerless and withdrew.

Sitting upon the earth, the prince at last found what he was looking for. He became known as the Buddha, the enlightened one. Buddha is from bodh, meaning "to know." He transcended the trials and tribulations that appear upon the spiritual path to realize truth and the meaning of existence. As all the primordial, instinctual forces of his own nature rose from his subconscious depths as well as from the collective mind, he was not shaken from his center. He watched with dispassion as thousands of lifetimes sprang forth from the storehouse of citta (subconscious mind) to be realized by the manas (conscious mind). Free from attachment or aversion, he observed with dispassion, whatever arose. For as it arose, it also passed away. Anicca, anicca—changing, changing.

In sitting, we observe whatever arises, including any pain of the lower body. If we can sit like the Buddha, with dispassion, that pain dissolves away … until the next sensation arises. We sit in the center of the pairs of opposites, not even identifying pain or pleasure but merely sensations that arise and pass away. This by itself is a powerful practice that can lead to self-revelation.

In the Vipassana tradition of meditation, we are asked to not move for one hour. This practice, known as insight meditation, can lead to amazing revelations. During Vipassana pains arise, stay for awhile, and then subside. The pains are temptations to change positions, and I began to observe that when something is uncomfortable, we want to fix it or stop it. But if we can come to the place of observation without reaction, whatever arises will eventually pass away, and then we see that everything—even the worst of our pains—is impermanent. Thoughts too are impermanent; they rise and fall. Like the temptations of Mara, they swirl around, absorbing the mind into their storms, taking us further away from the discovery of Self.

When the body becomes still and unmoving, deeper recesses of the mind are revealed and its oscillations move like waves, creating ripples of distraction. I have found that even swallowing can be a distraction of the mind during meditation. If the breath has too much friction, it too seems to create wavelike ripples in the brain. I've experimented with refining the breath, shortening the incoming and outgoing breath until they feed into one another. As the invisible link between mind and body, the breath is a reflection of the wavelike movements of the mind.

When I am able to find that place where I am not breathing but breath is, my mind becomes still and whatever reveals itself as karma bubbles up to the surface of the conscious mind. As we are taught in yoga, the invisible must become visible before it can be eradicated or transformed.

Samadhi

If meditation (dhyana) can be held for twelve breaths or twelve seconds, it automatically leads to the first stages of Samadhi. The term Samadhi is from sam, meaning to "sum it up" or "bring it together" and adhi, which is to adhere or to "stick to it." In this state, one would be immersed and bonded in a state of Oneness, no longer perceiving separative consciousness of body or mind. In this state, it feels as though there is a fusion of consciousness that transcends this world beyond the doing into a state of pure blissful being.

Samadhi, which some equate with enlightenment, seems far beyond one's reach. Over the years, however, I've found the first stage of Samadhi is not beyond reach. This stage is accessible when following the prescribed practices of yoga. We have only to create a space for the mind—through refining the breath and aligning to the earth and heavens—and we will create space for grace to enter in. In asana, we create the space where meditation can occur. We cannot make meditation or Samadhi happen through personal will. When the time is right and when we sit erect with an attitude of self-offering, we can find that still seed point or bindu within the asana, and it is surprising what may arise out of the unseen depths of mind.

One of my teachers, Dr. Haridas Chaudhuri, founder of the California Institute for Integral Studies, was a close disciple of Sri Aurobindo Gosh. Dr. Chaudhuri would ask students to sit and open the heart and crown of the head like a chalice to invite direct revelation of the Divine into one's being. He called meditation an act of self-offering, referring to Sri Aurobindo, who said the ascent (of consciousness) is followed by the descent (of Divine consciousness). Instead of creating personal effort or trying to awaken kundalini, he suggested that inviting grace would in turn gently awaken that bio- or psycho-nuclear force to reunite with the Creator.

This first stage is known as Savikalpa Samadhi or sabija. Sa means "with," kalpa means "time," and bija means "seed." Thus, in this beginning stage, Samadhi still has a seed in this dimension of time. In this stage of Samadhi, the seeds of the kleshas are not fully scorched. In Savikalpa Samadhi there is form, meaning that we can still be reborn upon the earth plane when our celestial merits run out. But if this stage of Samadhi is held for twelve seconds, and the breath is in Kevala Kumbhaka (not held through force or will), then we may merge into the higher stages of Samadhi, known as Nirbija (without seed) and Nirvikalpa (beyond time), beyond the prakriti or nature of this world or the celestial temptations of the next. These stages of Samadhi are considered more desirable because when the yogi transcends time, space, and causation, he or she is not be subject to rebirth, and consciousness is once more absorbed into the Source of all creation.

If Savikalpa Samadhi is held for twelve seconds, the fusion of the mind would organically flow into the higher or more expanded states of Samadhi. We cannot say "if it is held for twelve breaths" because in the first stages of Samadhi, the prana of the in-breath and the prana of the out-breath merge into one. When this happens, it feels as if the breath has stopped; we are not breathing, but breath is. This state is what all asanas and pranayamas are meant to bring us to, kaivalya kumbhaka, "the retention of that which is isolated and absolutely pure." This retention of the breath brings about a retention in the waves of the mind or, as Patanjali says in Sutra 1.2, Yogas Citta Vritti Nirodhah.

Meditation in Asana

Over the years, I've known several teachers who felt that the practice of asana and pranayama was not an end in itself, but was only a means to curb the restlessness of the body and help quiet the mind so one could sit for meditation. However, as I deepened my practice, I discovered that dhyana or meditation is not just a sitting pose but can be found in the center of all yoga asanas.

In asana, it is possible to shift from concentration (dharana), where subject and object are still separate, into meditation (dhyana), where the two become one. To practice concentration within a pose, one part of the body becomes the subject and the other the object. If we keep the mind focused on the breath and continue the self-offering of one part to the other while in the pose, the energy of these two parts can actually feel fused into One.

When Mr. Iyengar was staying in my home in California, he would stand on his head for one hour every morning before other practices. Once, I naively asked if he meditated. My question must have sounded impertinent, for he replied brusquely, "My dear lady, I have been standing on my head for an hour. What do you think I was doing?"

A year later, I traveled with Mr. Iyengar from Pune to Bombay, where he was teaching a weekly public class for his Indian students. There was a young boy in the class who attended with his family. Mr. Iyengar directed us into Kurmasana, Tortoise Pose. As we completed this and went onto other yoga postures, I noticed that the boy, who was next to me, did not move. He was still in Tortoise Pose. Seeing my puzzled look, Mr. Iyengar rushed over and slid the boy's small body under a table, whispering, "Don't disturb him. He's in Samadhi." It was in that moment I realized that meditation is not just found in a cross-legged sitting pose, but lies within the center of every asana … if we allow the consciousness to go deep enough.

There are eighty-four basic asanas with infinite variations on each. According to classical yoga traditions, however, they are all meant to bring us to one pose—Dhyanasana, the pose of meditation. In the Yoga Sutras, Patanjali offers only three sutras on asana. The first is Sutra 2.46 Sthira sukham asanam, which many commentators have translated as "Take any comfortable pose" or "motionless and agreeable form." Some commentators go on to describe cross-legged positions for meditation, with a straight spine and the breast, neck, and head kept erect. My Sanskrit teacher, however, interpreted this sutra as "Take any pose and be comfortable." With this translation, the objective is to find the center and stillness of the seated pose in every pose.

The next sutra on asana is a very beautiful one, giving us a guide into the inner sanctum of yoga postures: "By relaxation of effort and meditation on the Infinite, asana is perfected." Fixing the mind on the infinite, or on the surrounding void, also develops perfection of asana. The practice of keeping the body always at rest and effortless not only helps us progress in asana but also helps us to find the meditative state within the pose. As one sutra commentary affirms: "My body has become like a void dissolving itself into infinite space and I am the wide expanse of the sky."

When the crown of the head is aligned with the base of the spine, the polarities of the body align with the polarities of the earth, and whatever is to be will reveal itself.

Mudras

It should be mentioned in sitting poses that there is a thin line between sleep and Samadhi (the superconscious state of mind). Perhaps this is why ancients referred to the poses as mudras. The verb mu means "form," and dra is from drav, meaning "to flow." In mudra, one flows with form. Asanas are mudras where the mind expresses itself through the body. Whether via a hand position or yoga pose, emotional and mental states reveal themselves through the body.

If we take a sitting position with the promise of meditation but consciousness drifts away from the awareness of the moment, the citta or "mind stuff" withdraws itself from the central nervous system. The heart drops, the head droops forward, and the spine no longer holds itself erect—this would be considered a state of sleep. Even the chosen mudra of the hand may lose its alertness, revealing that the mind is drifting into sleep rather than experiencing the heightened and expanded states of awareness of dhyana or Samadhi.

Hand Mudras

In the meditative seated postures, the palms of the hands are usually turned upward in order to open the heart center as well as to receive prana from the pathways of the heavens into the heart. The cin mudra or blessing mudra is practiced with the back of the hand resting on the knee, palms turned upward. The three fingers are extended toward the earth as the thumb and index finger touch, closing the circuit of prana that would otherwise escape from the body through the fingertips. Prana is recycled back into the systems of the body when the thumb, symbolic of the universal or Brahman, and the index finger, representing the Atman, the individual soul, are joined together.

Some practitioners recommend bringing the index finger downward toward the first knuckle of the thumb as a gesture of humility, showing that the individual is not equal to the universal. Other teachers stress joining the tips of the thumb and forefinger, representing the equal joining of the Atman and Brahman, the essence of Classical Yoga.

A very simple hand position for centering is to rest the left hand on top of the right, resting them both in the center of the lap. The left hand represents the left side of the body and the parasympathetic nervous system, which correlates to ida nadi on the subtle level. The left side of the body is associated with the right brain hemisphere, which receives knowledge holographically; this is desirable in the meditation seat. Bilateral integration is important in all yoga practices. When we are engaged in linear left brain activity throughout the day, it is helpful during sitting for meditation that we engage the right brain to create more balance in practice as well as in life.

Assisting Seated Poses

In aligning any sitting pose, the most important thing to remember is that the knees should always be a little lower than the pelvic rim. To achieve this, many of us will need to elevate the buttocks by sitting on the edge of a folded blanket or firm cushion. The height needed will vary according to an individual's hip flexibility. Sitting on a blanket or cushion this way relaxes and elevates the spine, keeping it erect and preventing compression within the areas of the pelvic and abdominal organs. This also prevents anterior compression of the lumbar spine and helps to bring the head, neck, breast, and hips into a perpendicular alignment to the earth. Aligning the head over the base of the spine helps the mind to center itself between past and future, bringing it into the present moment, experiencing the "power of now." The essence of any sitting pose is to keep the spine as erect in its natural alignment as possible.

Once the pose is established, a partner or teacher can gently press down on the upper thighs to help lengthen the torso. Standing behind the student, the partner can move the side of his or her knee into the student's spine while holding the shoulders down. Then the partner can cup her fingers under base of the student's skull and draw the head upward, lengthening the neck as the shoulders are encouraged to relax downward. This aligns the head, neck, breast, and base of the spine, helping to create a thoughtless state of awareness.

Sukhāsana

Easy Pose

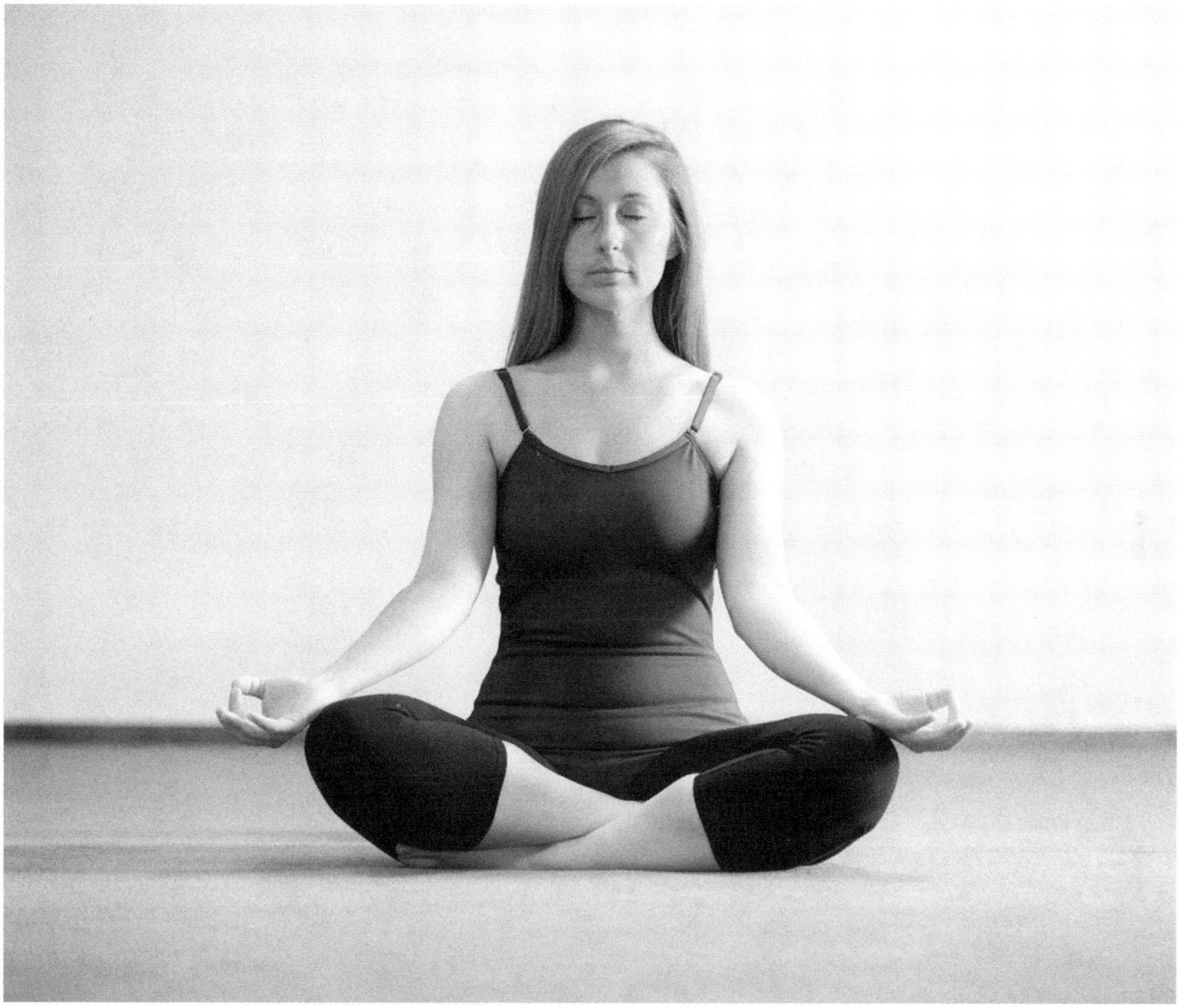

Many students use a blanket or a mudrā in Sukhāsana.

Sukha is like sugar. It means "sweet," "pleasant," or "comfortable." It also means going along with that which is pleasant or easy. In this case, it is a natural cross-legged position with the feet relaxed and resting under the backs of the thighs. People with stiff hips can practice Sukhāsana. This is not a traditional yoga pose because people who didn't have furniture many thousands of years ago had flexible hips.

Less flexible students can use a chair or, if using the floor, can raise the pelvis by sitting on a folded blanket. Adjust the blanket to the height where the knees are slightly lower than the pelvic rim. This elevates the spine and allows pelvic rotation, which relaxes the inner organs and preserves the natural curvature of the lumbar spine. When the spine curves naturally, the head is aligned over the base of the spine.

If there is pain on the inner knee(s), you can place additional blankets or pillows underneath the knees and thighs for support until the adductor muscles of the inner thighs can relax and release. There are a great many "trust issues" within these areas. Keep relaxing from the sides of the pubic bone to the inner knees, opening as if to the universal light above, below, and within your Being.

Samāsana

Balanced Pose

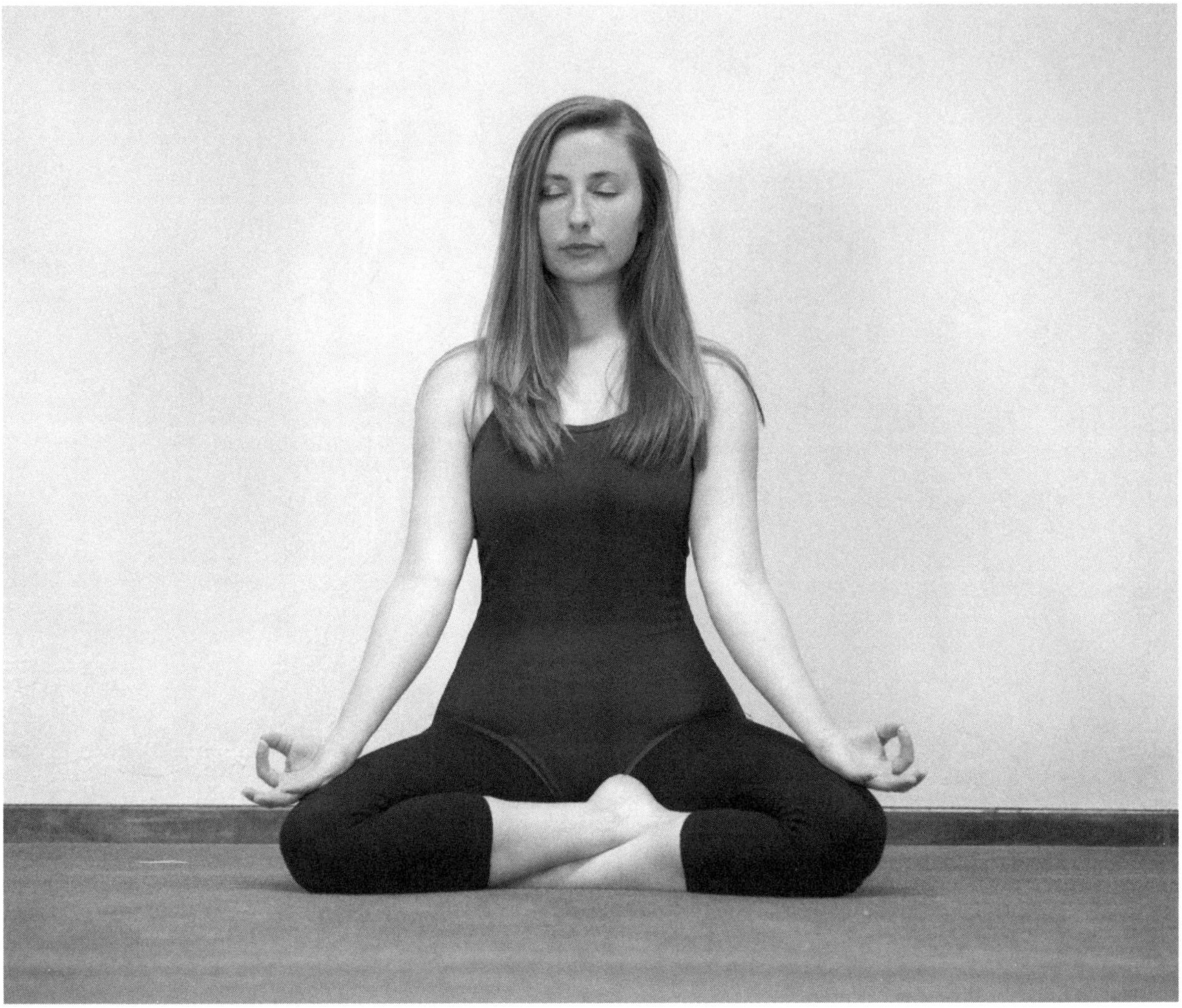

In Samasana, the student balances equally on the right and left buttocks, symbolizing the union of the poles of opposites.

The word *sama* means "the same" or "equal." In this pose, *sama* refers to both sides being the same or equal to one another. It is the pose of "sameness." In this sitting pose one heel is aligned in front of the other and both heels are in alignment with the pubic bone. The feet, of course, are relaxed. The heel of one foot presses into the pubic bone, and the other heel is directly in front of it.

Samāsana creates a feeling of openness and helps to lengthen the adductor muscles. It is a posture of equanimity and equality. In Samāsana, because we're balanced equally on the right and left buttocks, we can balance the left and right brain, and the *eros* and *logos* respectively. On a spiritual level, this pose symbolizes the unification of the poles of opposites.

In Samāsana we create equanimity between the polarities by balancing the right and left sides of the spine. This equalizes the autonomic nerves that run on the outside of the spine; the sympathetic on the right and the parasympathetic on the left. As one (the sympathetic division) constricts and heats and the other (the parasympathetic division) dilates and cools, the autonomic nervous system has been equated with Ha (the Sun or masculine) and Tha (the moon or feminine). Hatha Yoga is a way of balancing these two opposites within our own being.

Samāsana creates more balance than other sitting poses. If the weight is just in front of the buttock bones with equal pressure on right and left thighs, the brain hemispheres as well as the autonomic nervous system can come into alignment. This balance can even be felt in the way the breath equally flows through right and left nostrils. When this equality happens, we may feel a vibrational awakening of the bio- or psycho-nuclear energy that expands consciousness into the remembrance of our own Divinity.

When we sit in Samāsana, we create a triangle of energy. The head is at the apex and the triangle moves out to the knees. It is possible to feel the energy that goes from the lines of the knees to the hemispheres of the brain. It is as if we are seated in the triangular center of a yantra with unwavering equilibrium; we are connected to the base, as well to the dynamic upward movement that is lifting consciousness toward the Universal.

In contrast to Lotus Pose (Padmāsana), Samāsana requires more vigilance to keep the spine erect. If the weight of the hips is balanced just in front of the buttock bones and the lumbar spine is lengthened, the heart lifts. It is this lift that brings the head back into a meditative alignment where thoughts cannot take form. As Mr. Iyengar said, "When the heart becomes the extrovert, the brain and mind becomes the introvert.

Āsana II sequence

Siṃhāsana

Lion Pose

Siṃha is a lion, and this āsana can be associated with Narasiṁha, the lion man who was Viṣṇu's fourth incarnation. Viṣṇu took the form of Narasiṁha to subdue a demon that threatened to destroy the Universe. This half-human and half-animal form is symbolic of our own evolutionary rise above the primordial instincts that bind our consciousness to third-dimensional limitations.

Philosophical Introduction

Today, we call the lion the King of the Jungle. In Hindu mythology, the lion was a majestic vehicle for the great goddess Durgā, who was born from the gifts of the Lords of the Universe. The gods were not strong enough to slay a powerful demon, so they combined their gifts of power and light to create a magnificent, radiant, and invincible goddess. Durgā was created for the intended purpose of going into battle to slay the unvanquished demon. (All the battles in Hindu mythology are fought to subdue the demoniac urge of ego, which sees only separation and not unification.)

The lion depicts Durgā's power, grace, and courage. Durgā, like the lion, was invincible. Some stories say that Durgā was so powerful that she did not need to enter into battle with the universal demon, who was symbolic of the collective ego of human kind. Instead, she sent forth a ferocious smaller form of herself from her third eye. Durgā supplied the energy and "held the space" (as we would say today) while Kālī destroyed and vanquished the foe.

Kālī's form is enough to frighten anyone, even a demon. Her unbound hair and wild eyes symbolize that she has no boundaries or restraints. Her eyes turn up into her head, and her tongue is thrust fully out of her mouth, which is red from the blood of her enemies. She drinks their blood and wears their skulls like a garland around her neck. In yoga, the head represents the ego. When an aspect of the ego arises, Kālī cuts off its head and takes it upon herself so that its remnants do not fall and reseed to one day rise again. She is the all-compassionate mother because she lifts the burden of suffering by taking the pain onto herself. All of humankind is considered to be her child.

What does this have to do with Siṃhāsana? Kālī's mudra, tongue extended with eyes wildly rolling up into the head, is the position we take in Lion Pose. This pose was assumed by warriors in various cultures as a scare tactic to frighten and in turn weaken the enemy.

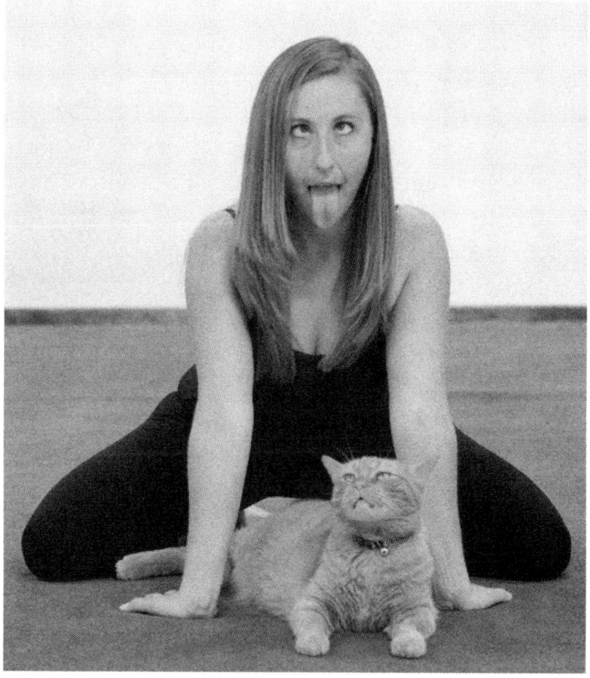

Simhasana, Lion's Pose, with inspiration from Lionheart the Temple Cat.

New Zealand's Maori warriors would thrust out their tongue, roll their eyes into their head, and even beat their chests when approaching the enemy in battle. Ferocious-looking Fu Dogs were placed at the gate of a Chinese temple or home to frighten away all evil spirits. Beloved Gaṇeśa, with his elephant head and boy's body, is also placed at the entrance of the home so that contractive forces cannot enter into the home. In subtle anatomy, Gaṇeśa guards the root cakra so that as aspirants embark upon a spiritual path, they will not be beset by their own primordial egoic natures, which hinder the unfoldment of expanded consciousness.

In Siṃhāsana, we see Kālī as a warrior who does not cower away from a battle and at the same time does not create it. When she sees injustice, she wants immediate retribution. She steps into a situation and takes on the suffering, pain, and grief of another because she can't bear to see others suffer. The Kālī nature passionately takes on a cause or another person's challenges as if it were her own. This very quality may exist in a family member, a friend, or within ourselves. Kālī is like mother lioness that will do anything to protect her offspring.

On the other hand, if we consider Siṃhāsana in the context of Durgā as the third-eye source for Kālī, we might recognize the Durgā energy as the "space holder." Durgā does not rush in to resolve a conflict but holds the bigger picture. She does not try to "fix it" as Kālī would do. Instead, Durgā might hold all parties in compassion and understanding so they may find their own answers. Durgā embodies the quiet compassion that the Dali Lama described as an equation: Love + Detachment = Compassion. Durgā is said to represent the ultimate in compassion because there are times we cannot prevent our children (all of humankind) from falling and hurting themselves. Instead of rushing in to help, like Kālī, Durgā holds them in her heart and consciousness, serving as the onlooker who sends a mantle of protection and love as her children learn life's lessons for themselves.

As Durgā, we might feel the suffering of another, but not take it on. Far from being indifferent, if we emulate this aspect of Durgā, we would feel the suffering of all humanity from a universal as well as individual perspective. Durgā gives the space for others to learn what they must and holds the space and love for all parties so they may draw upon their own inner resources to create a living and dynamic transformation.

Guidance

1. Begin by kneeling with the knees hip distance apart. Turn the toes under so the weight of the buttock rests on the heels and creates pressure across the balls of the feet (which in reflexology correspond to the chest, heart and lungs). Turning the palms down, place the heels of the palms on the upper knees. Stretch from the roots of the fingers to the tips, expanding the webs between the fingers, creating as much space as possible.
2. Inhaling, breathe across the back.
3. Exhaling, elongate the spine and bring it into the front of the body, lifting the chest.
4. Inhale into the back.
5. Exhaling, stick out the tongue as though you are trying to touch the chin with its tip. The tongue relates to the five lower cakras, from the tip (which relates to the root cakra) to the root (which relates to the throat cakra). This muscular extension helps to quiet the acidity of the mind that precedes the buildup of a cold or influenza.
6. Inhale across the back.
7. Exhaling, roll the eyes upward, directing your at the front crown of the head. With the tongue thrust out, begin to roar like a lion. Allow the sound to emanate on each exhalation.
8. On the inhalations, do nothing; there is no sound.
9. On the exhalations, produce the roaring sound, expressing the power of the lion.
10. When ready, slowly relax the tongue, eyes, hands, and feet.
11. Stretch the legs out and lie down, resting in Śavāsana and allowing the body to receive the benefit of the pose. This pose is far more intense and has more lasting effects than we may realize. It is a good pose to do once a day or once every other day, especially during cold or flu season.

Assist: If it is difficult to sit on your haunches like the lion, place a folded blanket between the buttocks and heels to help alleviate pressure on the knees and feet. If it is too painful to turn the toes under, simply sit in Vīrāsana or even on a chair. Although it is more effective to practice Siṃhāsana with the feet and toes engaged, the pose can be practiced in any comfortable sitting position.

Psychophysiological Benefits

Siṃhāsana opens the gates of the lymphatic system, stimulating drainage of the tonsils, which act to contain and protect the spinal cord from any infections. The Lion Pose also activates the adrenal glands, which dry out the mucus membranes, bringing the system into balance. This effect is especially helpful for those with what ayurveda considers a kapha imbalance. When the eyes roll upward, this stimulates the thalamus, hypothalamus, and pituitary glands, which in turn balance the entire endocrine system. The hyperextension of the tongue can eliminate toxins in the tonsils and stimulate the thyroid gland at the base of the throat, which speeds up metabolism, acting with the adrenals to dry excessive mucus production throughout the body.

Practicing Lion Pose clears the head when one feels foggy or confused. The movements of Siṃhāsana, especially of the tongue and eyes, have the effect of clearing breathing passages and airways. Sinus conditions may be alleviated, as practicing Siṃhāsana is beneficial to the passages of the ears and the frontal and maxillary sinuses.

In esoteric anatomy, the fingers and toes relate to the five prāṇas and corresponding five lower cakras. In reflexology, the fingers and toes relate to the sensory organs of ears, eyes, nose, and throat. In Chinese medicine, the meridians from the big toe to the little toe relate to the liver, stomach, gallbladder, and kidneys. The extreme extension of Siṃhāsana creates pressure upon the reflexes and accupoints, helping to relieve congestion by stimulating the pelvic plexus and the intestinal track. Stimulating these digestive organs help us to release any excessive undigested matter, including sensory overload. Siṃhāsana also opens and stimulates key lymphatic points to keep the lymph fluids moving, which also help us process all that we are taking in physically, mentally, and emotionally. It is also said to release negativity.

Siṃhāsana invokes the presence of its rider, the aspect of Divine Śakti known as Durgā. She is the protector in the face of negative and contractive forces. Where Durgā is present, it is said, negativity dare not go. We no longer have to fight the battles in life, because we become unattached to a result and feel compassion for every living being. With the rider of the lion, we can become inwardly victorious, even in times that may look like defeat. Siṃhāsana clears the channels of confusion and forgetfulness so that the Divine light can stream forth.

Eka Pāda Adho Mukha Śvānāsana

One-Legged Downward-Facing Dog Pose

Eka means "one." *Pāda* is "piece," "part," or "chapter." Pāda also refers to a leg, limb, or foot. *Adho* is "downward." *Mukha* means "face," and *śvāna* is "dog." The Sanskrit meaning tells us what we are supposed to do in the pose.

Philosophical Introduction

One of the greatest revelations is that love is the greatest power in the Universe. So much about love can be learned from dogs, who exhibit unconditional love to those who care for them. We can't call ourselves their masters or even their owners, for they are our teachers. Dogs teach through their presence and the love that they give freely and unconditionally.

The English word for canine is God spelled backward. In our country and other cultures of the world, there is a growing trend to treat pets as members of the family, and even at times like gods. How can we not? They give us love when we may feel unloved. They are there for us when we feel alone. They want to lick away the tears of sorrow and share in the tears of joy. They stay present at the deathbed of a loved one, and they act as silent confessors, listening to our rambling prayers without judgment and with the shining eyes of love. We are blessed that they cross life's path for the time they are meant to be with us.

My little "grand-dog" Obsidian will sweep into Adho Mukha Śvānāsana whenever someone says "Downward-Facing Dog." His back makes a beautiful crescent moon as his tail reaches for the stars. His heart center opens wide, for he doesn't seem to harbor any restrictions, resistance, or hardened corners of unresolved emotions in its chambers. He doesn't compress his neck by trying to bring his head up but humbles his head toward the earth, sometimes even touching his crown to the ground as if in prostration or prayer.

What is it that dogs can teach us about this variation on Downward-Facing Dog Pose? When it's time for Obsidian's walks, he struts along the red dirt paths around Sedona and anoints bushes and rocks when lifting his back leg. As his leg lifts, I've noticed that he does not keep the hips even but lifts one hip higher than the other, which allows for opening and stretching the belly of this upper side. His body weight tilts to the other side until he's finished and then the leg returns to earth.

In the basic Downward-Facing Dog position, we offer our tailbone to the heavens and the crown of the head to the earth. The base of the pole of the spine, which lies in darkness when we are upright, has a chance to lift to the light and receive the emanations of heaven through the base cakra. The movement of the spine allows for a non-muscular lift in the pelvic and solar plexus areas, creating a natural, organic, and effortless mūla bandha and uḍḍiyāna bandha. The navel is passive and elongated, allowing the prāṇa to flow freely to the heart center. We see this openness of heart not only in the way the dog moves its body when stretching, but also in its unconditionally loving nature.

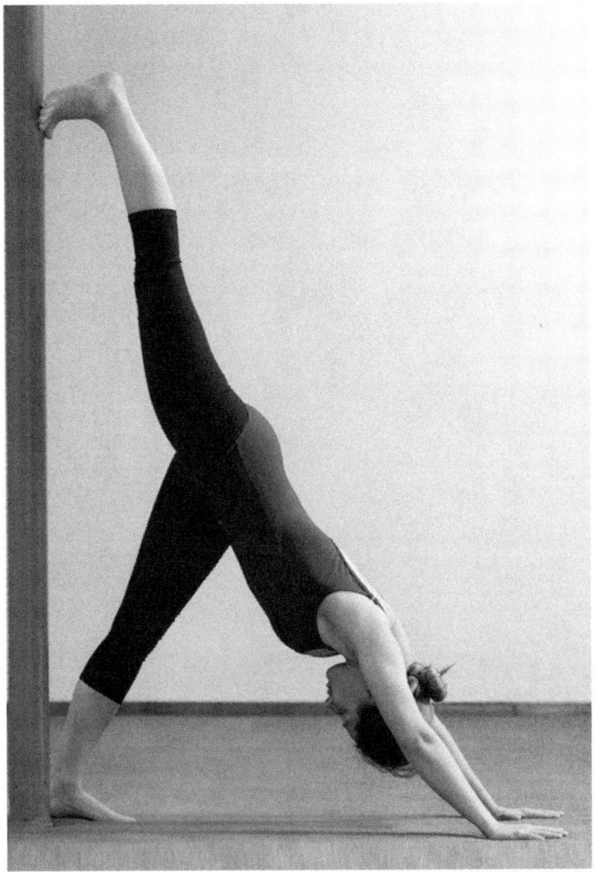

In Eka Pāda Adho Mukha Śvānāsana, we honor the polarities of earth and heaven.

I think there are times when it is not enough to lift the tailbone to the heavens and humble the head, the symbol of ego, to the earth in Adho Mukha Śvānāsana. At these times, my heart fills with so much love and gratitude for all aspects of creation that I want to offer more of myself to the light of the Divine. The way to express this is to expand the prayerful nature of the basic pose by lifting one leg and stretching into the sky as far as consciousness can go, coming into Eka Pāda Adho Mukha Śvānāsana. In this one-legged variation of Downward-Facing Dog, we again honor the polarities of earth and heaven through the physical and energetic body. The yantra of this variation adds a diagonal line to the triangular base of the torso and the bottom leg. This creates even more dynamism for invoking the Universal Śakti or energy into our Being. At times, it is possible to feel the sub-cakra of the upper foot come alive, as if thanking you for fulfilling the longing for light.

There is so much to learn from the dog, not just in "doing" this pose but as way of *being* in life. Can we give as freely as we are given to? Can we listen as deeply as we are listened to? Can we be compassionate when another is suffering and dry their tears with our own? Dogs teach us to keep our hearts open in the remembrance that love is the greatest power in the Universe.

Guidance

1. Begin in Mārjāryāsana (the cat pose). Inhale, bringing the breath into the back, rounding as much possible.
2. Exhale and bring the spine in like a backbend, straightening the knees and lifting the tailbone.
3. Inhale into the back from the shoulders to the hips, rounding with the breath.
4. Exhale as the spine comes in like a backbend. Raise the heel bone and come as high to the ball of the foot as possible. The heel is the extension of the tailbone.
5. Inhale, bringing the breath into the back while keeping the heel bone up to tilt the pelvic rim forward.
6. Exhale and, without dropping the tailbone, allow the heel of the standing foot to come toward (not to) the floor.
7. Inhale and allow the breath to round the back, still preserving the lift of the tailbone.

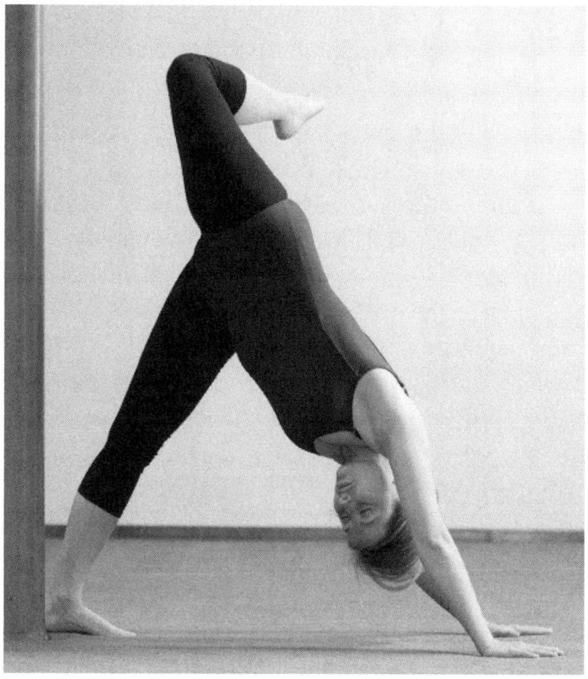

To prepare for the full pose, open the hips by bending the knee while keeping the naval passive.

8. Exhale and bend the knee of the upraised leg, opening that side of the pelvis and torso, keeping the navel passive. Equalize the weight between the right and left hands.
9. Inhaling, round the back with the breath.
10. Exhale and straighten the knee of the upper leg. Offer the sole of the foot to the heaven while maintaining the elongation of the upper side of the torso.
11. Inhale and pause. Relax as much as possible as you take the breath into the back.
12. Exhale; see if you can create a little more space within the pelvic organs and the digestive organs by elongating the back leg.
13. Inhale into the back body from shoulders to hips.
14. Exhaling, rotate the upper thigh internally and lift up out of the bottom hip, keeping the lift of the tailbone. Equalize the weight and pressure of both hands and arms. Biceps and triceps are activated equally to stabilize the weight upon the bones of the arms.
15. Inhaling, bring the breath into the back.
16. Exhale and offer the foot to the heavens as the crown of the head bows to the earth.
17. When you are ready to come out of the pose, bend the upper knee on an exhalation, keeping the internal space of the upper side of the torso as you lower the leg back to the floor.

18. You can rest and breathe in Child's Pose before taking Eka Pāda Adho Mukha Śvānāsana to the opposite side.

Note: In Eka Pāda Adho Mukha Śvānāsana, it is important to take time to open the upper side of the torso while the knee is bent. If you keep the knee bent (as a dog does), you have a wonderful opportunity to create space within the pelvic and digestive organs and open the heart center so the love that has always been there can shine forth. To create this space, we breathe while moving into the pose, while staying in the pose, and when coming out of the pose. When the torso opens, see if the upper leg can straighten without closing the space. Keep the navel passive and on an exhalation lift up out of the bottom hip as the upper thigh rotates internally. This brings the hips level to one another. However, it is important not to try to bring the hips level if the space that was created begins to close.

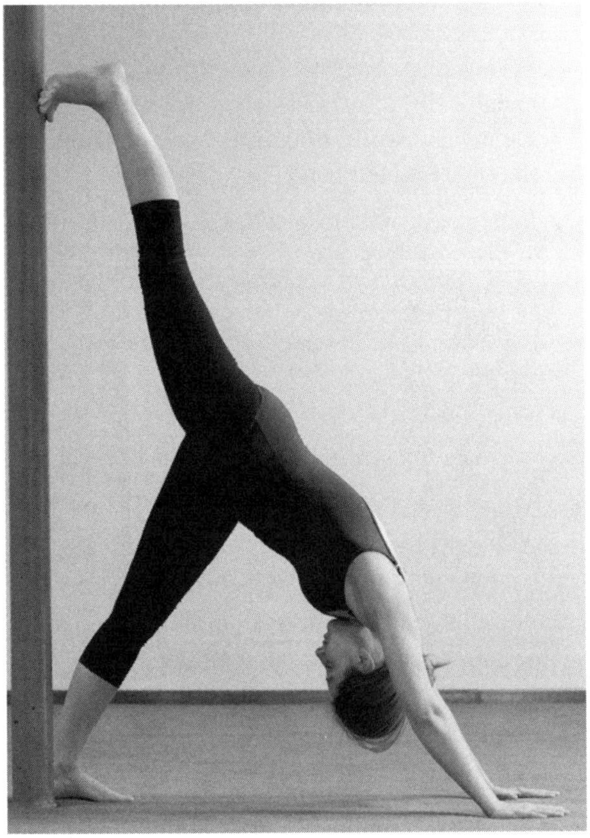

Working with a partner or using the support of a wall helps preserve the opening as you level the hips.

Assist: A partner or teacher can stand facing the student's back, holding the tops of the shoulders and lifting them, which takes pressure off the arms and helps the weight of the body to move backward toward the heels rather than forward onto the fingertips. Once you have established the opening of the side of the torso of the upper leg, your partner can step behind you so that you can place your upraised leg onto his or her shoulders. At the same time, he or she can lift the lower hip to give evenness and stability to the pelvis.

Psychophysiological Benefits

Since bones grow along the line of stress, in this pose we increase the bone density of the arms and legs. The natural lift of the mūla bandha and uḍḍiyāna bandha (see page 255) tones the inner core muscles of the torso. This not only aids in digestion by massaging the small and large intestines but also helps prevent pelvic prolapse. For women in particular, Eka Pāda Adho Mukha Śvānāsana is an excellent āsana for preventing prolapse of the reproductive organs.

The inversion frees neck tension that restricts the circulatory currents and the flow of the cerebral spinal fluid. The sacrum acts as a pump for the cerebral spinal fluid to rise against the gravitational pull. Bringing the leg up activates this flow and, if the neck is relaxed and not constricted, energy can reach the brain more easily. The increased energy from the inversion is excellent for preserving the nerve impulses that flow between the spinal cord and brain.

With the hands spread wide and the middle finger facing straight ahead, stretching the thumbs toward one another (as if spanning an octave on the piano) will aid carpel tunnel syndrome. This is excellent for the wrists, alleviating the repetitive strain injury so common from using computer keyboards.

Psychologically, Eka Pāda Adho Mukha Śvānāsana gives us greater trust in our own strength and balance. It humbles the snares of ego that can cause future pain. When we offer the leg to the heavens, extending and giving from that small area of our heel and foot, it is a reminder that there is a power greater than one's self.

If you have dogs at home, it's fun to practice this pose with them. Their perfection in this āsana may cause you to feel inadequate, but their presence helps you bask in the love of a heart that is open and unconditionally giving.

Sālamba Śīrṣāsana

Supported Headstand

Śirṣ means head. *Ṣa* is "with," and *lamba* means "support." This is the headstand with the support of the triangular base of the arms.

Philosophical Introduction

When my youngest child was born, her nine-year-old sister stood at her side and whispered into her tiny ear, "Tell me what it's like. It's been so long that I have forgotten."

Since then, whenever practicing this pose, I think of the infant whose pulse can be seen beneath the frontal fontanelle, the "soft spot" covered by membrane until the skull bones join at about two or more years of age. This is the area of the skull that we focus on when we practice the headstand. I have always wondered if the closing and hardening of the skull bones relates to the ego becoming more aware of itself.

One of the many reasons we practice Śīrṣāsana is to humble the ego, transforming it from its individuated nature into a unified field of consciousness. Perhaps this pose gives us an opening to return to that egoless infant state that is beyond the separative consciousness, bringing back the remembrance of that which the true Self has never forgotten ... that it is already one with the universal source.

In yoga, the ego is said to be the part of the human mind that fosters separation. It is the part of consciousness that seems to have a need to defend, compete, and project criticisms onto others. It is the part that creates borders and boundaries that separate nations, states, and people. The head symbolizes the ego. Wherever our head goes is where we think "we" are going. In inverted āsanas, when one humbles the ego to the altar of the earth and raises the feet, the symbol of humility, as an offering to the heavens, this new spatial orientation may at first confuse the ego.

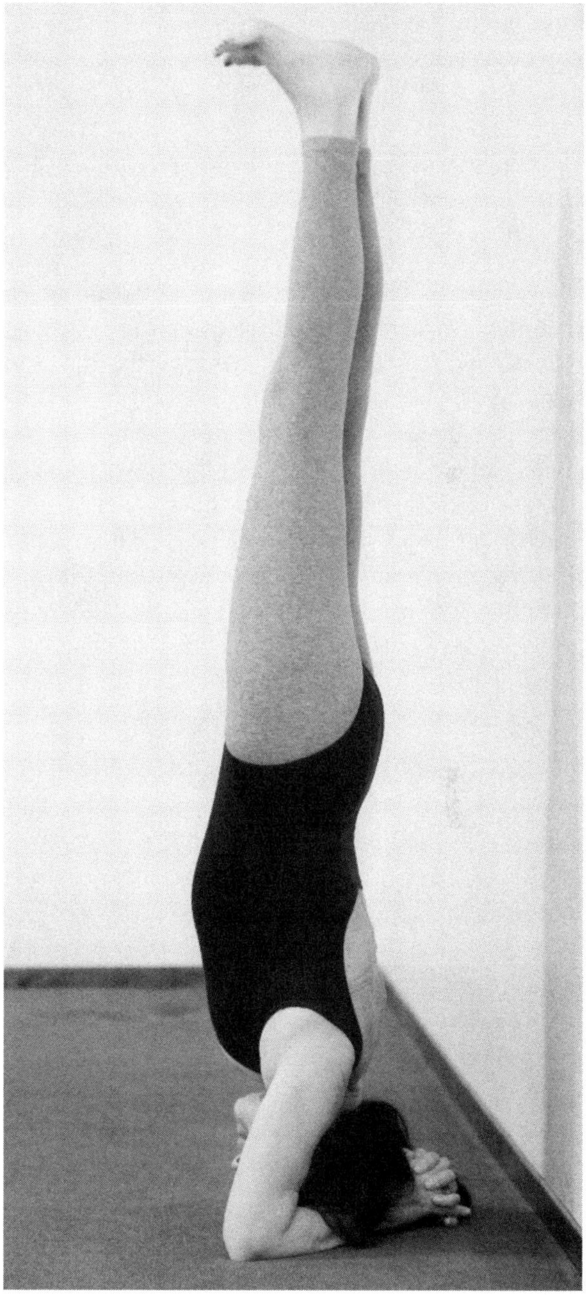

On an energetic level, the headstand opens the crown cakra.

On an energetic level, the headstand (often called the King of Āsana) opens the crown cakra or *Sahasrāra,* the thousand-petalled lotus. The crown of the head is considered to be the gateway of Brahmā, the creator, and when the crown cakra opens, it unfolds like lotus petals, revealing a unified field of consciousness. As the prāṇa rises from the sacral and coccygeal plexuses through the pathways of the cakras, the lotus within the head, whose petals were dropping downwards, are given new life and bloom upwards. Like the earthly lotus that unfolds with the light of the rising sun, the petals of the *Sahasrāra* unfold with the dawning of the Divine inner light. In this state there is no separation, only the remembrance of our Oneness with the Divine source of all creation.

The center of the crown of the head is said to be *śivaloka,* the mystical dwelling place of the Divine Union between Śiva and Śakti, which is the Supreme Yoga. Śiva and Śakti unite when Kuṇḍalinī awakens from her serpentine sleep and rises up the energetic channel of the spine. Kuṇḍalinī is the bio- or psycho-nuclear energy that dwells in the sacrum (which looks like the downward facing head of a serpent). By inverting the prāṇas and creating a pole shift of the spinal subtle nerve currents, the headstand helps awaken this dormant energy, which turns upward and flows up the spine, bringing clarity and light to the highest centers within the brain and in turn, the mind.

A more esoteric element of the headstand is that it stimulates the solar entrance of the crown cakra, known as the body's sun or *sūrya dvara,* which means "to fill with the sun god Surya." The heart is said to be the point of contact between the soul and the body. The current that flows from the heart to the brain is known as *suṣumnā*. It cannot be found in the physical body and can only be discovered through spiritual practices such as meditation, prāṇāyāma, and āsana. In the yoga sutras (III:27), Patañjali says, "By practicing Saṁyama [concentration, meditation, and samādhi] on the sun, the point in the body known as the solar entrance, knowledge of the cosmic region is acquired."

Śīrṣāsana clears the *nāḍīs,* or subtle nerve channels, for the dawning of the effulgent light. It is said that that the body has 72,000 nāḍīs, the channels in which prāṇa flows. The nāḍīs cannot be seen by the physical eye, but they are the currents of prāṇa or energy—the Śakti that gives life. Of these, 108 are important because they radiate out from the heart center in many directions. One such ray is the suṣumnā, which rises to the brain and has the ability to open Sahasrāra (the crown cakra), the thousand-petalled lotus. This is the solar region that can reveal the secrets of the cosmos. Suṣumnā is also the name for the central canal of the spinal cord.

Śīrṣāsana not only puts pressure on the sagittal and coronal sutures of the skull to soften the fontanelle but in turn, can lift and open the heart cakra so that the rays of effulgent light reveal the solar entrance. It is believed that focusing on this effulgent light that passes between the heart and brain, the knowledge of the entire Universe is revealed.

The yantra of headstand is twofold. The body forms a straight line, perpendicular to the earth. According to the laws of physics, a straight line taken into infinity becomes a circle. The arms form a triangle, one of the strongest bases in existence. As the back of the head is placed in the apex of the triangle, the energy created unites the pairs of opposites into a unified field of consciousness. The crown of the head in the center of this triangle is like the bindu, the seed out of which all creation flows.

Guidance

1. Begin in Mārjāryāsana, facing a wall. Bend the elbows, placing the forearms on the floor and clasping the hands, joining the roots of the fingers firmly together while relaxing the tips of the fingers. Place the hands one or two inches away from the wall with the elbows shoulder width apart. Grow down through the inner elbow and the bottom wrist bone.
2. Inhale, do nothing.
3. Exhale and straighten the knees, bringing the buttocks up in a modified Adho Mukha Śvānāsana, forming a triangular apex with the tailbone.
4. Inhale and wait, observing the breath while relaxing the neck.
5. Exhaling, keep the neck relaxed as you begin to walk toward the wall.
6. Inhale into the back and pause. Do nothing as the breath comes in.
7. Exhale and bring the spine into the front body like a backbend while continuing to step toward the wall.
8. Inhale and pause. Do nothing while breathing into the back.

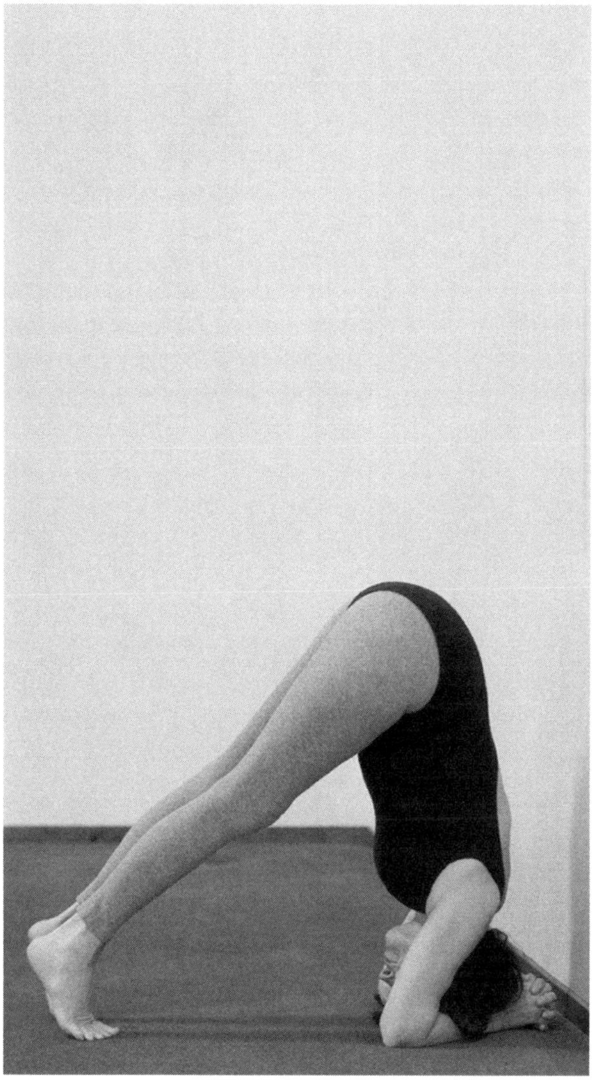

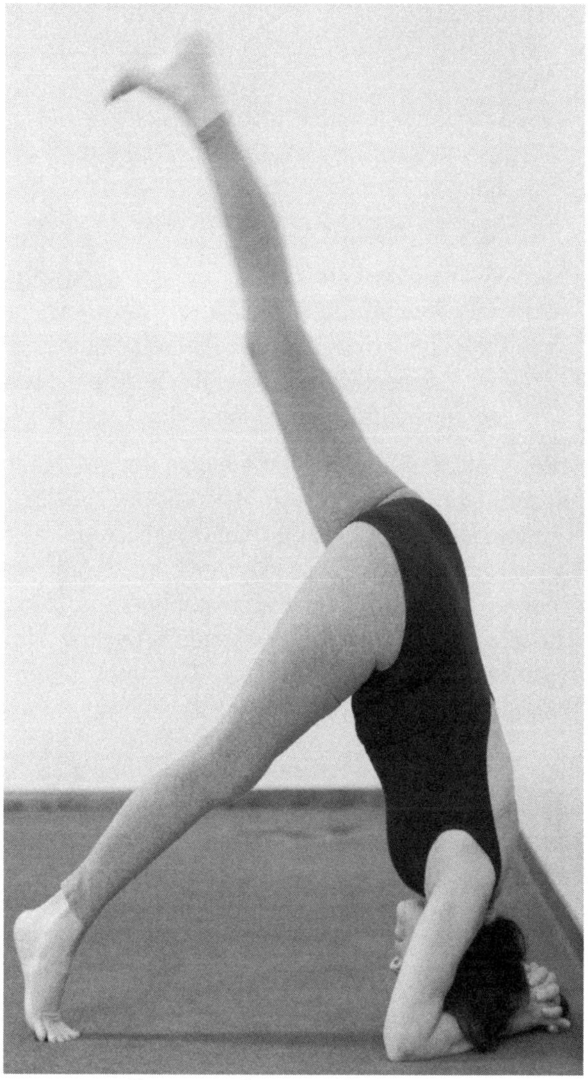

Placing the head into the apex of the triangle of the hands energetically unites the pair of opposites into a unified of consciousness.

9. Exhale and bring the spine in like a backbend, moving the armpits toward the ankles or shins as you walk a little closer to the wall.
10. Inhale and observe.
11. Exhale, lifting the shoulders and placing the top of head on the floor. (The contact point is not at the very crown, but a little closer to the forehead.)
12. Inhale and elongate the neck, creating space between the tops of the shoulders and the ears.
13. Exhale and lift the tailbone, coming onto the tops of the toes and bringing the spine in like a backbend.
14. Inhaling, feel a new spatial awareness being established.
15. Exhaling, bring one leg up to the wall and then let its extension lift the other leg.
16. Inhale and do nothing.
17. Exhale and move the thoracic spine in like a backbend, then elongate the lumbar spine by extending through the heels and the Achilles tendon. Then, without shortening the backs of the legs, offer the feet from the base of the big toes to the heavens.
18. Inhaling, maintain the elongation of the spine.
19. Exhaling, grow down through the forearms, the inner elbows, and bottom wrist bones to grow up through the spine, the legs, and the feet. Take care not to arch the lumbar spine as you continue to grow down in order to rise up through the backs of the legs. Make the backs of the knees as firm as the wall.
20. On the inhalations, do not take any adjustments but enjoy where you are.
21. On the exhalations, equalize the pressure between the forearms and head. If there is any neck compression, put more pressure on the forearms than on the head.

22. If the breath catches or becomes erratic, it is time for you to gently lower out of the pose the same way you came into it, bringing one leg down at a time. (Bringing both legs down puts more pressure on the neck and is a more advanced variation.)

23. When both feet touch the ground, gently lower into Child's Pose (Bālāsana), stretching the arms out above the head. Stretch from the kidneys or sides of the lumbar spine as the tailbone moves toward the feet. Stay in Child's Pose until the breath normalizes and becomes long and deep.

Note: Elongating the lumbar spine is important for preventing any compression in Śīrṣāsana. Take any adjustments on the exhalation. On the inhalation, stop the movements and allow the breath to renew and regenerate. If you can't keep the breath rhythmic, calm, and deep in the pose, take more time between poses to stabilize the breath once more. This in turn helps to stabilize the vṛttis or thought waves of the mind.

Assists: During the preparatory stages of Śīrṣāsana, a partner or teacher can sit on the edge of a chair facing the practitioner as he or she takes arm and hand position for Headstand. The partner supports and lifts the shoulders as the practitioner raises the hips into the variation of Downward-Facing Dog Pose sometimes referred to as Dolphin Pose. The head is not yet touching the earth as the shoulders are lifted. As the student walks in, the partner keeps lifting the shoulders and continues to do so even as the student's head comes down. The partner can use the side of his or her knees to gently press into the student's back. This is done to keep the armpits and chest from collapsing, which protects the neck.

If the student wishes to progress toward the full headstand, the partner can reach to support the student's hips as he or she lifts one leg at a time. Keep the hands on the student's hips, not on the legs. Remind the student to keep lengthening the lumbar spine, which draws the navel center toward the back to prevent any compression.

When ready, the partner continues to support the student's hips as he or she lowers the legs one at a time, coming back to Child's Pose. While the student is in Child's Pose, one or two partners can place their hands at the base of spine and the base of skull, creating space between these polarities with every exhalation.

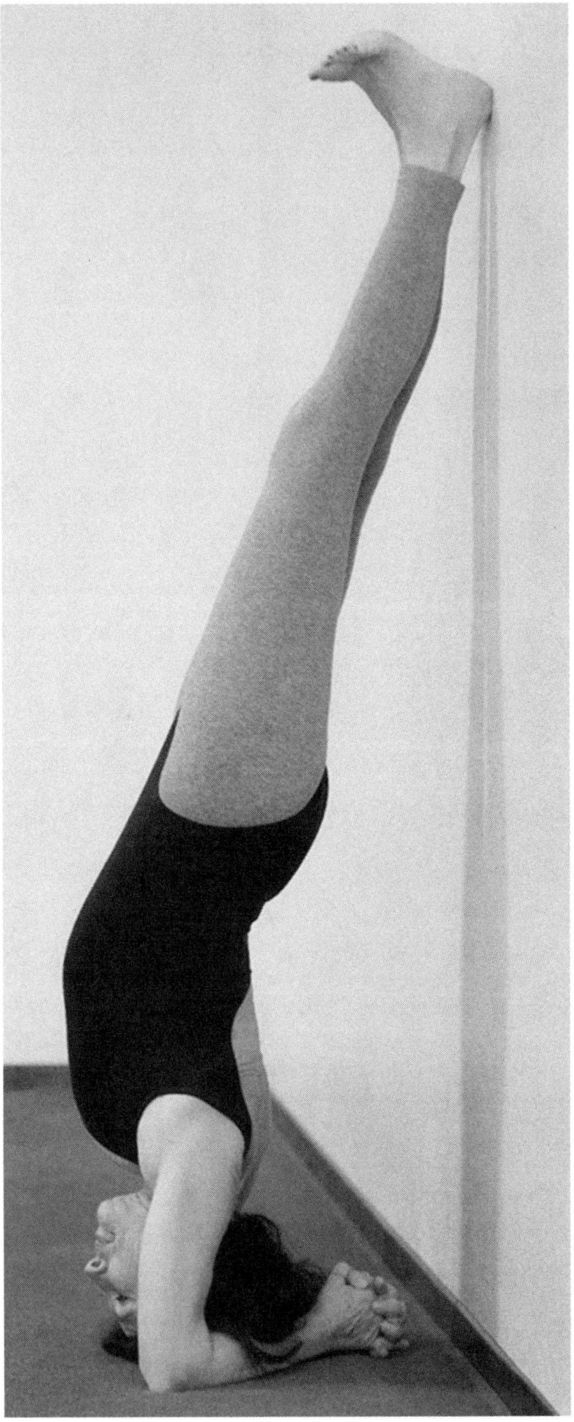

Press down through the forearms and lift up to release any compression in the neck.

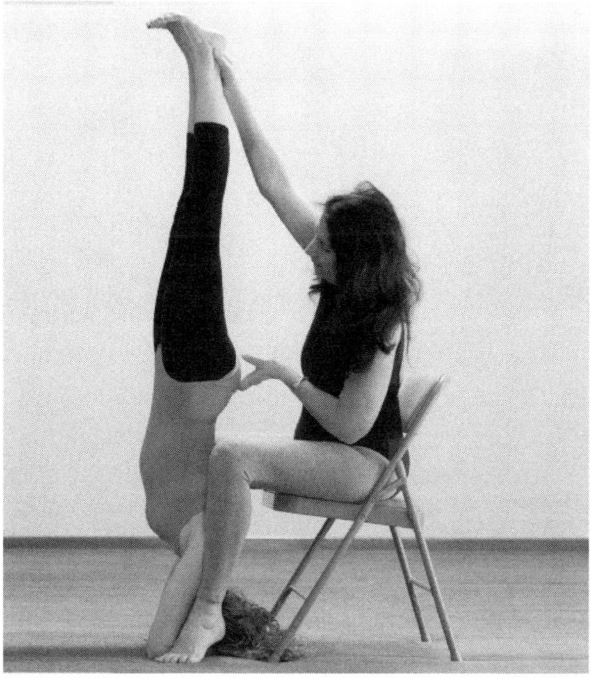

A seated partner or teacher can support the student as she progresses toward the full headstand.

Psychophysiological Benefits

The body is subjected daily to the gravitational pull. When we invert the body in Sālamba Śīrṣāsana, it is possible to prevent prolapse of the internal organs and enhance circulatory flow. If the emphasis is upon the breath and the pose is aligned appropriately, it helps alleviate and even eliminate neck tension.

The arms and hands form a powerful triangular base in this pose. When the head is placed in the center, it is like meditating under apex of a pyramid, which is said to slow the aging process, balance the metabolism, and renew, recharge, and rejuvenate one's energy and life force. The position of the arms and bottom wrist bones represent the union of right and left, or the masculine and feminine energies. This union also relates to the autonomic nervous system, with the activation of the sympathetic nervous system through the downward pressure of the right arm, and the parasympathetic nervous system through equal pressure to the left. This equalized pressure stimulates the hemispheres of the brain: the logical, sequential left brain and the intuitive, spatially aware right brain. To create balance, the head must be placed in such a way that the energy moves to the center, the corpus callosum that unites the two hemispheres. In this way, neural pathways and quick reflexes are preserved through this pose.

Śīrṣāsana affects the thalamus gland, considered by alternative health pioneers to contain a blueprint of every cell of the body. Just under the thalamus lies the hypothalamus. The hypothalamus regulates the pituitary (known as the "master endocrine gland"), affecting the entire endocrine chain, including the pituitary, pineal, thyroid, thymus, adrenal, and procreative glands.

Known as the king or father of all āsana, Śīrṣāsana has a masculine quality due to its influence upon the pituitary gland. The pituitary is close to the front of the brain, which is believed to be related to the conscious mind, the more projective or assertive part of one's self. If the head is positioned closer to the forehead in this āsana, it will have a more stimulating impact upon the pituitary, the thoracolumbar nerve roots associated with the sympathetic nervous system and, in turn, the adrenals. Practicing Śīrṣāsana with the head in this position has been known to relieve depression.

If, however, the head is placed slightly behind the point where the sutures of the skull join, it is known to stimulate the parasympathetic nervous system through the impact upon the cervical spine. This head position for Śīrṣāsana is especially recommended for those who are moving through stressful times, who have anxiety or difficulty focusing the mind, or who suffer from sleep disorders.

When we practice Sālamba Śīrṣāsana, we reverse the currents of positive and negative—the north pole of the crown of the head and the south pole of the base of the spine—to create an alternating current between the negative emanations of the earth and positive emanations from the heaven, renewing and recharging the pranic life forces in the subtle and

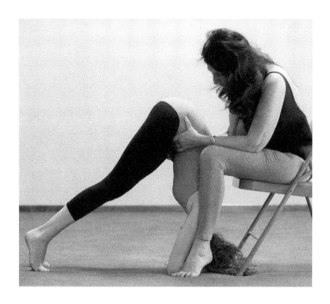

physical body. When I am practicing this āsana, it feels as though I am reaching for the center of galaxy with the feet, which are the extension of the spine. At times, I feel as if I'm holding the disk of the sun in the soles of the feet or, more accurately, the sub-cakras of the arches.

Practicing Śīrṣāsana is an excellent way to recharge brain cells and help prevent memory loss. However, the full potential of Śīrṣāsana is to help awaken or reawaken the remembrance that we are already one with the Divine source.

Śīrṣāsana represents a polar shift in body and mind, giving us a new perspective on life. It is a pose of empowerment—the experience of doing something we don't ordinarily do or thought we couldn't do. It helps us overcome the ultimate fear of the unknown. It teaches greater flexibility by helping us to adapt to a multitude of situations.

When practicing or teaching this pose, I think of the yoga sutra that alludes to āsana: s*thira sukham āsanam,* which means, "Take any pose and be comfortable" (II:46). This sutra does not say "take any comfortable pose." Taking Śīrṣāsana and even its preparatory stages, in which the feet do not leave the earth, helps us to break free from stuck patterns that no longer serve us. This āsana takes us out of old comfort zones and hardened belief systems to explore new perspectives and widen our parameters of life.

This makes Śīrṣāsana one of the more powerful poses to bring up saṁskāras, the deep psychic impressions created by previous experiences, from the latent subconscious depths of the psyche. It shakes up the sediment from the vaults of memory. "The invisible must become visible before it can be eradicated," or as we might say today, before it can be transformed.

Ardha Candrāsana

Half Moon Pose

Ardha means "half," and *candra* is the moon.

Philosophical Introduction

The story of the churning of the ocean of milk has several versions. This particular version is a prelude to the *Mahābhārata,* the great epic of India, and it highlights the importance of lunar energy and its relationship to Ardha Candrāsana:

Long ago, when the sea was milk, Nārāyaṇa (another name for Viṣṇu) said to the gods of heaven, "Churn the ocean, and she will yield *amṛta,* the nectar of immortality that is held in the cup of the moon. It will also bring forth precious gems and all manner of illusion and revelation."

So the gods placed the snowy mountain Mandāra in the middle of the milky sea. Its deep roots rested on the ocean floor; its summit rose high above the surface. The great serpent Śeṣa, whose hood is an island of jewels, stretched himself across the sea, his body wrapped endlessly round the mountain in the center. On one shore, his tail was held by the *asuras*, the dark, olden gods; on the other shore his neck was held by the *devas*, the mortal gods of heaven. They each pulled in turn, so that the mountain spun first one way then the other, while trees and stones were thrown off into the foaming sea.

First the mild moon rose from the milky sea, and then Lady Lakṣmī, bearing good fortune to all beings. Next came the smooth jewel adorning the breast of Viṣṇu, the maintainer of the Universe. As the churning continued, out of the ocean emerged the elephant of Indra, the god of the heavens; then Surabhi, the radiant and sweet white cow who grants any wish; and then the wishing tree of fragrance; followed by the nymphs and celestials. At last emerged Dhanvantari, the celestial physician robed in white, bearing the cup of the moon filled with amṛta, the essence of immortal life.

The chalice of the moon represents the fullness of our consciousness. The nectar of immortality is the remembrance that we are already one with the Divine Source—that there was never a time when we were not, nor is there a time that we will never be.

Some versions of this story identify Lakṣmī, the goddess who rises out of the ocean, as the bearer of the divine nectar. Lakṣmī, Viṣṇu's consort, is the post-Vedic queen of the waterways who is known for beauty, graciousness, and benevolence. She bestows success in all endeavors, liberation of consciousness, and enjoyment of life. In one of her four hands, she carries a white lotus, symbolic of purity of heart. Another showers gold coins upon her devotees. And in another hand, she holds the golden vessel of amrita.

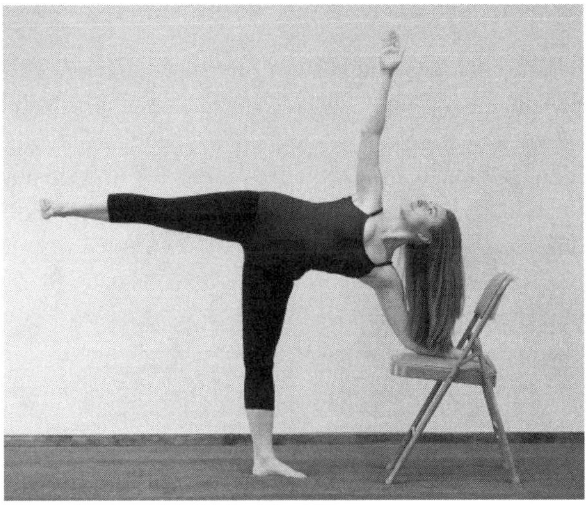

Using a chair for support helps open tight hips and hamstrings.

The details and variations to this story seem infinite and unending, like the changes of the moon that make the ocean rise and fall with the rhythms of the tides. Every aspect of Ardha Candrāsana relates to varying positions of the moon. The pose's bilateral movements represent the moon's waxing and waning. The full expression of Ardha Candrāsana, when the arm is brought to the side of the head, takes on the yantra or geometric pattern of the half moon.

The crescent moon is the symbol of the second cakra. This cakra, Svādhiṣṭāna, is associated with the water element and is significant in the practice of Ardha Candrāsana. The sacral center holds our reproductive essence and our experiences of pleasure and sweetness. (The Sanskrit word *śukra* refers to the reproductive tissue. It also means "sweetness," and it is the root for the English word "sugar.") Through this cakra, we experience the powerful urge for procreation, which can be sublimated into the higher centers for the co-creative union with the Divine.

In ayurveda, the reproductive essence is called *ojas,* and it is considered to be the refined nectar of our nutrition. Ojas is the physical life force, the foundation of our strength and immunity, and the lunar fluids in the body. Ojas is the procreative seed with the power to create new life. Ojas is further refined into *soma.* Soma, another word for the moon, relates to the cerebral spinal fluid, which allows for expansion of consciousness and awareness. In some Sanskrit texts, soma is said to be the nectar of immortality, which drips down from the head and gives a sweet taste to the saliva during bliss states. It is said that eight drops of soma (refined ojas) live in the heart, responsible for periodic feelings of intense joy and love.

Soma must be equal in strength to *agni,* the fire element in the body that burns, consumes, and transforms food and thought impressions. Without the balancing lunar influence, too many fire practices can burn out the tissues and the nervous system. (An ayurvedic teacher from India has said that with our current fixation on fire practices, we don't need sun baths ... we need moon baths.) The sun (ha) and moon (tha), represented by agni and soma, must be balanced for us to move into the higher states of consciousness.

Ardha Candrāsana activates the lunar, feminine energy of the moon. The divine masculine energy expresses the creative life force of the lower centers, releasing the ojas outwards as a gift to the divine feminine. She receives these juices and transforms them into soma, which travels up the spine and radiates from the heart back into the world to be recycled again.

Guidance

1. Begin Ardha Candrāsana by standing with the feet three feet apart. (Ardha Candrāsana is commonly taken from Utthita Trikoṇāsana, but I like to sequence it after headstand because it is an excellent pose for releasing neck tension.) Inhale across the back.
2. Exhaling, move the skin up the neck and down the back to create greater length between the shoulder and the ear.
3. Inhale and expand the breath horizontally across the back, from shoulders to buttocks.
4. Exhaling, turn the right foot out 90 degrees and the left foot in 30 degrees.
5. Inhaling, allow the breath to once more expand across the back.
6. Exhale and bend the right knee, keeping the hips open. Bring the right hand down to the floor or, if this closes the hips, to a block or to a chair. Using the seat or back of a chair helps to open the pelvis.
7. Inhale, breathing in across the back.
8. Exhaling, move the spine into the front of the body like a backbend and straighten the bottom knee, lifting up from the top of the kneecap to the top of the thigh.
9. On the inhalation, remain steady as you take the breath into the back, rounding slightly.
10. Exhale and rotate the bottom leg externally to open the upper hip.
11. Inhale and do nothing, allowing the breath to organically fill the back.
12. Exhaling, reach the upper leg back away from the head, giving the leg as much attention as the upper body. This helps lengthen the lumbar, preventing compression.
13. Pause on the inhalations.

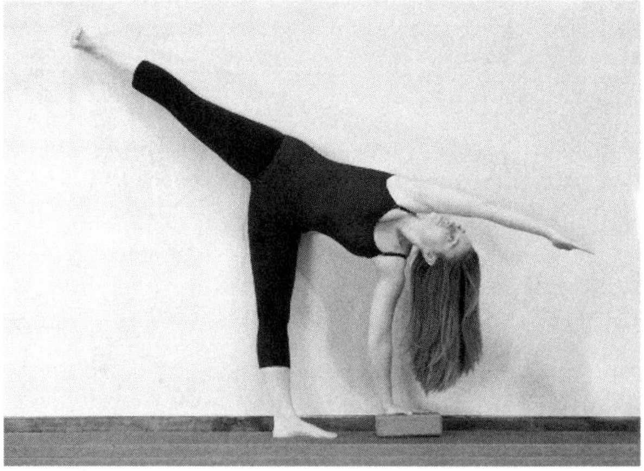

With every exhalation, open the heart center and allow the rotation of the head to follow.

14. With every exhalation, open the heart center toward the light and allow the rotation of the head to follow the rotation of the base of the spine. Rotate the neck only as far as the lower spine will allow. It is important to relax the neck, as this in turn relaxes the lower back, allowing the pelvis to open and the energy to flow from the lower cakras to the upper cakras.

Note: By moving into the fullness of the pose on the exhalation rather than on the inhalation, the breath helps the mind to become calm. If there is any neck tension, relax the elbow of the upper arm. If possible, bring the arm behind the ear rather than in front. The neck rotates as a result of the rotation at the base of the spine. Rather than turning from the neck, move by opening the upper hip.

To lift out of the bottom hip, rotate the bottom thigh externally to help open the groin area. In order to move the top hip, one first must move from the base. If there is strain on the back of the knee, the weight is too far forward toward the toes. If there is strain on the hamstrings, the weight is too far back on the heels. The key of the pose is to adjust the weight equally between the heel and ball of the foot, lifting the arch as the ball of the big toe rolls downward.

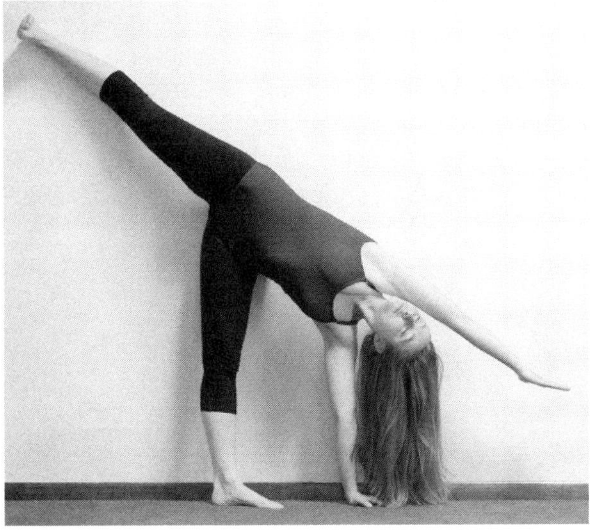

Every aspect of Ardha Candrasana relates to varying positions of the moon.

Assists: This pose can be entered from Utthita Trikoṇāsana (Triangle Pose), using a wall as support for the back body. The bottom hand can be placed on one or two blocks to help keep the hips as even as possible. Students with tighter hips and hamstrings can bend to the side, bringing the bottom hand to a chair. The upper hand can be brought to the back of the upper hip to help preserve the length of the lumbar spine.

A partner or teacher can place one hand at the back of the student's upper hip and buttock, moving the hip toward the upraised heel, as the other hand gently lifts the upper hip to help open the inner groin or psoas muscle. A partner can also help support the student's head and neck. As the neck releases in the pose, the mid and lower back will relax and in turn open as well as lengthen.

If the pose is practiced without the support of a wall or chair, a partner can stand behind, giving support, holding the student's upper arm or drawing the shoulder downward as the student lifts the arm to the side of the head.

Psychophysiological Benefits

Ardha Candrāsana opens the pelvis and releases pressure on all the pelvic organs. It helps to release compression in the mid-torso and the digestive organs, including the ascending, descending, and transverse colon. Because it affects the parasympathetic division of the nervous system, it increases bodily secretions, including digestive juices and hormones.

In Ardha Candrāsana, as in other inversions, the reproductive essence of the second cakra is not inhibited by the gravitational pull. It can more easily travel up the spine to the crown cakra, bypassing the fires of the navel, opening the heart, and merging with the divine. Ardha Candrāsana represents the feminine aspect of this divine union, the transformation of ojas from procreation in the annamaya kośa (the sheath of the body) into Soma of the ānandamaya kośa (the Bliss sheath beyond the body).

The Soma in the head is like a magnet for the Kuṇḍalinī Śakti to rise upwards. This is referred to extensively in Vedic texts and mythology. In the story of the churning of the ocean of milk, the celestial physician (Dhanvantari) arises, carrying with him the chalice of the moon, the soma or nectar of immortality. When we start to churn our spine in forward bends, backbends, twisting poses, and inverted poses, we awaken the latent energy. And if we practice Half Moon fully, it opens up all the channels, from the base cakra or earth element through the third cakra.

Brahmā, the creator, is said to reside in the first cakra, but what follows creation is that which maintains and stabilizes creation. The second cakra, therefore, associated with the element of water and the sense of taste, is said to be the dwelling place of Lord Viṣṇu, the sustainer, who presides here with his consort Lakṣmī.

Viṣṇu is the spiritual power that is in every atom, cell, molecule of our body. It is the energy the pulses through the procreative centers of all species. It is the prāṇa of our breath, the beat and rhythm of our heart. The word Viṣṇu means all pervasive. It is the all-pervading prāṇa or life force that maintains the substratum of the Universe. It is said that Viṣṇu holds the balance between Brahmā, the creator at the base of the spine and Śiva, the destroyer or transformer the energy that dwells in the crown pole within the head. Viṣṇu represents balanced living and like his later incarnation of Kṛṣṇa, symbolizes the cosmic līlā, the Divine play of life.

The milky ocean represents the subconscious mind and its vast storage of cellular memory. As the spine moves omni-directionally in Ardha Candrāsana, that which is stored in the latent depths of the psyche arises up to the surface of the consciousness. The story of the churning of the ocean alludes to a poison that might have destroyed all creation. Śiva, the Lord of Yogis, was called to come down off his mountain to drink the poison that arose from the milky sea. He held it in his throat and his neck turned blue, iridescent as a butterfly's wing.

In Ardha Candrāsana, the poisons that arise are the mental and emotional toxins that must surface before the gems that represent insight and wisdom come forth. As these long-stored toxins are released, the subconscious also unfurls, bringing with it the darshan of the celestial beings who give their blessing to life's journey. Śiva's drinking of the poison represents calling for Universal help and intervention, or consulting a friend or therapist to help us understand the healing reaction and to support us in our continuing practice.

At times, we all need reminders to keep up our yoga practice, even though toxins may periodically rise to the surface of the mind. If āsana is appropriately practiced, it does not create pain but simply (or not) reveals the pain that is already there. Afterward, the beauty and wonders of that which lies in the hidden depths of the psyche can rise to the surface. The celestial goddess Lakṣmī, representing spiritual and material abundance, graces us with her vision and bestows her blessings. The Celestial Physician finally emerges from the bottom of the ocean. In the cup of the moon, he carries Amṛta, the nectar of the soul's immortality, which is a balm to soothe any wounds inflicted from life's journey.

The story of the churning of the ocean of milk is the story of Earth's creation, the beginning of time. It reminds me of a verse in the Mahābhārata: "Wherever land ends, there the sea dances with the uplifted hands of its waves, wide as space and vast as time."

Vīrabhadrāsana I

Warrior I

For the Sanskrit translation, refer to Vīrabhadrāsana II (page 75).

Philosophical Introduction

Vīrabhadrāsana I, II, and III all represent the salute to the Gods and Goddesses of the Ten-Sided Universe. In the Warrior series, we honor the eight directions of east, west, north, south, northwest, northeast, southeast, southwest, as well as the external and internal center of one's Being.

In Vīrabhadrāsana I, the forward leg forms the yantra of the square while the back leg and foot move in a diagonal line from earth to heaven, giving śakti to the static qualities of the square. Without the diagonal momentum and the firmness and stability of the back leg, the pose could become tamasic or lethargic, where energy becomes stuck in old patterns and puts a strain on the forward hip and knee.

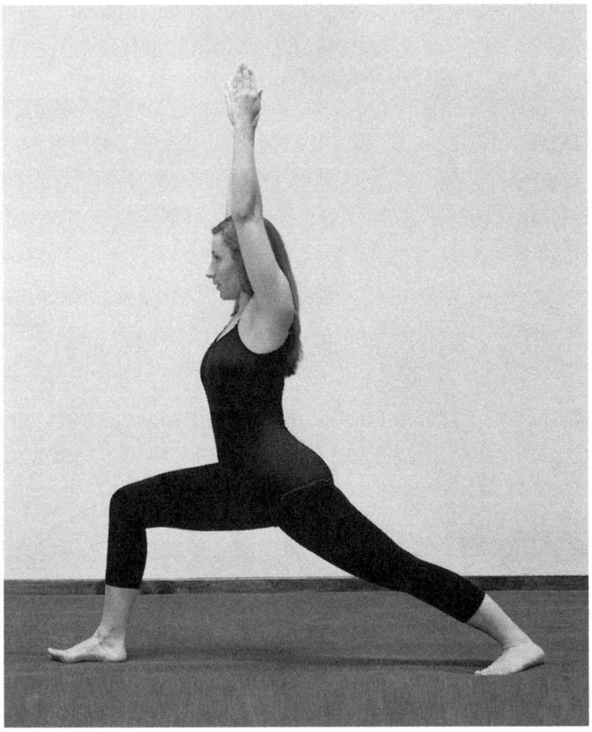

In Vīrabhadrāsana I, the forward leg forms a square, the yantra of Gaṇeśa.

By bending the knee of the forward leg to create a right angle, we form the yantra of Gaṇeśa, who is known as the elephant god of good fortune because he has great strength to remove obstacles, both spiritual and material, from our path. Vedic astrologers invoke Gaṇeśa because he is said to hold the keys to understanding the language of the skies. As the lord or presiding deity of astrology, Gaṇeśa knows the destiny of all living beings. He is the overseer of karma, allotting the results of all previous actions.

Gaṇeśa acted as scribe for the sage Vyāsa, completing the celestial dictation of the Mahabharata, the Great Epic of India. Gaṇeśa is usually depicted with one tusk; the missing tusk was used to write the scripture. His vehicle is the mouse, the one creature elephants fear, according to folklore. One of Gaṇeśa's hands is raised in *abhaya mudrā,* the gesture that represents fearlessness. Gaṇeśa subdues the fears that arise in the first cakra, and removes the fears that are obstacles in our spiritual life. He is the macrocosm of the Universe, and the mouse is the microcosm of the ego that keeps the mind and consciousness in the illusion of separation.

When the body forms Gaṇeśa's yantra in Vīrabhadrāsana I and II, we invoke the energy field that the symbol of Gaṇeśa represents. Doing so helps us not to destroy the ego but to master and transcend the ego and enlist it in service in our realization of the Divine. In Vīrabhadrāsana, we reflect Gaṇeśa, this gargantuan macrocosmic form who has conquered his fear of the microcosmic mouse and now rides upon it as his vehicle in life. The tiny mouse, symbolic of the contractive egoistic self, is now the support and carrier of its own transcendence, the remembrance of our expanded Universal Self.

I often remind students that we can lift our hearts without lifting the ego. This is the key to practicing this version of the Warrior Pose. In the Bhagavad Gītā, a warrior is not attached to the result of his or her own actions: "Do the action for its sake thereof without attachment to its fruits" (II:47). This reminds us not to buy into culturally competitive ambitions that take us further from rather than bring us toward our own center. A spiritual warrior does not enter into battle because of anger (which can disempower), but steps in without attachment to the results. The spiritual warrior enters into the battlefield of life because *dharma*—destiny or life's purpose—has brought him or her to the field.

The battlefield in the Bhagavad Gītā is known as Kurukṣetra. *Ku* means "darkness," *ru* is the light, *kṣe* means "destroying," and *tra* means "in order to transcend." In ancient scriptures, the warrior moves from the darkness to the light, destroying in order to transcend. What is it that is destroyed? The ego. The individuated consciousness that keeps us from remembering that we are not just this body, mind or passing personality but that we are One with the Universal Source. We are all warriors upon the field of life, and this pose can be a vibrant reminder that bravery does not mean that we are without fear; it means that we have the courage to face our fears.

Guidance

1. From Tāḍāsana, step the feet approximately five feet apart.
2. Turn the right foot out 90 degrees and the left foot inward 60 degrees so that the heel of the right foot is in alignment with the arch of the back foot.
3. Exhaling, rotate the torso and hips to the right, rotating the back leg internally. In establishing the base, it sometimes helps to use the hands to draw the hips down to elongate the lumbar spine. This also frees the ribs and upper torso to lift to the light.
4. Inhaling, allow the breath to expand across the back (even rounding it visibly), lifting up the back ribs.
5. Exhaling, keep lifting the back ribs as you lift the side and front ribs toward the head.
6. Inhaling, bring the breath into the back from shoulders to buttocks.
7. Exhaling, make the back leg firm as if the back of the knees were expanding vertically and horizontally. Bring the back heel into the earth, lifting up the back inner arch. If there is strain in the back knee, rotate the back foot to 70 or 80 degrees.
8. Inhale and again allow the breath to fill the back body.
9. Exhaling, draw the shoulders down away from the ears as the arms fly out and up effortlessly, not just from the heart but from the base of the ribs and the kidneys.
10. Inhaling, fill the back with breath, keeping your awareness firmly on the back leg.
11. Exhale and maintain the firmness of the back leg as you bend the forward knee. Bend the knee only as far as the back leg will allow. Eventually the forward hip will become level to the knee.
12. Inhale, holding steady while bringing the breath into the back, even rounding it a little.
13. Exhale and offer up from the heart center while extending the back of the neck. The chin stays parallel to the floor.
14. Inhale, filling the back with the breath.
15. Exhaling, elongate the spine a little more, creating even more space between the rib cage and the pelvis.
16. Inhale and expand the breath horizontally across the back from shoulders to buttocks.
17. Exhaling, preserve the length you've created as you straighten the forward knee, keeping the back leg firm and unwavering.
18. Without losing the awareness of the breath, come out of the pose the same way you went into it. Repeat on the opposite side.

Note: It is not important to bring the hips level to one another. In the past few years, it has become a trend to bend the back knee to bring the hips into alignment with one another. However, in trying to do so, it puts strain on the lumbar spine, the knees, hips and creates a loss of stability and centeredness within the pose. If one loses the diagonal śakti of the back leg, the energy of the pose becomes static. When the back leg is firm and unmoving, the psoas muscles slowly elongate, freeing stuck energy within the sacroiliac joint.

Assist: A partner can stand behind the student and use a belt or his or her hands or thighs to clasp the back of the student's thighs. The student's back thigh skin can be rotated slightly internally to help free the back hip, allowing that hip to move a little more forward. The partner can hold each side of the student's sacrum and bring the buttocks down, encouraging the student's spine to rise up as he or she bends the front knee. This helps to prevent spinal compression and brings the internal pelvic organs back into their natural alignment. If the lumbar area collapses, bring the buttocks down a little more and encourage the student to lift the back ribs upward during the exhalation. Alternatively, the partner can hold the tops of the student's shoulders down as the arms reach out to the side and then fly up.

Vīrabhadrāsana I can also be practiced by placing the back heel on a wall to help give leverage to the back leg. This is the key to the spinal lift.

Psychophysiological Benefits

In this pose, the buttock muscles (gluteus maximus) become firm and space opens in the hip joint, preserving the synovial fluids that maintain the flexibility and youthfulness of the hips, knees, and ankles. Through the strength and opening of this pose (and in Vīrabhadrāsana II), the secrets of the first and second cakra begin to reveal themselves.

At the same time, if the back of the neck is lifted rather than compressed, we free the prāṇa of the heart cakra to flow through the subtle nerves of the vijñana nāḍī, which relates to the carotid arteries. This opens the channels for the prāṇa to flow freely, allowing the brain to receive the light of illumination through the crown cakra. The yoga sutras say that it is through the crown cakra, the Sūryavara (also known as Sahasrāra, the thousand-petalled lotus) that the knowledge of the Cosmos reveals itself.

When the front knee bends, we erroneously think we are going down. Instead, every vertebra of the spine is going up, lifting to the light. As we do this, we eventually free the back of the heart center, allowing the spine to offer itself into the front body and lifting the base as well as top of the sternum, to receive the grace of the Gods and Goddesses. However, if the head lifts with the heart, we engage the ego. When the face lifts, the heart region has a tendency to collapse, and the back of the neck becomes compressed, restricting the circulatory flow from moving freely between spinal nerve roots, peripheral nerves, heart and brain.

As the spinal axis remains in the center of the forward and backward movement of the legs, the mind is brought into the NOW, into the present moment. It no longer lunges into the future with anticipation, hesitation, or fear (reflected in the tension of the toes). The energy from the top of the buttocks is given equal attention as it grows into the earth from the back heel. It is this momentum that gives dynamism to the pose and prevents any compression in the lumbar spine. This equality of movement of front and back brings the mind into the present moment.

As the arms rise, the shoulders drop down, creating ever-growing space between the tops of the shoulders and the earlobes. Since the arms are the extension of the heart, it is helpful to reach out of the heart center to the fingertips as the arms rise. Allow them to lift effortlessly, without tension in the neck or arms. Move and hold the arms from the heart center and, if possible, even down to the kidneys. It is important not to bring the hands together prematurely, a common tendency for most practitioners. Maintain the space between the earlobes and the shoulders and preserve the lateral expansion of the clavicle bone: Do not bring the hands together, but keep the arms shoulder-width apart or even wider if you have tight or muscular shoulders. As the fingers extend from their roots to the tips, the energy of the heavens streams into the heart center.

When the back leg extends from the buttocks through the heel down into the earth, we become that warrior who is deeply connected to the source and the ground of Being while performing the aspiration of his or her own dharma, moving with equanimity through life, centered within Oneself in the midst of all life's actions and interactions. In this pose we adjust the forward movement of reaching into the future with the backward movement that could be reluctance or fear that keeps us stuck in past patterns that no longer serve us.

By honoring the Center of our Being in this pose, there is a tension between the forward lunge and the firm unchanging quality of the strength of the back leg. The pose is the balance of Puruṣa and Prakṛti, the changeless, eternal and the play of life. When there is equal balance, front and back, right and left, inner and outer, the pose feels light, sattvic, and serene. We may feel that we can stay in it indefinitely. As the head, neck and breast come into alignment, it is possible for the mind to come into a thoughtless state of awareness. In this state of consciousness, we would be in what Patañjali calls Dhyanāsana, or the meditative seat.

The meditative seat can be found in every āsana and its variations, not just by sitting cross-legged. All āsana poses help to remind us that we are already one with the Universal light. As we open the space of the darkened corners of mind and emotions through our body, we come into that remembrance. A spiritual warrior is one who draws strength from the remembrance of the Source and, in offering all actions to the Divine, finds the "inaction within the action."

Vīrabhadrāsana III

Airplane Pose

For the Sanskrit translation, refer to Vīrabhadrāsana II (page 71).

Philosophical Introduction

This variation of the salute to the gods and goddesses of the ten-sided universe is popularly known as Airplane Pose, but when this pose was brought forth upon this earth, there were no airplanes as we know them today. Instead, consider this āsana in terms of older times. The pose honors the directions of a yantra, which are different than a global map. While they honor north and south, the torso, upper leg, and arms form a parallel and horizontal relationship to the earth that stretches out to all humanity. The bottom leg is perpendicular to the earth plane, offering to the gods of the east (pūrva) and west (paścima). This perpendicular line can be seen as the vertical ascent of Universal Consciousness. When we rise up out of the bottom hip and leg as the heel and ball of the foot grow down into the earth, we caress the earth like a bhakti yogi, experiencing the spiritual fullness of the pose through the body.

This variation of Warrior Pose springs out of Vīrabhadrāsana I. The length of the front of the torso is preserved and even more energy is taken into the back leg and heel as the torso comes to rest upon the forward thigh. So as not to create strain or fluctuations in the mind, even more awareness soars from the back buttocks to the heel as the torso and arms are brought forward. This creates a diagonal line, which transforms the yantra of the square formed with the forward leg from a static to a dynamic expression of the pose as an offering to the gods and goddesses of the ten-sided Universe.

As the forward propulsion of the torso and arms automatically lift the back leg, one comes effortlessly into Vīrabhadrāsana III, a pose that evokes interdimensional planes of consciousness—the airplane. Here the planes of air or airplane represent the various planes of existence from the netherworld regions below the earth plane to the many celestial realms where the gods of varying degrees of consciousness are said to dwell.

It is said that the etheric space within the nucleus of an atom—between the protons and neutrons and the electrons that dance a million times a minute around its center—is like the gap between the planets and the sun. It is believed that if one contemplates this Ākāśha or space, or something as light as cotton wool, the body will assume an aura of light and lightness.

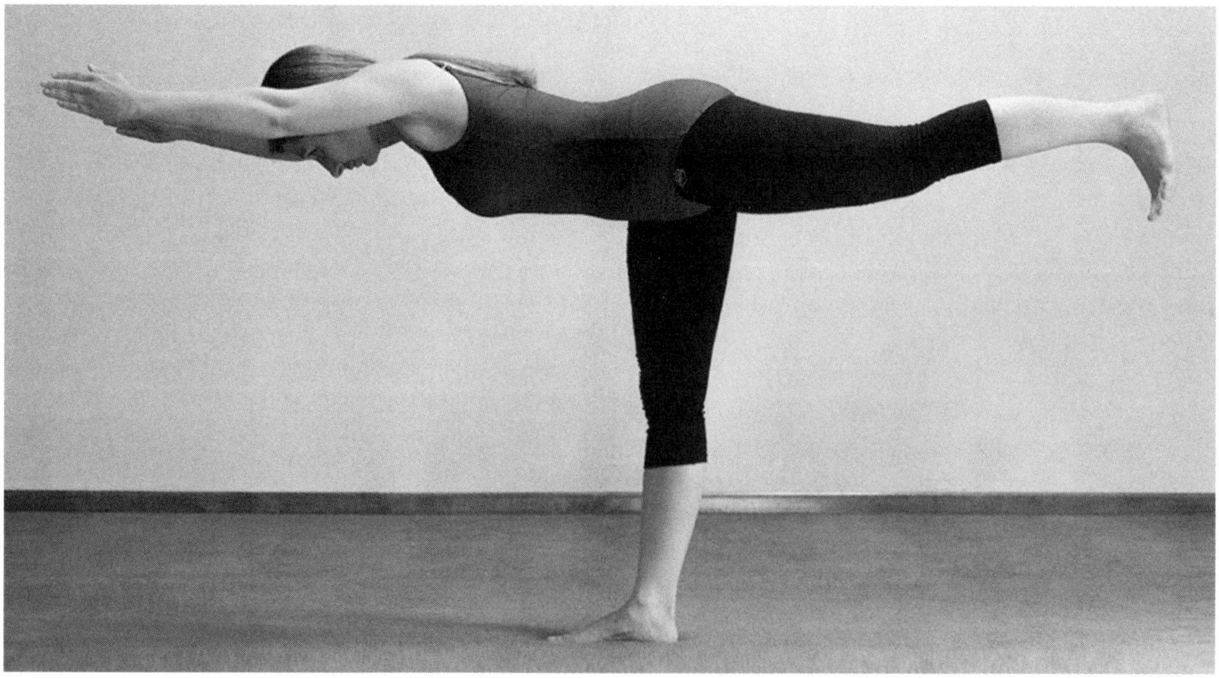

The forward propulsion of the arms and torso in warrior III effortlessly lift the back leg.

Airplane Pose is a wonderful āsana in which to practice this lightness. Weight in yoga means force that moves towards the center of the earth. As the bottom leg in Vīrabhadrāsana III grows down into the earth, the horizontal plane of the torso, arms, and leg grows up out of this gravitational force, giving lightness to the particles that constitute our body. As one commentary on the Yoga Sutras says, "Our Ego acting on the materials constituting the body shapes them into the form of a body and makes it feel heavy. By concentrating on the relationship between the body and Ākāśha or ether it is possible to transform the ego."

Or, as I like to tell students, "We create space in the body so spirit can reveal itself."

Guidance

1. Begin in Vīrabhadrāsana I, inhaling across the back of the torso.
2. Exhaling, place the torso upon the forward thigh.
3. Inhale into the back.
4. Exhale, allowing the spine to surrender to the front of the torso creating the sense of a backbend while in a forward bend.
5. Inhaling, wait and center the mind while breathing into the back body.
6. Exhaling, elongate the front of the torso as the spine comes in to meet the front body.
7. Inhaling, allow the breath to round the back.
8. Exhaling, grow back with the back leg with as much attention as the force that is propelling the torso and arms forward.
9. Inhale and bring the breath into the back, keeping the extension of the back leg.
10. Exhale, allowing the extension of the torso and arms to effortlessly lift the back leg, and then straighten the front leg, lifting up out of the hip joint.
11. Inhale, bringing the breath into the back as much as possible.
12. Exhale, living in varying dimensions simultaneously—vertical and horizontal—aware of the back (upper) leg and foot, the spine, the arms and fingertips, and the standing foot, leg, and hip.
13. Inhale and hold your consciousness on etheric space or the lightness of cotton wool. The bottom leg descends into the gravitational field of the earth as you use it to transcend gravity.
14. Exhaling, reach back with the upper leg as the lower leg bends, bringing the torso to the thigh once again. Come out the same way you moved into the pose. Repeat on the opposite side.

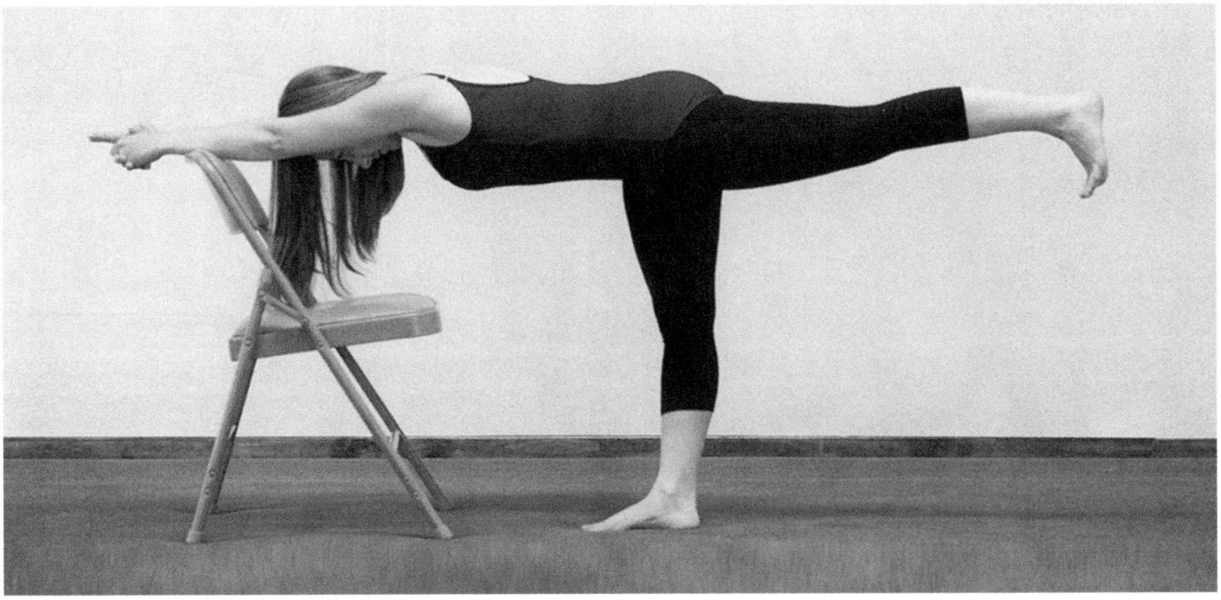

Supporting the arms on the back of a chair aids in balancing and gaining greater extension.

Assist: Support your arms on the back of a chair and/or stand in front of a wall and use it to support and extend through the back foot. You can also work with a partner, who will support your arms while you gain greater balance and extension within the pose.

Psychophysiological Benefits

Standing poses use gravity to transcend gravity. They lengthen and elongate the spine, stretching the limbs from the seed center of bindu, the point out of which all creation flows. In the standing poses, the bindu is the seed center within the pelvic plexus. The Vīrabhadrāsana series, like other standing poses, are prayers. They reflect an evolving psyche that can now transcend rather than sink into old patterns.

Psychologically, this pose gives a growing sense of security and trust in one's own inner strength. We don't have to "lean" or rely on others as we find an inner strength radiating out, reflecting the new balance and strength within the body and Being. Physically, this pose strengthens quadriceps of the front thigh while lengthening the hamstrings of the back thigh. It strengthens the areas surrounding the knee while creating space and increasing strength within the joint of the hips. By concentrating on "lightness" within the pose, the body feels lighter as it lifts above the gravitational field to create a growing confidence in oneself.

The pose invoking the "air plane" relates to the third chapter of Patañjali's Yoga Sutras: "By practicing concentration, meditation on the relationship between the body and Ākāśha (ether) and by concentrating on the lightness of cotton wool, passage through the sky can be secured" (III:43). In his commentary on the sutras, *Yoga Philosophy of Patañjali,* Swami Hariharananda Aranya elaborates: "The Yogin becomes light and can move through the sky. By meditation on cotton wool or other light things down to atoms, the Yogin becomes light. By becoming light, the Yogin can then walk on water, then on cobwebs and on rays of light and move to the sky at will."

Prasārita Pādottānāsana

Wide-Legged Forward Bend

Pra means "to bring forth." *Sa* means "with," and *rita* is from *ri,* "to rise upward." Prasārita can also be translated as "to spread apart." *Pād* means piece or little part. In this instance, pad would refer to the foot or leg. The Sanskrit verb *tān,* which is found in many āsana names, means "to go beyond" or to stretch intensively. The word *tanu* is used in the Yoga Sutras in reference to the kleshas, life's painful afflictions, and in this instance it means "to thin."

Philosophical introduction

The name of the pose gives us instructions as well as the possible benefits of the pose. In Prasārita Pādottānāsana, we spread apart the feet and legs, rising upward and going beyond our self-imposed limitations. How can we do this, we may wonder, if the head and torso are moving down? The answer is because this pose creates a different spatial orientation as the body offers itself in all directions, including heaven and earth.

In Prasārita Pādottānāsana, the horizontal pressure of the legs honors the right and left sides, or the masculine and feminine aspects of our being. The head, the symbol of ego, is usually dominant over other areas of the body, including the heart, but in this pose the head humbles itself to the earth. The tailbone represents humility. When we are upright, the tailbone lies in darkness, always facing the earth. Now the tailbone has an unusual opportunity—to face upward and draw upon the energies of the heaven. Prasārita Pādottānāsana, like other āsanas, is a prayer in which we offer the upper body to the earth and the lower body to the heavens.

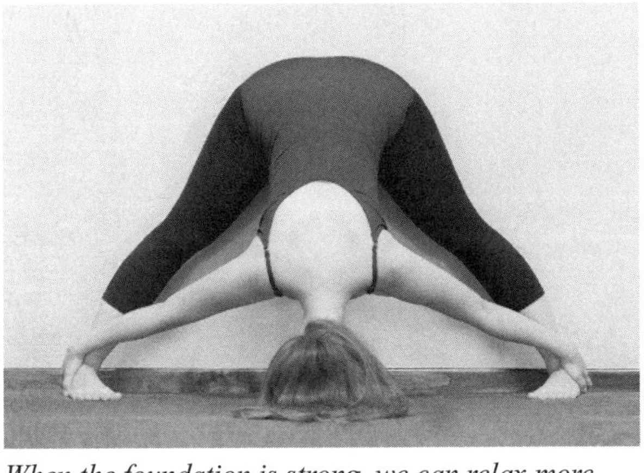

When the foundation is strong, we can relax more deeply into this pose of yoga, and ultimately, all the poses of life.

If the foundation (the feet and legs) is firm and strong, we can relax more deeply into this pose of yoga, and ultimately, all the poses of life. Patañjali says: "Through the relaxation of effort and meditation upon the Infinite, āsana is perfected" (II:47). As the feet are firm and the inner ankles uplifted, the adductor muscles of the inner thighs elongate. By resisting the inner thighs away from one another, space is created within the sacroiliac region. We assume a backbend while in a forward bend—the counterpose within the pose. The tilt of the pelvis is important in relaxing the spine and, due to the inverse gravitational pull, releasing subtle blockages within the spine, which allows prāṇa to flow freely between the base of the spine base and the crown of the head.

If the feet and legs remain firm and unwavering, this allows for fluidity of prāṇa within the spine and its spiritual center, the Suṣumnā. When unblocked, the light of spirit moves through unimpeded to the crown cakra, Sahasrāra, the seat of the thousand-petalled lotus. This pose is excellent for learning the natural and effortless bandhas or locks that allow prāṇa to flow freely between lower to higher centers within the body. Mūlabandha is the first bandha affected in this pose when the Mūlādhāra, the base support of the lifted tailbone, receives the light of the heaven. Mr. B.K.S. Iyengar used to say: "Let your buttock bones shine like the rays of the disk of the sun. Let them cast their light in every direction simultaneously. They have been hidden in darkness; now let their light be seen."

If the next bandha, at the navel or solar plexus, is relaxed and elongated without muscular contraction, it begins to fly upward like its namesake, the great bird Uḍḍīyāna. Prāṇa flutters into the heart cakra, Anāhata. On each exhalation, the spine is offered into the heart center, allowing prāṇa to heal any stuck, dark, or hardened corners within the heart.

As the spine continues to elongate with each exhalation, prāṇa continues its journey to the throat cakra, the Viśuddhi. The bandha within the throat is known as jālandhara. *Jāla* is a network, grid, or lattice. *Dhara* means "support." In the subtle or pranic body, the throat center—the point of the finest element, ether—has the strongest knot, or *granthi.* This keeps us on the earth plane.

In Prasārita Pādottānāsana, if the throat, neck, lower jaw, and face remain totally relaxed, the prāṇa can move through to the crown cakra. Alternatively, we can contain prāṇa within the spine by bringing the heart center toward the chin, elongating the front of the throat without tensing the neck or chin.

Prasārita Pādottānāsana not only inverts the spine and brain but also, when practiced with the breath, lengthens and thins the waist, softening and releasing the solar plexus. This helps release the subconscious storehouse of impressions from the depth of the psyche. When the kleśas—the reasons for our afflictions and suffering in life—are brought to the surface, they can be released and transformed.

Guidance

1. Begin in Tāḍāsana. Step the legs four and a half to five feet apart. Place the hands on the hips.
2. Breathe into the back body, allowing the inhalation to round the back.
3. Exhaling, bring the spine into the front of the body, elongating it upwards. Turn the toes in to a slightly pigeon-toed position to internally rotate the thighs and open the spaces between the right and left buttocks and the sides of the sacrum. Lift the inner ankles to strengthen and preserve the inner arches of the feet. Relax the toes, creating space between them as you grow down through the outer heels.
4. Inhale across the back, from shoulders to the ribs and then to the hips.
5. Exhale, growing down firmly through the outer edges of the feet and lifting the tops of the knee caps. Press the hands against the thighs and bring the spine in like a backbend to create space in the front body and anterior spine while bending forward. Bend from hips, not from the waist, keeping the spine as straight as possible.
6. Inhale, pausing in the movement of bending forward. Focus on breathing into the spine and the back body.
7. Exhaling, bring the spine toward the front body as you continue the descent of the upper body, lifting the tops of the kneecaps and bringing the fingertips to the floor while rotating the pelvis forward. Lengthen from the top of the pubic bone, offering the navel (not the head) to the earth.

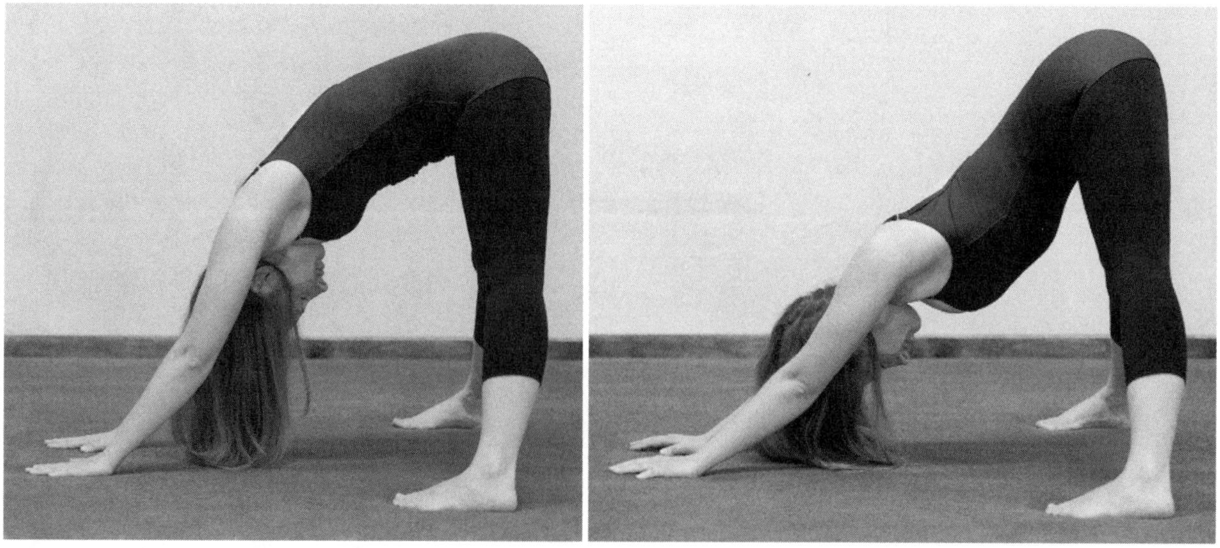

Let the breath round the back on the inhalation. Exhaling, elongate the spine, bringing it in like a backbend.

8. Inhaling, let the breath round the back, allowing the head to relax to follow the curvature of the spine.
9. Exhaling, press down with the fingertips for leverage and elongate the spine, bringing it in like a backbend while rotating the upper arms externally to roll the skin from the upper shoulders down the back.
10. Inhale and let the breath (not the mind) round the back, allowing the head to drop slightly to relax the neck.
11. Exhale and grow down with the outer edges of the heels and the ball of the big toe, lifting the slack out of the top of the knee caps. This raises the quadriceps (front thigh muscle). At the same time, relax the hamstrings. As the calf muscles move toward the earth, the knees lift, and the hamstrings gently rise up. Soften the mind to soften the hamstrings.
12. Inhaling, stay in the pose while the breath fills the back body.
13. Exhaling, grow down into the earth with the outer edges of the feet. Lift the knee caps without straining, soften the hamstrings, and let the head and spine descend toward the earth as the tailbone and buttock bone rise with intensity, like the morning sun.
14. Inhaling, hold the pose and allow the breath to flow into the back.
15. Exhale and proceed more deeply into the posture, bringing the back spine into the front of the body.
16. Inhale, holding steady, allowing the breath to fill the back.
17. Exhaling, bend the elbows, moving them back (not out to the sides) and bringing the spine into the front body, like a backbend. Allow the tailbone and buttock bones to rise up to the heavens and the head to descend to the earth.
18. You may take a variation within the pose. Inhale do nothing, and then exhale, bringing the spine into the front body and stretching the arms out to thin the midline of the torso. Keep the head and neck passive and elongated. (Do not raise the chin and compress the neck.)
19. Whichever variation of Prasārita Pādottānāsana you have chosen, keep the mind quiet and still on the inhalations. On every exhalation, move the tailbone back as the torso elongates and the neck and skull extend away from the shoulders.
20. Come out of the pose on an exhalation, moving the feet and legs closer together and then rounding the back to come up. Come back into Tāḍāsana.

Note: To alleviate any existing neck condition, on every exhalation roll the shoulders down the back, away from the ears, and keep elongating the neck forward without raising the chin or compressing the neck. The extension of the hands and arms is excellent for relaxing and stretching the lateral muscles of the back. The thinning of the waist helps to release past subconscious impressions that can build up in this region.

Throughout this pose, the head is relaxed. As the student progresses in this āsana, the head comes toward or to the floor. If the head comes down too far, creating compression in the neck, then the legs have to come closer together. The further apart the legs are, the easier it is for students to come toward the floor. More flexible students can bring the legs a little closer together and then tilt and elongate from the pelvic region.

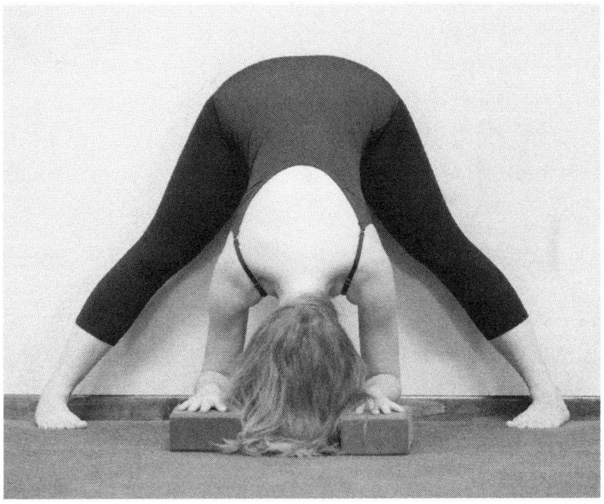

Use blocks until the hamstring muscles lengthen adequately.

It is important to make sure the spinous processes are not protruding when bending in this pose, for this indicates compression in the anterior (front) spine. The front and back body are equal to one another. If the back is rounded, place the hands on a higher surface (such as blocks or a chair) to help straighten the spine until the hamstring muscles begin to lengthen.

Eventually, as the hamstrings lengthen, the elongation of the spine can be maintained in the forward extension. Eventually the hands can touch the floor and move closer to align with the feet. Ideally, the palms will come to the floor in a perpendicular line from the shoulders, and the fingertips will align with the toes.

Psychophysiological Benefits

More than other standing poses, Prasārita Pādottānāsana strengthens the adductor muscles of the inner thighs. Practicing Uttānāsana with the legs together or hip distance part stretches the two outer of the three hamstring muscles, but Prasārita Pādottānāsana affects the inner hamstring muscle, the semimembranosus.

This pose also opens the hips, preserving the flexibility as well as the strength of the hip joint. To aid in hip opening, it is important to elongate the spine, creating space between the pelvic rim and the thigh in order to release the lumbar and in turn the psoas muscles of the inner groin. The pose will create space in the back of the hips at the sacroiliac joint, where the pelvis joins the sacrum. The pose releases compression on the lumbar spine and between the five fused vertebrae of the sacrum and the four fused vertebrae of the coccyx (tailbone).

Even though the feet never leave the ground, Prasārita Pādottānāsana is considered to be an inversion, increasing circulation to the head and brain. It has a stimulating affect upon the thalamus and hypothalamus, which is the master endocrine gland. This in turn impacts every other endocrine gland, from the thyroid in the throat to the thymus, the immune center associated with the heart cakra. It in turn influences the balance of the adrenals, which sit above the kidneys, as well as the kidneys themselves. Due to the intense stretch or elongation of the midline of the body, it not only helps reduce the buildup of belly fat but also has a stimulating affect upon sluggishness by releasing compression within the liver, gallbladder, pancreas, spleen, and stomach.

When we practice this āsana, we live in two polarities simultaneously. We experience an expansion, not just a shift, of consciousness. When we focus on one part, we don't forget the other parts, instead moving the awareness from one part of the body to the next. We expand the periphery of consciousness as we hold intense strength from the feet, planted not just on but into the earth, as the back of the legs release upward to the heaven. We expand consciousness by holding the strength of the lower body while totally relaxing the upper.

As the breath carries us into the āsana, the head is relaxed. This gives the cells of the brain an opportunity to open like the petals of a flower to receive the energy of the earth. At the same time, the buttock bones receive the energy from the heavens. Near each ischial tuberosity (the base of buttocks) is the sciatic notch, where the branches of the sciatic, the largest nerve in the body, pass through into the legs. This nerve has a tendency to hold an accumulation of saṁskāras, the deep psyche impressions that are stored as a result of our past experiences. Prasārita Pādottānāsana is powerful in its ability to release the bubbles of saṁskāras as they come to the surface of the conscious mind. This is known as the "thinning of the kleshas" or as *tanu,* going beyond self-imposed limitations.

This pose has many physiological effects, but the depth of experience may be felt at sub-cakra levels. There are seven major cakras, but through the practice of this āsana, I have sensed the openings of the sub-cakras, the energy centers that help guide prāṇa from one cakra to the next. This experience is like discovering the notes between the notes on the musical scale. As the base of the buttocks becomes alive, we may feel the spiral-like movements of the sub-cakras. There are sub-cakras in the palms of the hands, the bottoms of the feet, and the backs of the knees that can be unlocked through the descent of the lower body in this pose, creating an ascent of prāṇa through the upper body.

The great Indian master Sri Aurobindo Gosh said of meditation, "The ascent is followed by the descent." As we invoke and invite the Divine light into the individual Being, the bio-energetic field or Kuṇḍalinī energy rises upward to meet the descending energies. Prasārita Pādottānāsana is a beautiful pose for practicing this meditative principle. As we offer the feminine (Prakṛti) at the base of the spine to the light above, the head (the masculine pole or Puruṣa) offers itself to the darkness within the earth. The descent of Divine energy through the lower body brings forth (*pra*) an ascent of our consciousness through the crown cakra. Through this, we create a balanced equilibrium and a new relationship to the world and universe around and within us.

Ūrdhva Prasārita Pādāsana

Leg Lifting

Ūrdhva is "upward," and *pra* means "to bring forth." *Sa* means "with," and *rita,* "to rise upward." In this pose, we are lifting the legs and bringing them toward the head, then lowering them as if we were in Śavāsana (Corpse Pose), relaxing throughout the duration of the posture.

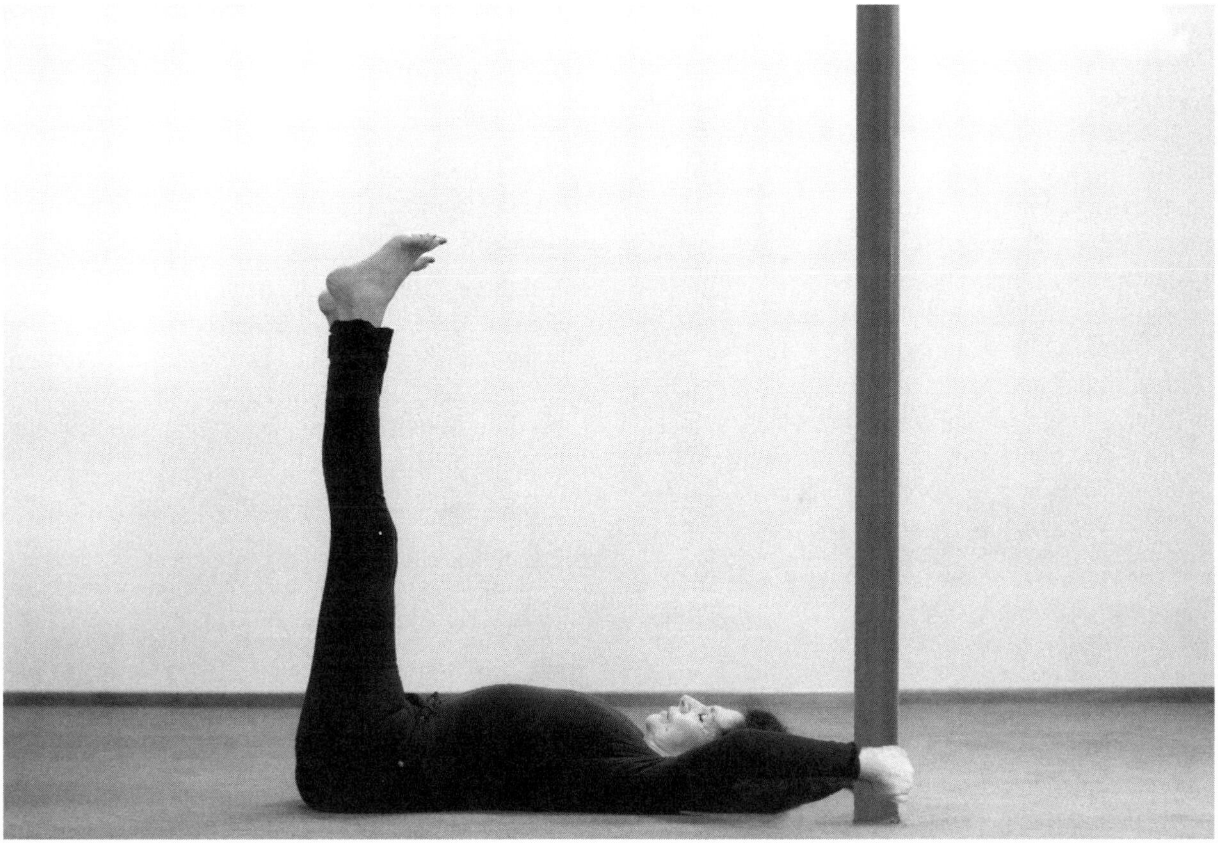

Ūrdhva Prasārita Pādāsana is one of the best poses to build true inner strength.

Philosophical Introduction

In the fitness world, so much emphasis is placed on exercises to build core strength. This pose—in terms of both yoga and fitness—is one of the best to build *true* inner strength. Ūrdhva Prasārita Pādāsana goes deeper than the lateral core muscles of back and abdomen, penetrating to the deepest center of the body and the Being.

All yoga āsanas emphasize the spine, which many refer to as the Meru Daṇḍa—the mountainous staff or the central axis of creation. Yoga poses revolve around the spine and the nerve roots of the autonomic nervous system, which runs along the outside of the spinal vertebrae. Āsanas also emphasize the main energy conduit, the central canal known as the Suṣumnā, which relates to the physical spinal cord. This is, as the Bible calls it, the pillar of light—the most important channel in the subtle body—where the light of illumination, if unimpeded, can flow through.

So many speak of enlightenment, but so few can withstand the intensity of the light as it pours through the subtle channel of the body and the Self. If the nervous system is not prepared, this in-pouring of energy can have a drying, overheating, and weakening effect within the physical as well as subtle nervous system.

Leg lifts strengthen the abdominals and, in turn, the lower back, but Ūrdhva Prasārita Pādāsana does far more. If practiced appropriately, the posture will give great inner strength, both physical and emotional, as it strengthens both the autonomic and central nervous system. The effects of Ūrdhva Prasārita Pādāsana penetrate deep below the core muscles of the torso, strengthening the spinal ligaments and the erector spinae muscles, as well as the nerve roots that extend from the spine to the periphery of the body. The pose also strengthens the myelin sheaths of the nerves: This not only prepares the nervous system to withstand the light of illumination, but also insulates the nerves. raising the threshold for stress and giving great inner strength.

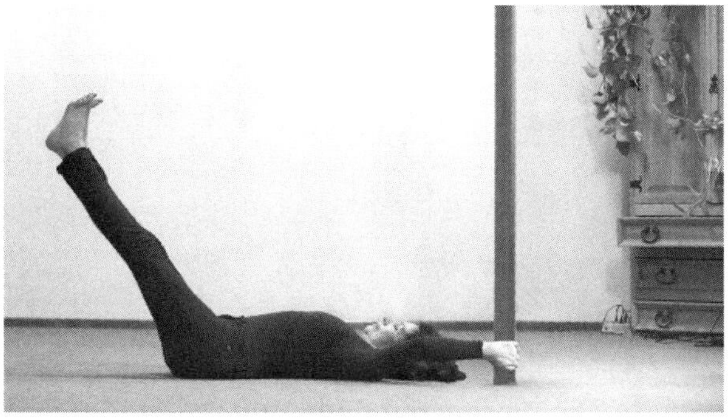

Relax the navel center keeping the abdomen hollow and continue lowering the legs if there is not strain.

As we develop inner strength by practicing Ūrdhva Prasārita Pādāsana, we also gain serenity of mind. We can stay centered within ourselves regardless of what is happening in the world around us. As we grow in this deep inner strength, we have an opportunity to soften our defenses to people and situations around us.

If we are strong in the deepest core of our being, we will not have to armor ourselves by tightening the outer muscles, which display a defensive stance to the world around us. With deep inner strength, even the skin becomes softer. The solar plexus, which reveals our defenses, can also soften. When this occurs, the adrenals—usually in a fight or flight mode when we are defensive—can come to a more relaxed state.

When we have that deepest core strength to rely on, we can allow ourselves to become more flexible, listen more to others, even if their views may be different then our own. With deep inner strength, negative situations that might have entered our field at one time may drop away. We eventually develop an unseen energy field that does not allow negativity to penetrate. And if it should, it will not have the same impact and will soon dissolve, no longer having power over the mind or emotions. With this deep inner core strength, we grow in our faith in a higher power and feel more deeply connected to the Source of all creation.

Guidance

Begin in Śavāsana, for this pose is an extension of Śavāsana. In the beginning, hold onto the leg or edge of a heavy chair or couch with the hands. Bend the elbows out to the side and relax neck tension by drawing the shoulders down from the ears.

1. Inhaling, allow the breath to fill the back of the body from the shoulders all the way down to the hips, if possible.
2. Exhaling, lengthen the neck and spine as much as possible. Bend the knees, bringing the feet to the floor, hip distance apart. Place the hands on the upper thighs and, while exhaling, push the thighs away from the hips, giving greater length to the lumbar spine.
3. Inhale horizontally across the entire back body.
4. Exhale, bringing the arms back over the head and bending the knees into the chest while keeping the length of the front of the torso.
5. Inhale horizontally across the back body and relax the lumbar spine, navel, neck and face.
6. Exhaling, bring the feet to the sky (or ceiling) while keeping all other parts relaxed.

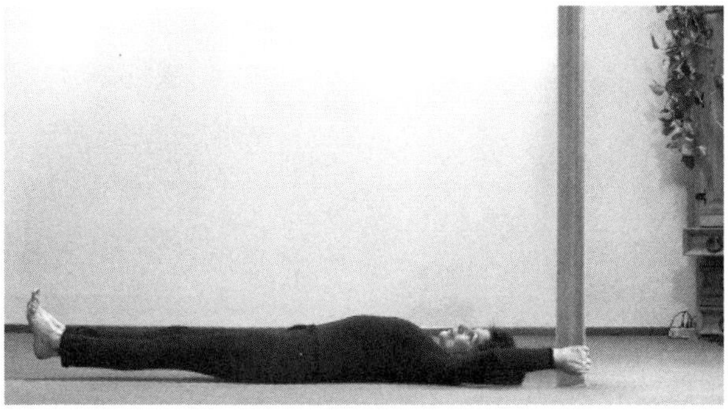

Until deep inner core strength increases, practice this pose with props or partners to protect the lumber spine.

7. Inhale, spreading the breath across the back, still keeping all parts as relaxed as possible.
8. Exhaling, soften the navel, neck, and face while bringing the legs slowly toward the floor. When the breath stops, stop the movement.
9. Inhaling, hold the pose where it is relaxing the legs.

10. Exhaling, continue bringing the legs toward the earth, wiggling the hips away from the head to lengthen the lumbar. If the navel puffs out, stop. Relax the navel center and solar plexus. If there is no strain, continue lowering the legs to the floor (only if the lumbar is in contact with the floor and the navel plexus is soft and relaxed). If there is any strain on the lumbar, stop and bend the knees before continuing to lower the legs.
11. To repeat the āsana, on an exhalation, bring the legs away from the floor. If the lumbar arches and the navel center is not relaxed, then practice Ūrdhva Prasārita Pādāsana by focusing on bringing the legs down before attempting to lift them away from the gravitational field.
12. To complete the practice, bring the feet to the floor to relax the back and belly, and then slowly—keeping the heels on the floor—slide the legs out back into Śavāsana.

Note: Sometimes people will inhale the legs up and exhale them down. However, to deeply strengthen the nervous system and prevent overarching and compression of the lumbar spine, I highly recommend using the exhalation for both movements. This helps to keep the navel area passive and relaxed, sinking back toward the spine. This in turn lengthens and strengthens the lumbar spine.

Assists: Until deep inner core strength increases, practicing Ūrdhva Prasārita Pādāsana with partners or props can help protect the lumbar spine. It is important (when bringing the arms up overhead) to hold onto something firm, such as a piece of heavy furniture. Using a wall is helpful for gradually building inner core strength while protecting the lumbar area. Bring the heels to the wall, keeping the lower back connected to the floor. The distance between the wall and hips depends upon the strength of the abdominals. The pose becomes more intense when the hips are farther away from the wall.

Assistance from a partner or teacher is helpful. The partner stands an arm's length from the student's head, the partner's feet and legs a little more than hip distance apart. The student clasps the partner's ankles for leverage, bending the elbows outward to create space between the top of the shoulders and ears, which helps to keep the neck and face relaxed.

The partner may also bend forward, bringing his or her thumbs and forefingers to the top of the student's pelvic rim, the fingers reaching to the back of the hips to move the hips down away from the upper torso when the student's legs are lowered or lifted. This helps the lumbar spine elongate and remain in contact with the floor.

Another partner assist is to support the student's feet and legs as they are lowering. During this assist, the partner watches the student: When the face contracts, the navel puffs out, and/or the lumbar begins to arch, the partner will hold and support the legs. At this point, while the feet are held, the practitioner can focus on relaxing and lengthening the lumbar. The partner can draw the legs toward her to help release compression in the hips and spine.

Psychophysiological benefits

When the abdominal muscles are weak, it puts stress on the lumbar spine. It is important to keep the abdominals strong for the health of the back and the spine. Ūrdhva Prasārita Pādāsana strengthens the abdominals, which in turn protects the lower back. It is one of the most powerful poses for strengthening and rebuilding the nerve sheaths of the central and autonomic nervous systems, which relate to the subtle channels of Suṣumnā, Iḍā, and Piṅgalā. These are the three most important nāḍīs, which correlate to the nerves but are not the nerves. They are the main pathways of enlightenment or self-realization.

Ūrdhva Prasārita Pādāsana is an extension of Śavāsana. The head, neck, throat, and jaw are to be kept passive and relaxed whether bringing the legs down or lifting them up. The key to the pose is preserving the elongation of the lumbar, even during the leg lifts. If the spine arches and lifts from the floor during leg lifts, the lumbar spine may be compressed.

Another major component to this āsana is the relaxation of the navel area. There should be no willful muscular contraction. If the navel puffs out, this means there is stress on the lumbar spine. Throughout this pose, the elongation of the torso helps the navel to recede toward the backbone rather than tense and puff out. If the spine arches, the pose produces more tension, stress, and weakness rather than deep inner strength.

When the navel pushes out and the solar plexus tenses, it indicates that the ego is engaged in the pose. To practice āsana in an egoless state—allowing the poses to be done through us and not from us—it is important to keep the navel relaxed. This is true in all poses, and especially in Ūrdhva Prasārita Pādāsana.

On a more esoteric level, if the mind focuses on the relationship between the body and space (ākāśha), it is possible to transform the ego. This is a great way to meditate on light and lightness.

The weight of the legs will be felt whether lifting them or lowering them, but we can counter this weight with the deep inner strength of the physical spinal nerves as well as with the unseen channel of suṣumnā. Weight means force, and this gravitational force moves toward the center of the earth. In Ūrdhva Prasārita Pādāsana, we are moving against this downward force.

In the first chapter of the Yoga Sūtras, the first word Patañjali gives to quiet the mind waves is *abhyāsa.* It is commonly defined as continual practice; however, it is can also be defined as "checking the downward pull." This refers not only to the body's physical posture but also to the downward pull of mind and emotions.

Thus, Ūrdhva Prasārita Pādāsana is a wonderful pose for practicing this Sūtra (I:12): a*bhyāsa vairāgyābhyāṁ tannirodhaḥ.* Again, *abhyāsa* means continual practice or checking the downward pull. *Vairāgya* means nonattachment, dispassion. *Tan* means going beyond or thinning, and *nirodhaḥ* means to quiet the storms or noise or turbulence of the mind. However, it should be noted that there is a thin line between detachment and indifference. As one of my teachers used to say, "Before we can know true nonattachment, we must first know attachment. Until then all is indifference."

Practicing Ūrdhva Prasārita Pādāsana, even though it may be difficult, can help us find that neutral place within ourselves that brings us to the Buddhi state of mind, also known as the Over-mind or as the detached (not indifferent) observer. As we breathe out while elongating the spine, we go to a deeper place within and hold the mind in a state of detached observation. This helps us to be in the serenity of the Buddhi mind when faced with challenging postures of life.

Gomukhāsana

Cow Face Pose

Go means "cow" and *mukha* is face; this is Cow Face Pose. The cow is considered sacred in India. It symbolizes innocence and purity. It is the giver of the life force of milk, and in turn butter, ghee, curds and whey, and cheeses of many varieties. The cow nurtures and placidly gives all of itself, asking nothing in return.

Philosophical Introduction

In the Bhakti tradition of yoga, it is said that the devotee should long for God the way a mother cow longs for her lost calf. The great Indian epic, the Mahābhārata, extols the purity and innocence of the white cow in its opening story about the churning of the ocean of milk. After crystals, gems, and celestials emerge from the swirling waves of the sea, Surabhī the magnificent white cow emerges. Through her milk, she banishes old age, sickness, and death.

Surabhī, the wish-fulfilling cow, arose from the ocean of milk to grant wishes for the devotees who were hungry for knowledge and wisdom. This beautiful creature is said to exist on a subtle level, either within the Soma cakra—a sub-cakra between Ājñā cakra (the brow center) and Sahasrāra (the crown cakra)—or within the Shunya Maṇḍala, the void within the hollow space where the right and left hemispheres of brain meet. This is known as the tenth gate of the body.

Yogins meditated upon Soma cakra to stop the process of aging and remain ever youthful and even immortal while in the body. When the procreative seed of the lower cakras is brought upward to the Soma cakra, it is known as Ūrdhvaretas (*Ūrdhva* is "upward," and *reta* means "stream" or "flow"). Soma, which is associated with the moon, is also known as amṛta, the sought-after nectar of immortality that inspired the story of the churning of the ocean of milk. Resting within the Soma center is the crescent moon of Śiva, which is the source of soma or the nectar of immortality.

In Gomukhāsana, the body assumes a position with one thigh crossed over the other and one arm rising up and dropping behind the back to clasp the bottom hand. The legs, arms, and torso assume the face or head of a cow, but more significantly this pose brings about an emanation of light, like the radiance of Surabhī that shines through the endless grace of giving. Practicing Gomukhāsana removes psychophysiological impediments in the physical and subtle heart.

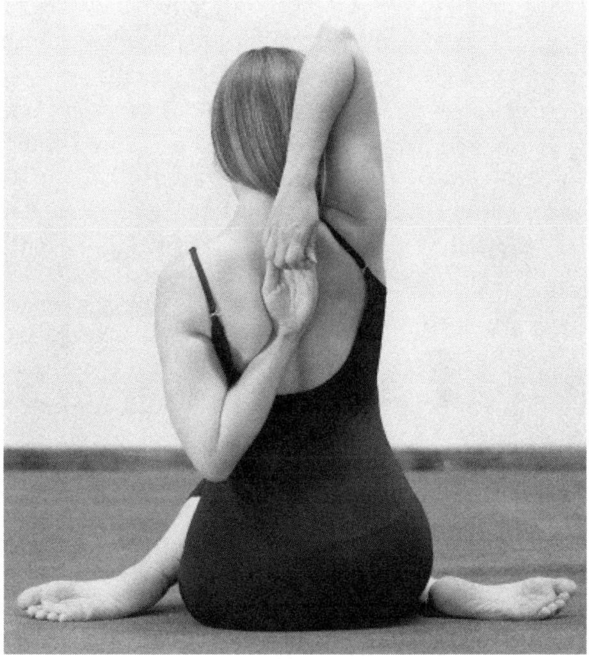

Practicing Gomukhāsana removes impediments in the physical and subtle heart.

It opens the channels for the radiance and effulgent light to flow into Vijñana nāḍī, the subtle correlate to the carotid arteries, which run from the heart through the sides of neck into the brain, and the vagus nerve. In ancient times Vijñana nāḍī was known as the "pathway of shining light." Contemporary neuroscientists refer to the vagus nerve as the "compassion nerve." Its pathways enervate the heart as well as the intestines, viscera, and lungs.

As we release old pockets of hardness from beneath the shoulder blades, we open the rays of light that emanate from the Suṣumnā, the central nāḍī that flows between the heart and the brain. This illumines the mind and heart as we release past emotional blockages. As we allow this effulgent light to flow to the highest gateways of the body, the face takes on a luminous radiance. As we move through past restrictions within the subtle as well as physical heart, it is possible to release past hurts and learn to trust and forgive. In releasing past grievances, there is a lightness to body and mind helping us to feel more youthful, as if we have taken a sip of the nectar of immortality.

Like Surabhī, we all have the potential to become more loving and giving. We are not giving for the sake of getting something in return but for the sake of giving and serving alone. This is the innocence and purity that the white cow represents. The Cow Face Pose relates to the first niyama, *śauca,* which means purity. This is not just purity of body but purity of heart, the purity of being motiveless. As this relates to practicing Gomukhāsana or any āsana, it means that we undertake the practice for its sake alone, not because we are trying to get somewhere or something from the pose.

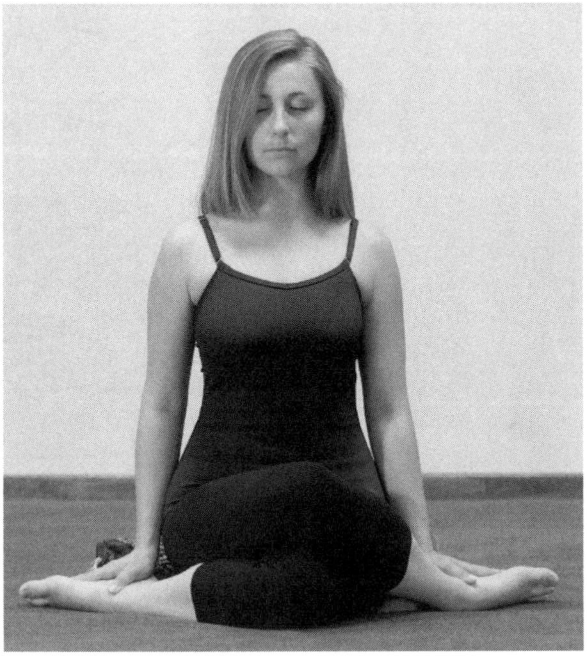

Press on the feet to lift through the spine.

Guidance

1. Begin seated with one thigh crossed over the other. If the hips are tipped back, sit on a folded blanket so that the tops of the hipbones are level with the knees. Fold the legs as tightly as possible. You can sit on the edge of a folded blanket to elevate the hips; the knees are approximately the same height as the pelvic rim.
2. Inhale into the back, rounding it, allowing the head to bow toward the heart center
3. Exhale and bring the back in as if trying to do a backbend.
4. Inhaling, spread the breath as far into the back as possible from shoulders to hips.
5. Exhale and reach the left arm out to the side as far from the sternum as possible.
6. Inhale into the back.
7. Exhaling, bend the left elbow, bringing the arm behind the back with the hand reaching to the back of the heart. Widen the expanse of the clavicle bones as well as the shoulder blades.
8. Inhale, rounding the back with the breath.
9. Exhale and bring the spine into the front of the body like a backbend. Externally rotate the upper left arm to open across the clavicle bone (where the lymphatic fluid drains) and bring the left inner shoulder blade into the heart center at the left side of the spine.
10. Inhale and do nothing; just breathe.
11. Exhaling, bring the right arm up over the head and bend the elbow, taking the forearm behind the back as far as comfortable. Observe: Do the hands touch? If not, gently work with the bottom arm, bringing the hand up the back as far as comfortably possible. If the fingers touch, hold them together. Those who are supple in the shoulder blades may clasp the wrist with the fingers of the other hand.
12. Inhale and exhale, continuing as long as the breath is rhythmic and calm without overdoing or straining. This is very deep emotional work; move slowly, and in your own time. On the inhalations, do nothing. On the exhalations, gently ease yourself deeper into this pose.
13. Release the pose on an exhalation. When you are ready, take the opposite side.

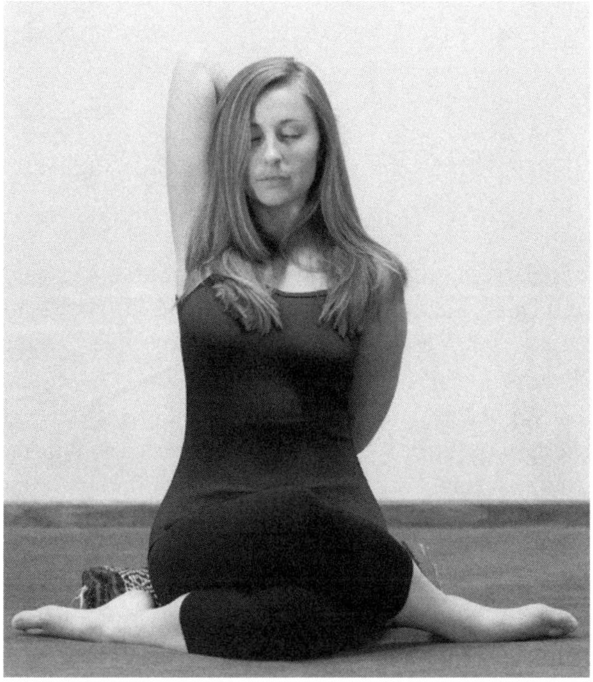

Continue practicing the pose as long as the breath remains rhythmic and calm.

Assist: A teacher or partner can gently press down on the crease of the student's thighs (where the thighs meet the hip joints), which gives the student leverage to elongate by lifting out of the base of the pelvis. As the left elbow bends and the forearm is brought behind the back, the partner can gently rotate the student's upper arm externally. Touch the inner scapula (the edge of the shoulder blade nearest the spine), guiding it forward toward the heart center. The outer edge of the shoulder blade comes back. Lift the skin on the student's inner upper arm and—without strain or effort—let the elbow bend and the forearm release behind the back. Eventually, the upper arm can be brought behind rather than in front of the ear.

Psychophysiological Benefits

On a physical level, Gomukhāsana helps preserve the flexibility of the hips. It is also a marvelous pose for relieving shoulder and neck tension, but most important it opens our physical and subtle heart. Energetically, the position of the legs brings the procreative fluids up to the Soma cakra, a process known as Ūrdhvaretas. The pranic stream of energy that flows downward and outward is in this pose drawn inward and upwards. The position of the arms behind the heart center continues to bring this seed up through the opening channels of the heart center to ride upon the beam of light that radiates out of a pure and open heart.

A healthy heart releases trapped emotions and becomes more loving, tender, and compassionate with one's self and with others. This is a heart that no longer opens to one and shuts to another but radiates its rays in every direction simultaneously, like the rays of the sun. With this opening, it is possible to transcend the limited belief systems of the past and go beyond physical and psychological boundaries. The love that has always been can now shine through and reveal itself. A healthy heart has a beautiful rhythm, like a melody—a heartsong. An unhealthy heart has an unharmonious and discordant sound. Perhaps this is why Anāhata (the heart center) is known as "unstruck sound." The heart's sound is a vibration that already flows within us, a sound produced without friction or disharmony.

Whenever I think of Gomukhāsana, I think of Lord Kṛṣṇa, the playful, mischievous incarnation of Lord Viṣṇu, who maintains and sustains this world. Just as Lord Rāma came to be the example of dharma, Lord Kṛṣṇa, Viṣṇu's later incarnation, is said to have come to this earth plane to teach us love. When the gopis and gopas—the cowherd girls and boys—hear the enchanting sounds of Sri Kṛṣṇa's flute, they drop their milking pails and their staffs, leave their homes, and run toward the sound of the flute. Intoxicated with love of the Lord, they rush to the rendezvous with their beloved. They join hands and together dance the Rasa Līlā, which is the joyful dance of the circle of creation that reminds us of the sweetness of the play of life. Even the cows gather under the night sky, swaying to and fro with the celestial sounds of the flute.

Sant Keshavadas, one of my Bhakti Yoga teachers, once said, "Some of the great Gnani Yogis and Rishis had to be reborn again as gopis and gopas."

"Why," I asked.

He replied, "They had great intellectual wisdom and knowledge, but they came back to learn to open their hearts and love."

How wonderful it would be if we could hollow ourselves like Kṛṣṇa's flute, releasing egoic feelings of separation so that the sounds of creation can be heard flowing through us. As the gopis and gopas join hands and enter into the circle dance of the Rasa Līlā, it is a reminder of the play of life and love in a circle that has no beginning and no end.

Eka Pāda Sālamba Sarvāṅgāsana

One-Legged Supported Shoulderstand

Eka is "one," and *Pāda* refers to a foot, leg, piece, or part. This variation of Sālamba Sarvāṅgāsana is therefore known as the One-Legged Supported Shoulderstand.

Philosophical Introduction

The same philosophy and psychophysiological benefits associated with the Supported Shoulderstand apply to this pose as well. Eka Pāda Sālamba Sarvāṅgāsana is a more advanced extension of Sālamba Sarvāṅgāsana and can be sequenced after Setu Bandhāsana and before Halāsana. This variation is actually a good preparation for Halāsana because it is easier to extend one leg at a time rather than both legs.

Over the years, I discovered that the ways our limbs move and unfurl into a multitude of variations in āsana is like Prakṛti, the primordial śakti or feminine principal of creation. The word *prakṛti* (activity) means "to bring forth doing." In turn, I discovered that there is a seed point or bindu in every pose that remains unmoving, unchanging. This can be compared to Puruṣa ("to fill with the dawn"), the masculine principal of creation, which is that point of stillness that is changeless and eternal. Puruṣa is the remembrance that we are not this body, mind, or passing personality. Rather, we are beyond form; we are Immortal Beings.

In this Eka Pāda Sālamba Sarvāṅgāsana, the upper leg remains stable and thus can be seen as Puruṣa, the substratum of creation that is unchanging, stable, timeless, and eternal. Puruṣa is not subject to evolutionary change and is beyond the evolutionary process. In this pose, the upper leg is still and unmoving, like the proton and neutron within the center of the atom. The movement of the bottom leg can be seen as Prakṛti, and compared to the electron that elliptically whirls a million times a second around the atom's stable nucleus. Like the dancing girl of many veils, Prakṛti, the female śakti, is said to dance and circle around the unchanging center of being. It is said she beguiles us and tempts us in the forgetfulness of our Source.

In practicing variations of an āsana, there is a tendency to get caught up and focus on the part of the body that is moving rather than the part that is stable. In this variation of shoulderstand, if we can hold our focus equally upon both, it brings us into the balance of polarities between the Puruṣa and Prakṛti, the Being and Doing. The variations in this pose help our mind to transcend duality and hold the transcendent light of consciousness within the play of life's polarities. These polarities can be seen in sun and moon, day and night, masculine and feminine, success and failure, compliments and criticisms. As we learn to hold the stable center within this pose, we learn that—even though life's variations may play around us—we can hold to the unchanging center within.

The yantra of this pose can be seen in the perpendicular alignment of the torso and upper leg, which is symbolic of desire, activity, and dynamism as well as of our vertical connection to the Divine. The bottom leg is a diagonal angle that also brings greater dynamism to the sacred geometry of the pose.

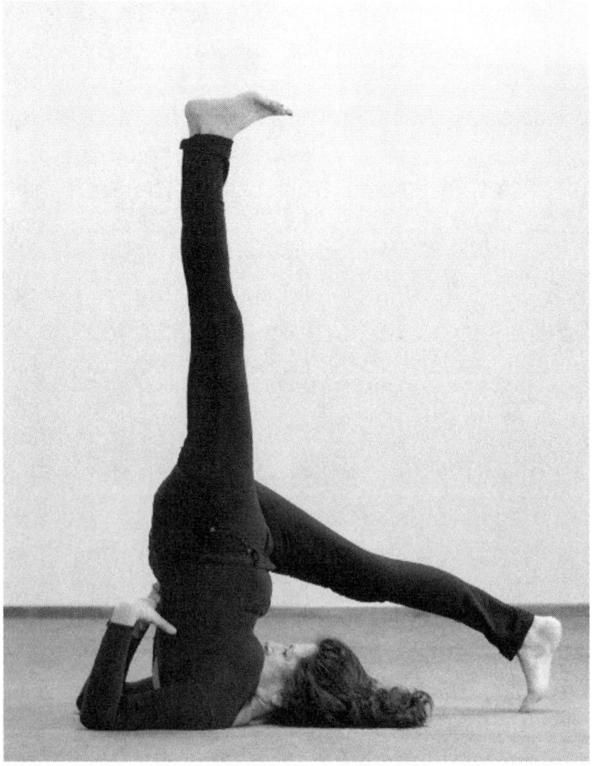

Practicing this variation of the shoulderstand strongly affects the medulla oblongata, the principal entry point of prana.

In this variation of shoulderstand, the medulla oblongata at the base of the skull is affected even more than in Sālamba Sarvāngāsana. The medulla connects the brain with the spinal cord and its nerve roots. All communication between the brain and spine involve tracts that ascend or descend through the medulla. The medulla, measuring only about one inch in length, also contains vital reflex centers, including the cardiovascular, which adjusts the heart rate, the strength of cardiac contractions, and flow of blood through the tissues. The medulla is a respiratory rhythmicity center, setting the pace for movements of breath. The medulla is part of the cerebrospinal system, which controls the entire functioning of the human body as well as the psychic centers. This is an ancient system that is said to develop at conception.

Swami Parāmahansa Yogananda, the founder of the Self-Realization Fellowship, called the medulla the seat of the soul:

> The medulla is the principal point of entry of the life force (prāṇa) into the body; it is the seat of the sixth cerebrospinal center whose function is to receive and direct the incoming flow of cosmic energy. The life force is stored in the seventh center (sahasrāra) in the topmost part of the brain. From that reservoir it is distributed throughout the body. The subtle center at the medulla is the main switch that controls the entrance, storage and distribution of the life force.

Swami Yogananda equated the center or "eye" of the medulla with the third eye of the pineal gland. He said that the pineal and the eye of the medulla are one and the same. It's interesting to note in Sālamba Sarvāngāsana and in this one-legged variation, stability in the pose draws the energy of the pituitary gland (which is attached to the optic nerve), backward and slightly upward to meet with the subtle energy of the pineal gland. Practicing shoulderstand or this variation of shoulderstand seems to unite these two energy fields of the endocrine system—the pituitary and the pineal—which represent polarities.

The pituitary projects its energy forward, and the pineal draws energy into the back of the brain. The pineal is deprived of prāṇa during times when there is more frontal brain stimulation: when using cell phones or computers, or when working late into the night, or when experiencing insomnia. The pineal is benefited each time we close our eyes, especially in āsana. It is the sleep gland that manufactures melatonin. If the pineal is balanced, on a subtle level it draws prāṇa into the back of the head at night and helps us to sleep deeply. The pineal gland seems to correspond to parasympathetic activities, whereas the pituitary corresponds more to the sympathetic ganglia of the autonomic nervous system.

When the pineal gland is activated through this pose, the medulla and the two physical eyes unite in the mystic union of maithuna, and the energy of pituitary and pineal meet in the center of the brain to awaken Ājñā cakra, known as the third eye. In Eka Pāda Sālamba Sarvāngāsana, this can be achieved by concentrating on the point between the two eyes. From the pressure and elongation of the area of the medulla and the pons, the relay center where the spinal cord meets the brain, the two eyes become one. One can then see the medulla reflected as only one light. In the Bible (Matthew 6:22) it says, "If thine eye be single, thy whole body shall be full of light."

In Eka Pāda Sālamba Sarvāngāsana, we experience a bifurcation of consciousness in which we practice dharana, concentration. In this case, the one leg becomes the object and the other leg becomes the subject, and we are the witness in between the two polarities, like the Buddhi, the higher mind that sees differences but does not compare or favor the differences. In this pose, one leg is rising upward, offering to the heavens, and one leg is coming downward, offering itself to the earth. It's a bit like living in both dimensions at the same time. This is like holding two or more perspectives simultaneously, which is helpful in any situation in life. When perspectives differ, we can more easily hold our own center while listening to the perspective of another. This is the essence of Yoga, staying centered in the midst of polarities.

This pose helps us to become inter-dimensional in our consciousness so we can be in two places at the same time while holding the center in the midst of change. When the bottom leg drops, we need to keep our awareness in the upper leg. What happens when we lose the stabilizing point of focus on the upper leg? The upper leg droops, the bottom hip collapses, and the torso and hips come out of alignment. This may indicate how we run our lives. We put our attention on one thing and then lose the focus on another thing. This āsana teaches us to be able to expand the periphery of our consciousness to embrace equally whatever presents itself in our lives.

Guidance

It is recommended that one remain in shoulderstand with calm rhythmic breathing for at least five minutes before taking the variations.

1. Begin in Sālamba Sarvāngāsana, the shoulderstand. Keep the weight to the outer edge of the elbows and keep the torso uplifted on the exhalations for five minutes or more.
2. Exhaling, drop one leg back behind the head, while keeping the other leg steady and stable. Keep the upper leg perpendicular to the earth even if the bottom foot does not touch the floor.
3. Inhale, breathing into the back. This is a time to do nothing but to restore and renew the energy.
4. Exhale and press down with the top of the big toe of the bottom foot to raise the hip of the bottom leg until it is equal to the opposite hip. The hips need to be aligned to hold the center and the physiological balance of the pose.
5. Inhale and do nothing except to observe the incoming breath.
6. Exhale, press down again to lift the hip while relaxing the psoas muscle of the inner groin. Without forcing the stretch, relax and allow any tight areas of the hamstrings and calf muscle to soften and release.
7. Inhaling, breathe into the back.
8. Exhaling, move the spine in like a backbend. Lengthen the front body to be equal to the back body. This equalizes the anterior and posterior nerves of the spine, which in turn equalizes the awareness to the frontal and back brain, the pituitary and pineal glands, the cerebrum (front brain) and the cerebellum (back brain).
9. Inhale and breathe into the back.
10. Exhaling, move the spine in like a backbend, open the inner thigh, and draw the buttock back away from the head. At the same time, lift the bottom hip and the spine upward.
11. Inhale into the back, feeling the breath within the palms of the hands.
12. Exhale and, from the top of the calf, move toward the heel and press down through the tip of the big toe or the ball of the foot to preserve the arch of the foot. As the heel moves back, the buttock moves equally in the opposite direction.
13. Inhaling, breathe into the back.
14. Exhaling, moving the calf toward the heel, keeping the back of the knee neutral and firm, if possible. If necessary, bend the knee to keep the spine straight and the bottom hip (the hip of the lowered leg) in alignment with the top hip.

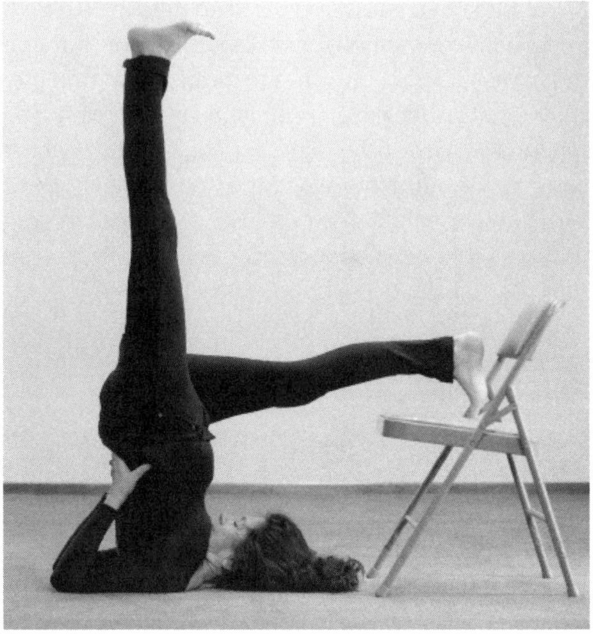

Use a wall or chair to help keep the spine elongated.

15. Inhale, allowing the breath to spread across the spectrum of the entire back.
16. Come out of the pose on an exhalation, raising the upper leg to bring the bottom leg up to meet it. Stay in Sarvāngāsana and breathe before taking the pose to the other side. When you have completed practicing Eka Pāda Sālamba Sarvāngāsana on both sides, exhale and come out of the pose the same way you went into it.

Note: The same principles described above will apply to Halāsana, only with both legs.

Assist: Not everyone can get the foot down to the floor without collapsing the front body. It is important to keep the spine straight and elongated, so it's helpful to place the foot on a block, a chair, or even a wall. Goal orientation (i.e., touching the floor) pulls people out of alignment. Ideally, the big toe of the upper leg aligns with the inner corner of that eye. A teacher or partner can support the student's bottom hip and keep it lifted, helping to give the student a feeling of lightness as she lowers the leg and lengthens the spine on the exhalation, drawing the buttock back away from the head.

Psychophysiological Benefits

One of the greatest gifts yoga has given to the world is the shoulderstand. If we can do only one pose a day, it is recommended that it be the shoulderstand. Sālamba Sarvāṅgāsana and its variations benefit every bodily system and have subtle, unseen correlates to the cakras, koshas, and prāṇas.

One of the greatest benefits of this pose is to keep the thyroid gland in balance. The thyroid is an emotional gland that is impacted by sorrow, grief, and repressed feelings of not expressing or speaking out. It is also affected by electromagnetic fields in the atmosphere. The thyroid produces three major hormones, one of which helps to regulate calcium levels in the blood. The production of thyroid hormones is regulated by the higher gland in the endocrine chain, the pituitary. The thyroid governs a number of important metabolic functions. It accelerates energy consumption and increases oxygen consumption of all tissues. When thyroid functions are depressed, we feel fatigued.

The thyroid also governs carbohydrate metabolism and the assimilation and absorption of glucose from the intestines. There seems to be a relationship between the thyroid and blood sugar, either high (hyperglycemia) or low (hypoglycemia). The thyroid governs the heart rate, which increases when there is hyperthyroidism (an overactive thyroid) and decreases with hypothyroidism (an underactive thyroid).

The shoulderstand and its variations help bring the metabolism into balance. They do not speed up the metabolism, as in backbends, or slow it down, as in forward bends. The shoulderstand balances the metabolic functions of this most important gland that reaches out to affect our entire body, our emotions, and our energy levels.

Eka Pāda Sālamba Sarvāṅgāsana is exceptionally beneficial for the lymphatic system, which cannot pump lymph fluid on its own. In Eka Pāda Sālamba Sarvāṅgāsana, the movement of the legs activates lymphatic flow. Lymph nodes are located throughout the body, even on the outside of the intestinal tract. The movement of the clavicle bones in this āsana affects the lymphatic flow within the chest cavity, lungs, and breasts, helping lymph fluids to drain and circulate.

Cerebrospinal fluid, which normally is pumped upward from the sacrum against the downward gravitation pull, is greatly benefited by the inversion and counter-body leg movement of Eka Pāda Sālamba Sarvāṅgāsana. The sacrum has five vertebrae that fuse at puberty, and the coccyx has four that also fuse at puberty. This fusion seems to protect the essence of the Kuṇḍalinī Śakti or bio nuclear energy within the human system. The movement of the legs in the Eka Pāda variation gently awakens this dormant energy by emulating the action of walking. Combined with the inversion of Sālamba Sarvāṅgāsana, this pose becomes superior to walking for getting the lymph and cerebral spinal fluid to circulate. When we move our legs, we are also decongesting and opening the lungs.

For the same reason, this is also an excellent pose for the heart. This inversion puts no strain upon the heart muscles, and is actually beneficial for the heart. This pose benefits the vagus nerve, a cranial nerve that passes into the carotid sheath, contributing to the innervation of the heart as well as the intestines, viscera, and lungs. A University of California at Berkeley researcher, Dascher Keltner, suggests that the vagus nerve is "a bundle of nerves that are devoted to trust and social connection. When it is activated, it feels like humming vibrations." Thus, researchers now refer to the vagus as the "compassion nerve."

The vagus is the physical correlate to the Vijñana nāḍī, a subtle passageway that runs from the heart to the brain. It is also known as Sūryavara, meaning "to fill with the light of the sun." This passageway can be opened through Sarvāṅgāsana and its variations when consciousness expands beyond the granthi, or knot, of the throat cakra to rise on a ray of effulgent light to Sahasrāra cakra, the uppermost center in the brain.

Sarvāṅgāsana and its variations elongate and compress the carotid sinuses, preventing any undue rise of blood pressure. The carotid sinuses are very sensitive baro-receptors that help to regulate respiration, heart rate, and circulatory pressure. The natural chin lock created in shoulderstand is used in prāṇāyāma retention to engage the parasympathetic nervous system, which dilates rather than constricts blood vessels. The carotid arteries and carotid sinuses are known as consciousness producers. The brain requires a very high amount of oxygen and glucose for its functioning and both are supplied by the carotids. Through āsana and prāṇāyāma, the yogin can regulate his blood pressure and heart rate. In the field of yoga therapy, carotid-stimulating positions are known to help patients with high blood pressure. The stimulation to the carotids also helps to draw consciousness from the external to the internal world.

Trapped emotions can influence our thoughts, create pain, malfunction, and eventual disease. Āsana increases psycho-physiological coherence. When we move closer into the center of a pose such as Sālamba Sarvāṅgāsana, we move closer to the center within ourselves. Through this Eka Pāda variation, we learn to hold that center in the midst of change.

Eka Pāda Sālamba Sarvāṅgāsana can expand awareness and lead the soul back to the Divine through the crown of creation locked in the secret chambers of the human brain. As the highest inner temple of life and mysticism open, they reveal the hidden secrets of the universe where the Ancient One looks into space and there beholds his own image.

Halāsana

The Plough

This āsana, when done as a backbend in the forward bend with the feet turned toward the head and the heels reaching to the earth, looks like a hand plough or *hala.* The hand plough has been used throughout the centuries in many countries and cultures.

Philosophical Introduction

One rainy and stormy night, I sat with other yoga teachers who had gathered before a fire to listen to Sant Keshavadas, a radiant moon-faced saint of India. He told us inspiring stories of kings and demons, princes and warriors, sages and saints. As each story unfurled into the next, yoga poses would come to my mind. During one story from the Rāmāyana, I was reminded of Halāsana, the Plough pose:

King Janaka had no children. He wanted to perform a great fire sacrifice. According to the scriptural injunction, he had to Plough a piece of land with a golden furrow. As he was ploughing, he came across a thousand-petalled lotus in which he found a transcendental baby girl crying, "Om, Om." Because she was discovered while the king was ploughing, she was named Sītā, which means furrow. King Janaka and his kingdom all rejoiced at the manifestation of the Universal Power of God in the form of that divine child. Sages declared her to be the avatar of Lakṣmī, the goddess of prosperity and spouse of Viṣṇu, the maintainer of the Universe.

Sītā grew up hearing the divine discourses given by great masters at the spiritual assembly in her father's court. She became versed in the Vedas and Upaniṣads. When she was five years of age, a miracle happened. King Janaka saw Sītā playing with the time-honored, mighty bow of Lord Śiva. She was lifting and twanging the bow, known as Sunabha, a feat that was impossible even for thousands of strong warriors. This convinced the King and his people that she was Viṣṇu Śakti or the power of Viṣṇu, the stabilizing force of the Universe.

Plough Pose reminds me of this story of Sītā, who became the wife and consort of Lord Rāma. The name Sītā, which means furrow, signifies fertility, or tilling the soil for the seeds of creation to bring forth the new life force.

While in Afghanistan, I had the opportunity to observe a farmer ploughing his small plot of land. His hand plough became a teacher to me, instructing how to align and lift in the pose. The plough was more angular than rounded, a triangle shape with an apex that actually looked like the buttock bone. In the fullest expression of Plough Pose, we find the yantra of a triangle with the tailbone at its apex, and the bindu or seed point in the procreative plexus.

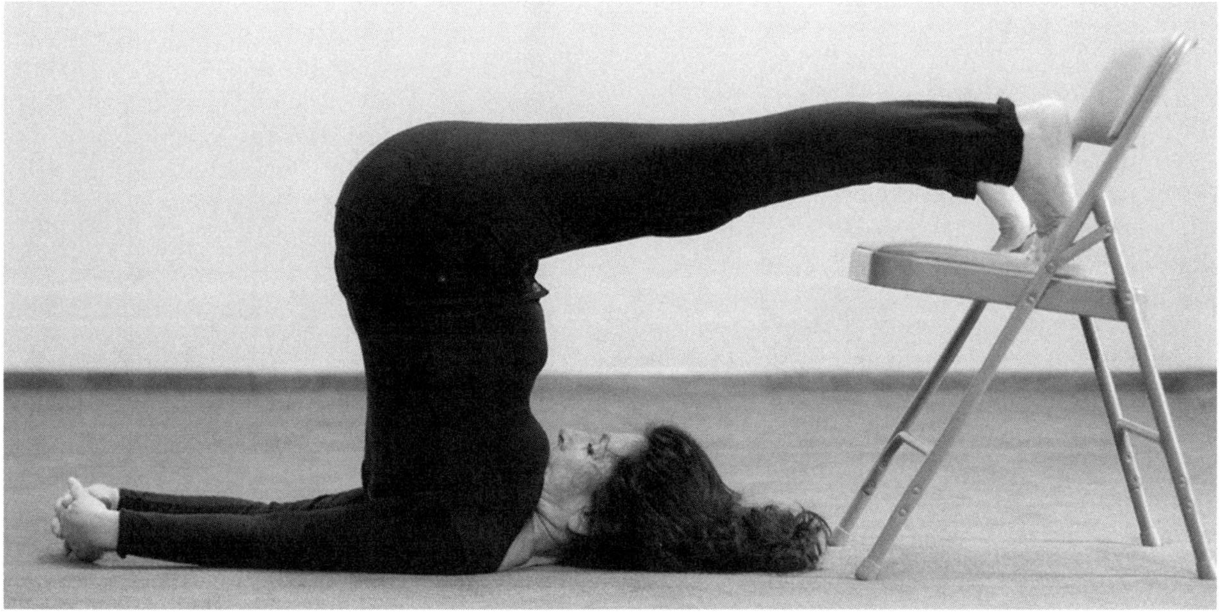

When the hamstrings are tight and the back rounds, use a chair to preserve the elongation of the spine.

Halāsana, in which the tailbone is offering itself to the heaven, aids the seed known as Ūrdhvaretas to rise upward in its transmutation of sexual energy into mental power. This is the ascent from earth's elemental plane at the base cakra into transcendency. As in nature, with the right conditions the seeds we have planted will sprout and bloom, bringing forth a new birth that springs from the elements of earth (the base cakra) and water (second cakra) to rise upward to the Lotus of the Heart. Sītā represents Viṣṇu Śakti, the energy of manifestation and preservation, where energy transforms itself from the procreative to the co-creative plexuses in the upper cakras, where Śiva and Śakti meet.

Practicing Halāsana awakens the fertile parts of our Being in the reproductive plexus. These become like the golden furrows of the earth in which we can plant the seeds that will one day become an out-flowering of the Divine awakening.

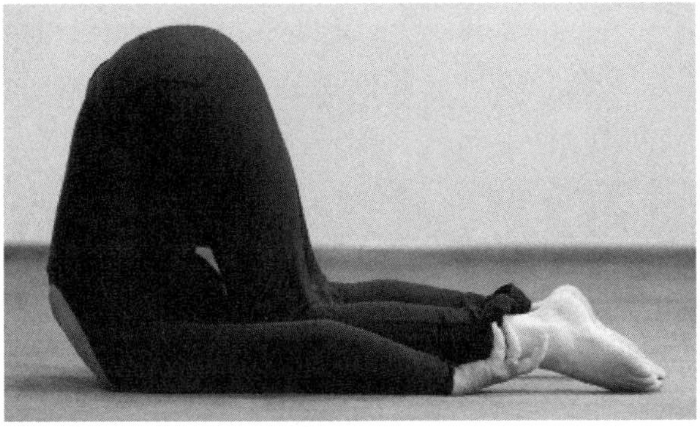

In the variation of Halasana known as Karna Pidasana, we can withdraw from the external to the vast universe within.

Guidance

1. Halāsana usually originates from Sālamba Sarvāngāsana, the shoulderstand. Inhale and use the support of the hands to lift the spine, bringing it in like a backbend.
2. Exhaling, drop one leg down.
3. Inhale and let the breath fill the back from the top of the shoulders to the buttocks.
4. Exhale and drop the upper leg. If the toes touch the floor, press down on the tips of the big toes to lift the spine and move it in as much as possible, as if you are trying to do a backbend.
5. Inhale and relax the head, neck, lower jaw, tongue, and mind. The head is in Śavāsana.
6. Exhale, growing down through the outer edge of the elbows and gradually bringing the hands up toward the center or upper shoulder blades, supporting each side of the spine.
7. Inhale into the back, slightly rounding it with the breath, keeping the relaxation of the head, shoulders, and mind.
8. Exhale and see if the buttock and tailbone will lift toward the heaven as an offering.
9. Inhaling, breathe into the back.
10. Exhale and divide the legs at the knees, moving the calves toward the heels and elongating the Achilles tendon, while at the same time allowing the hamstrings to move from the back of the upper knee toward the buttock.
11. Inhale, bringing the arms up over the head.
12. Exhaling, round the back, stretching the buttocks and legs as far back over the head as possible.
13. Breathe and relax in the pose. When the breath becomes erratic or shallow, the mind is no longer quiet, indicating that it is time to come out of the pose.
14. Exhaling, hold the ankles, keeping the legs as close to the torso as possible as you slowly lower out of the pose, rounding the back and keeping the head on the floor. Do not bring the legs straight down, as this puts strain on the back. Coming out of the pose with straight legs is appropriate only in advanced stages of yoga practice.

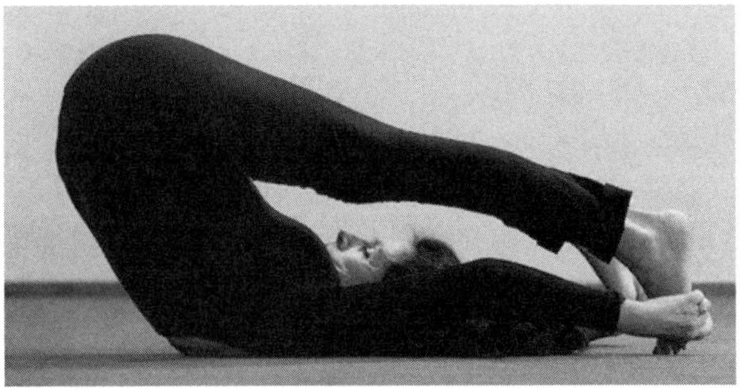

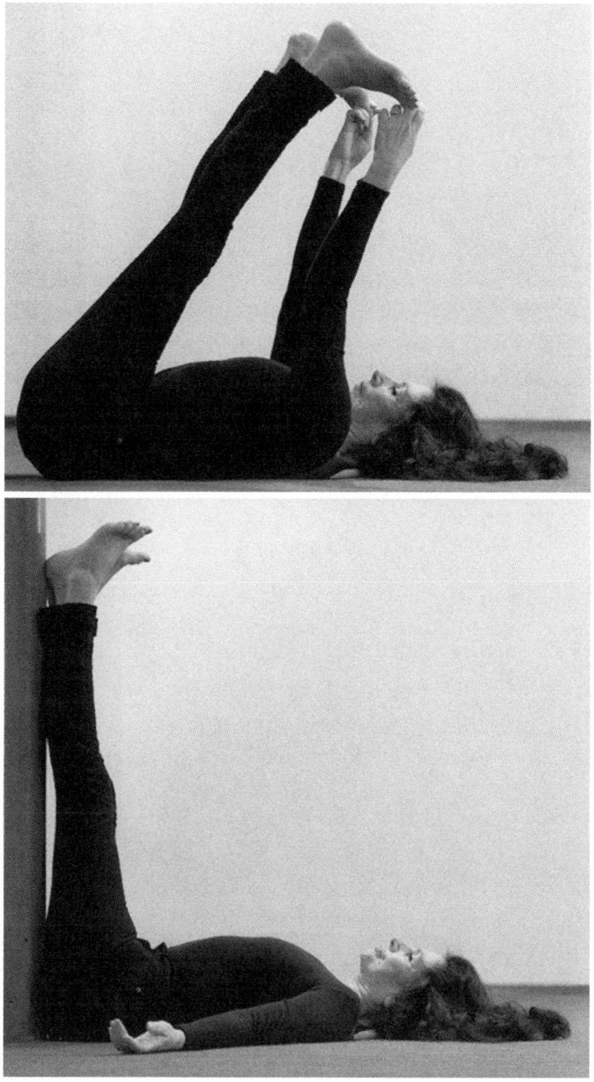

Continue elongating the spine as you come out of Halāsana.

15. Inhale when the hips touch the floor, and then exhale, bending the knees and bringing the feet to the floor. Rest in Śavāsana, observing the breath. With every exhalation, allow the lumbar to rest more and more deeply into the earth.

Assist: Place a chair about an arm's length away from the top of the head. When you are ready, moving from shoulderstand, bring one foot at a time onto the chair. Keep the legs and back straight. Bring the back spine into the front body to strengthen the erector spinae and abdominal muscles. On the exhalations, lift the hips and bring the spine into the front body like a backbend. Instead of using a chair, you can practice with a wall behind the head. Lower the feet to the wall and press them into the surface of the wall to give leverage for the spine to ascend.

A partner or teacher can lift the student's thighs to take pressure off the neck. The partner observes the student's spine, allowing the feet to move toward the floor as long as the spine does not round or collapse.

Psychophysiological Benefits

Like the shoulderstand and its variations, Halāsana elongates the carotid regions of the neck, helping to lower or stabilize blood pressure. As an extension of the shoulderstand, Halāsana has similar benefits, especially to the thyroid and parathyroid, which are responsible for our metabolism and assimilation of calcium. However, Halāsana seems to give even greater stimulation and relaxation to the adrenals and kidney area, and beneficially affects the digestive organs.

In Plough Pose, the lower cakras are lifted above the upper centers, increasing circulation, lymph, and hormonal flow, while opening the heart from the nerve roots and plexuses at the back of the thoracic spine and sacrum. This strengthens and revitalizes the procreative organs that feed the higher cakras, increasing fertility in both male and female practitioners while helping to sublimate sexual energies and bring the energy into the heart, throat, and upper two cakras within the head. Halāsana awakens and balances the procreative forces, distributing them equally throughout the subtle energy centers, bringing luminosity and radiance to the practitioner.

The sacral-occipital alignment in Halāsana stimulates the parasympathetic nervous system, which dilates blood vessels and in turn cools and quiets the brain and neuromuscular system. This cooling and quieting affect can be helpful in reducing constriction and inflammation. Plough Pose and its variations bring the pranic energies of the frontal brain into the back brain, where the entire nervous system can rest. Practicing Half Plough over a chair is excellent for alleviating insomnia and headaches.

While in Halāsana, we can withdraw from the external world to the vast universes within. This is especially so when the knees are bent next to the ears and eyes are closed. This variation is wonderful for preparing the practitioner for pratyāhāra, the withdrawal—or better yet, integration—of the senses.

Dhanurāsana

Bow Pose

Dhanu is the bow, and when I practice Dhanurāsana, I think of the story of Śiva's bow, which gives this āsana great significance.

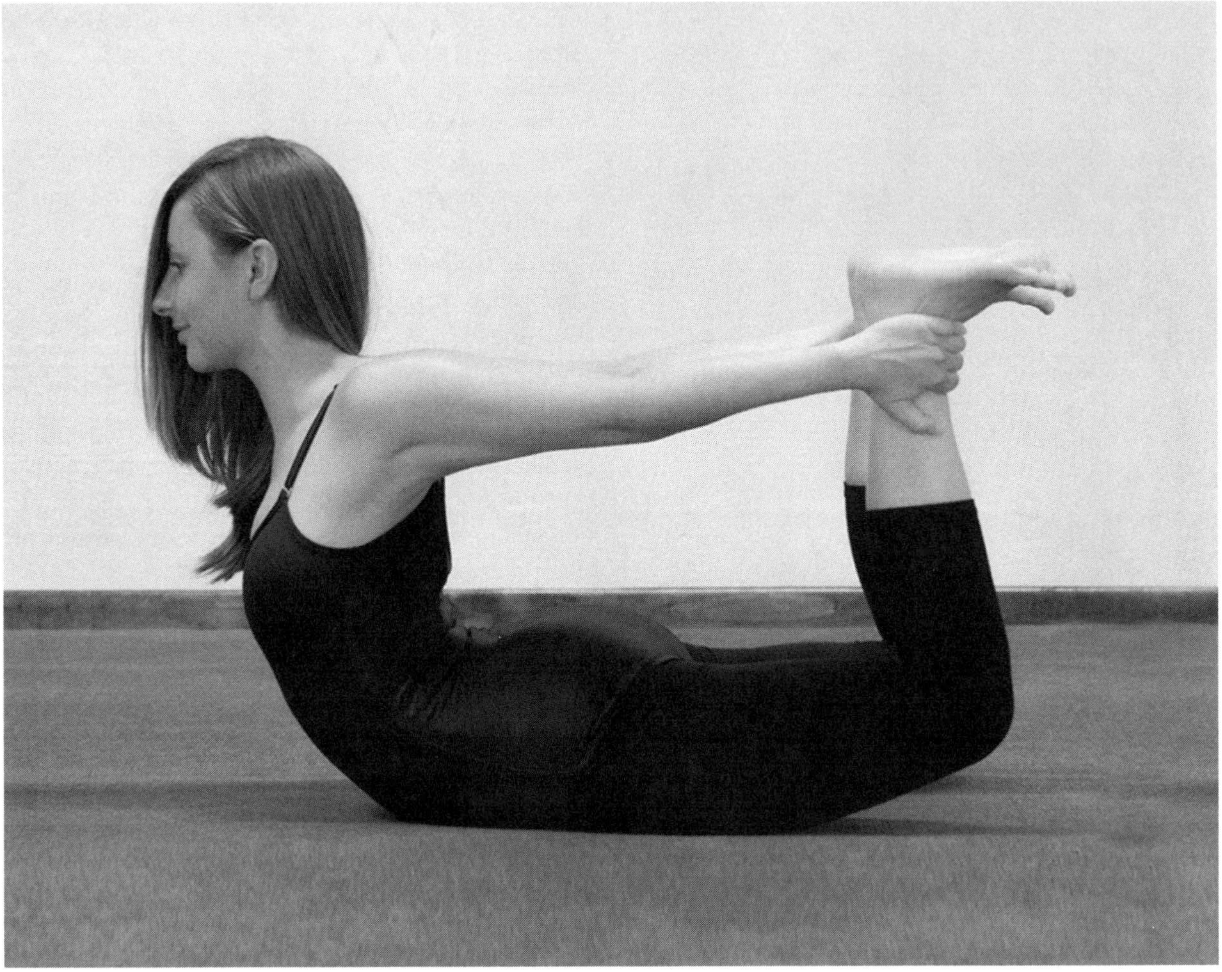

Dhanurasana represents the tension between two polarities.

Philosophical Introduction

One night long ago, several yoga teachers and I gathered for satsaṇg with Sant Keshavadas, one of India's beloved contemporary saints. He told us the story of Śiva's bow from the Rāmāyana: King Janaka of Mithali had a daughter named Sītā, who was renowned on earth and in the celestial realms for her luminous beauty and graceful presence. When she and Rāma, the handsome prince of the kingdom of Ayodhyā, met by chance in the royal gardens, they instantly fell in love.

King Janaka had a bow that originally belonged to Lord Śiva, which neither man nor gods could lift. The King promised his daughter's hand in marriage if the young Prince Rāma could lift and string the bow. On the appointed day, it took five thousand men to drag the bow before Rāma. To everyone's amazement, Rāma lifted the bow with ease. With the strength of the gods, he bent it back into a great arc. When he released the tension of Śiva's bowstring, the sound shook the earth and heavens with a resounding vibration.

Dhanurāsana represents the tension between the two polarities in the body, which are a reflection of the planetary axis. The upper torso and lower pelvis form the arc of the bow, and the arms create the tension and extension between the upper and lower body. If the head and neck elongate out and down, the tension formed with the arms becomes the string of the great bow.

Guidance

1. Begin by lying on the stomach, placing one hand on top of the other and resting the forehead on the hands.
2. Inhaling, bring the breath into the back from the shoulders to the hips
3. Exhale, extending the back of the neck and offering the spine into the front body as if offering the torso into the earth.
4. Inhale into the back, lengthening the neck and spine toward the top of the head as the legs extend out of the hips in the opposite direction.
5. Keep inhaling and exhaling in this way to elongate and give space to each vertebra of the spine before progressing more deeply into the pose.
6. Exhaling, bring the hands under the shoulders with palms down. Draw the spine forward, pushing up into a sphinx position.
7. Inhale, bringing the breath into the back and allowing the breath to round the back. Lengthen the neck as the head drops forward slightly.
8. Exhaling, keep the elbows bent with the forearms on the floor. Pull the belly and rib cage forward as the feet and legs crawl backward, giving greater length to the lumbar and thoracic spine. Keep lengthening the spine on every exhalation, pausing on the inhalations.
9. When ready, exhale and begin to straighten the elbows, coming into a semi Cobra Pose.
10. Inhale and do nothing.
11. Exhale and bend the knees, bringing the heels as close to the hips as possible.
12. Inhale into the back, widening the back horizontally.
13. Exhale, bringing the spine into the front body. Do this without arching the neck. Stretch the back of the neck forward, bringing one hand at a time to the ankles.

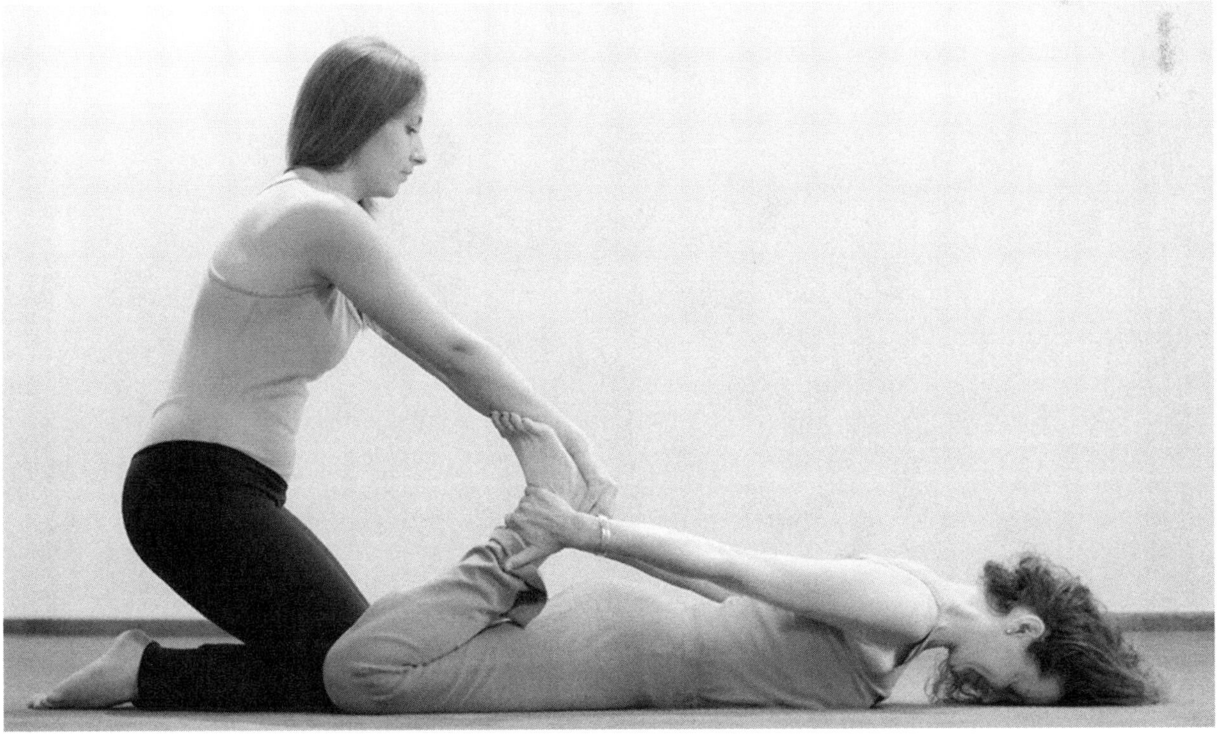

Elongate the neck, keeping the thighs on the floor to prevent lumbar compression.

14. Inhale into the back of the body without lifting the head or arching the neck.
15. Exhaling, keep the knees as close to the floor as possible as you bring the spine into the front of the body, elongating the back of the neck and relaxing the head forward to release neck tension.
16. Inhale, staying where you are in the pose, bringing the breath into the back.
17. Exhale and bring the spine into the front body a little more while drawing the tailbone toward the knees to prevent overarching in the lumbar spine. Try to bend more from the thoracic spine.
18. When ready, come down slowly, release the ankles, and return to the starting position.
19. Let go, breathing in and out and allowing the body to receive the benefits of the pose.
20. Exhaling, move into a counter pose such as the Cat Stretch (page 46), Child's Pose (page 43), or Downward-Facing Dog Pose (page 49).

Assist: If it is impossible to reach the ankles, hold onto a cloth or strap. You can also place a rolled towel or small blanket under the front of the rib cage, which helps to lift the upper torso. A partner can hold the student's heels, drawing her feet back as she keeps the knees on the mat to prevent overarching in the lumbar spine. When your partner is ready to come out of the pose, slowly help lower her down, and then take the feet and ankles, drawing the legs out to elongate the lumbar spine before she takes a counter pose.

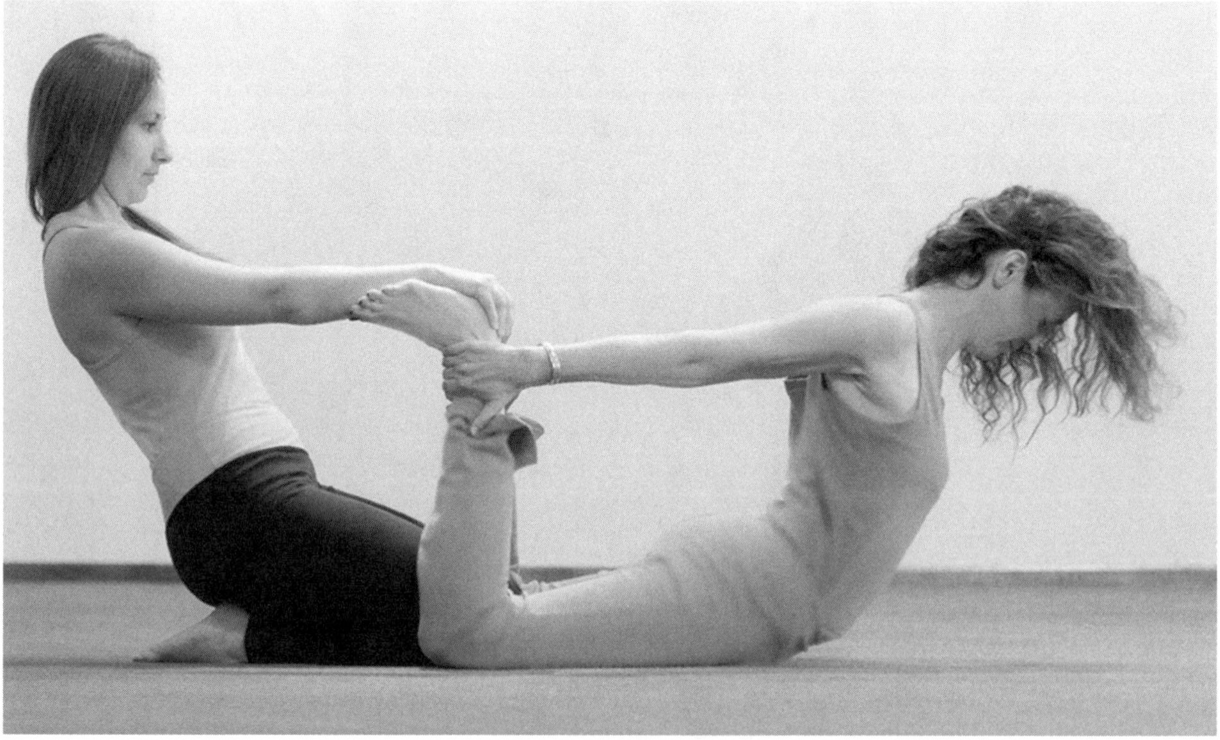

Partner assists, best learned from an experienced teacher, can help students find greater extension and relaxation in asana.

Psychophysiological Benefits

"We are only as young as our spine is flexible" is an oft-repeated phrase in yoga. One of Bow Pose's many physiological benefits is to preserve the health, strength, and flexibility of the spine. The equal arching of the back in Dhanurāsana maintains flexibility of the spinal nerve roots and strengthens the bones of the pelvis. Bow Pose is excellent for lengthening contracted psoas and quadricep muscles and, if done appropriately, it can relieve neck and shoulder tension.

Dhanurāsana is also excellent for preserving the balance and health of the female organs. It strengthens the adrenals and in turn preserves the health of the kidneys. When one rocks back and forth in Dhanurāsana, placing pressure on the abdomen, this stimulates the peristalsis of the small and large intestines.

However, there are subtle and esoteric reasons for practicing this pose. Dhanurāsana helps open the main channel for revelation and realization, the Suṣumnā. This is the central and most important nāḍī or subtle tubular vessel, which correlates to the center of the spinal cord. The ancient yogis believed that suṣumnā is fixed in the heart, forming a point of contact between the soul and the body and marked by the current of subtle feelings flowing up from the heart to the brain. In later texts and teachings, however, suṣumnā was located in the central canal of the spinal cord, the most protected area of the physical as well as subtle body.

Suṣumnā exists on a subtle plane and cannot be seen by the physical eye. Its channel cannot be found in the gross physical body but can only be located and experienced through meditation. It also can be experienced and opened through āsana. To do so, it is important that the breath is coordinated with the pose.

Suṣumnā is associated with the sun (as is the warrior king and archer Lord Rāma), and it is also known as the solar entrance. Like the sun, suṣumnā has innumerable rays, of which one goes directly to the solar region, opening the pathway of experience of the effulgent light that is always within and around us. This open channel clears the way for knowledge of the entire universe. One commentary on the Yoga Sūtras says that because of the similarity of the microcosm and the macrocosm, the suṣumnā and the solar region of the universe are related. Backbending poses, especially Dhanurāsana, are meant to open this channel where the knowledge of the cosmos reveals itself.

Dhanurāsana also reminds me of a passage from Khalil Gibran's *The Prophet*:

> You are the bows from which your children as living arrows are sent forth. The archer sees the mark upon the path as the infinite, and He bends you with His might that His arrows may go swift and far. Let your bending in the archer's hand be for gladness; for even as he loves the arrow that flies, so He loves also the bow that is stable.

Eka Pāda Rājakapotāsana I

King Pigeon Pose

Rāja means "regal" or "king." *Kapota* refers to a capon or pigeon.

Philosophical Introduction

Pigeons can be seen as a nuisance or a blessing. Just as all āsanas represent the spectrum of all creation, the pigeon is a life force that is symbolic of what we as humans can learn. The pigeon's life force can be seen in the prominent uplift of its chest as it struts through public parks with a confident air. A pigeon's heart has not pulled in and down because of hurts of the past. It seems to have no need to protect or close down as it walks lightly upon the earth or takes flight to the sky. What a great lesson the pigeon gives, teaching us to keep our hearts open in all situations. In Rājakapotāsana, we offer our hearts upward to transcend the pains of the past in the remembrance of the light of the Universal love.

Guidance

1. Begin in what is commonly known as "the yogini sitting posture" or Deer Pose, one leg bent with the knee pointing outward (externally rotated) and the other leg turned inward, as in Vīrāsana.
2. Exhaling, bring the Vīrāsana leg back, straightening the knee and leaning forward over the forward bent leg. Place the hands where they are supportive and comfortable, under the shoulders or one hand on top of the other under the forehead.
3. Inhale, bringing the breath into the back of the neck and shoulders.
4. Exhaling, extend the neck out of the shoulders and allow the shoulder blades to offer themselves into the earth.

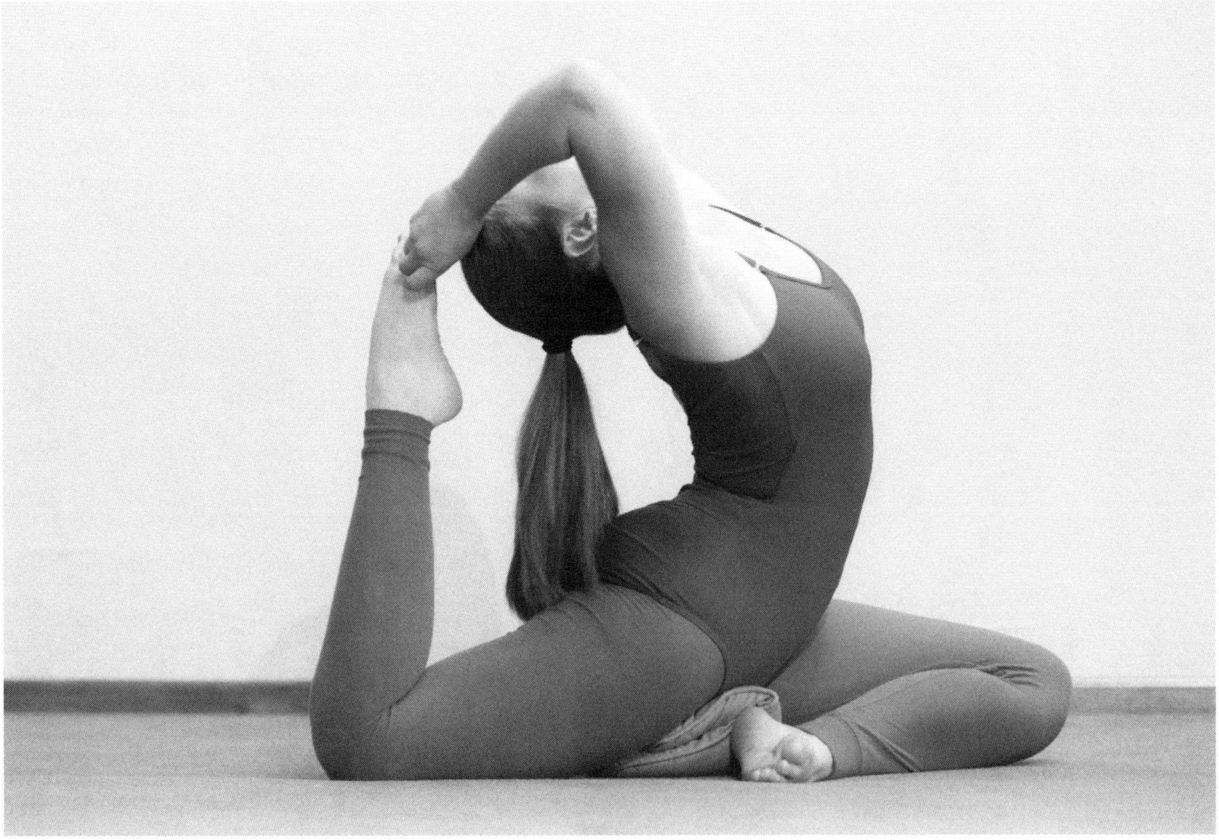

Eka Pāda Rājakapotāsana teaches us to keep our hearts open.

5. Inhaling, bring the breath into the lower area of the ribcage.
6. Exhaling, lift the back ribs toward the head and lengthen the front of the torso, lifting the floating ribs towards the chin.
7. Inhaling, bring the breath from the shoulders to the lower back ribs to the lumbosacral area of the spine.
8. Exhale and lengthen the back leg, turning the toes under and extending the heel to give greater leverage. Can you equalize this backward momentum of the leg with the forward extension of the spine and torso?
9. Inhale into the full spectrum of the back and spine.
10. Exhaling, place the forearms on the floor (as in Sphinx Pose) and slowly bring the spine in as you gradually elongate, coming up into a backbend (as in Cobra Pose). Keep extending the back leg to prevent any compression in the lumbar spine.
11. Inhaling, stay where you are, simply allowing the breath to fill and round the back, relaxing the head and neck.
12. Exhaling, elongate the spine, moving it into the front of the body like a crescent moon. Lengthen the back of the neck without raising the chin. By elongating the back of the neck, compression of the neck is prevented. The pigeon does not raise its head, but the back of its neck is long, upright, and majestic.

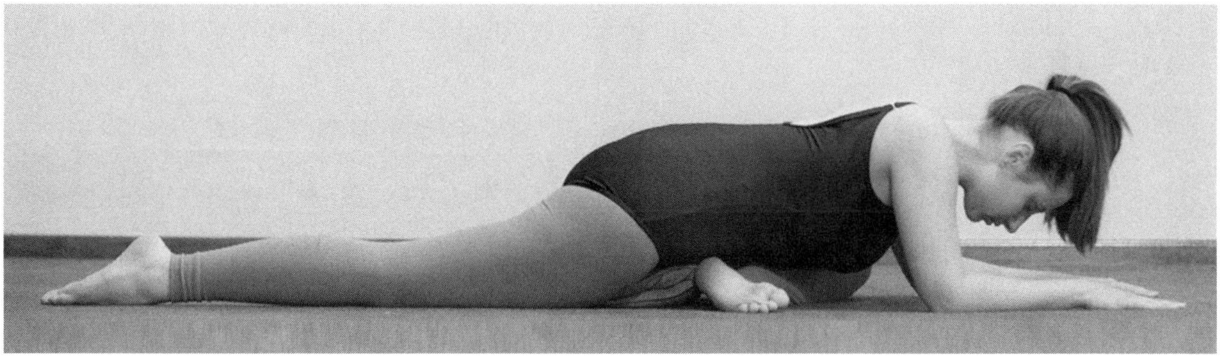

Inhale and exhale with in the arms in Sphinx position to lengthen the spine.

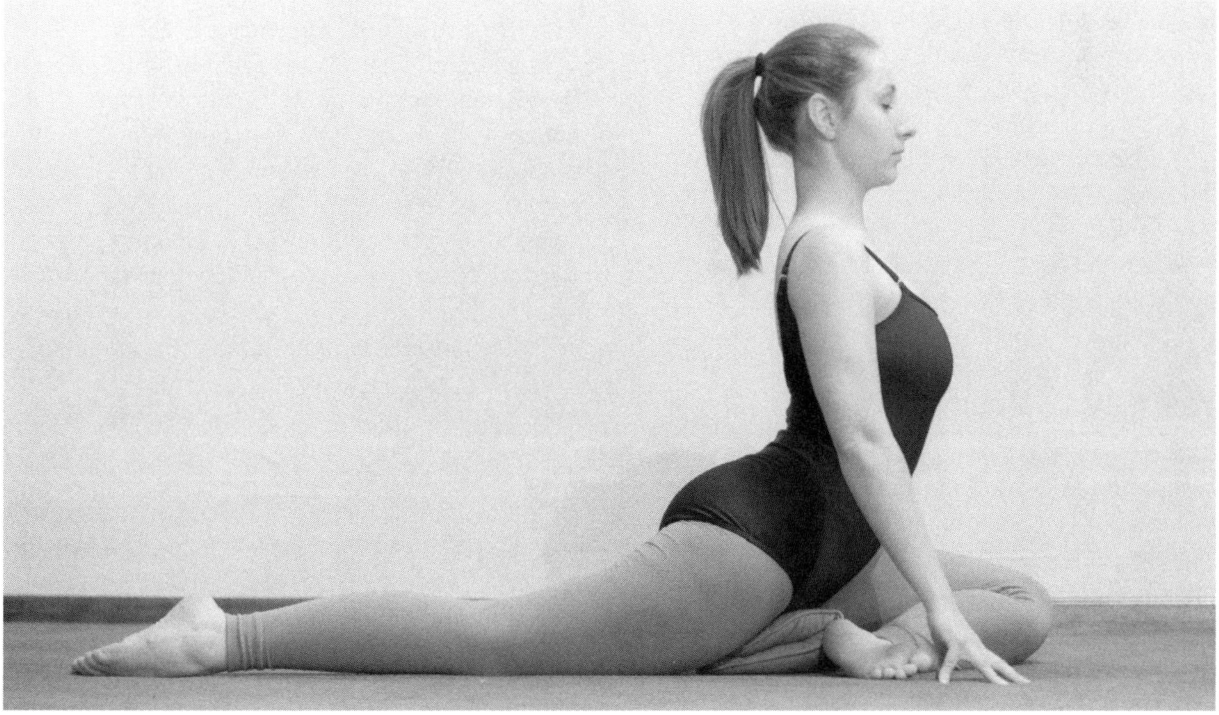

Lengthen the back of the neck while pressing into the fingertips, which emulate the feet of a pigeon.

13. Inhaling, allow the breath to spread throughout the back.
14. Exhaling, elongate the spine by offering the back spine to the front body. Offer the chest and heart center up toward the light, coming up onto the palms of the hands, if possible.
15. Inhale, allowing the breath to fill the back body.
16. Exhale, and if you would like to take the pose a little further, bend the back knee, rotating the upper thigh slightly internally and reaching back with the hand of that same side to clasp the ankle, if possible.
17. When you are ready, slowly come out of the pose the same way you went into it, moving on the exhalations and pausing on the inhalations. Extend the torso out across the forward bent knee, lengthening the spine before slowly rolling to one side. Repeat on the opposite side.

Note: Another way to enter the pose is through Adho Mukha Śvānāsana (Downward-Facing Dog), by stepping one leg forward. To exit Pigeon Pose, step back into Downward-Facing Dog and then go into Cat Pose (Mārjāryāsana) before taking the counterpose of Bālāsana (Baby or Child's Pose).

Assists: Build up a blanket under the hip of the forward bent leg to make the hips level to one another. A partner or teacher can help guide the breath with her hands, first placing her hands on the student's shoulder blades, and then the lower ribs, to increase the intelligence of the breath at these points. Finally, she can move her hands to the student's hips to help make that denser area of the torso more sensitive to the breath. As the āsana progresses and the student's torso begins to rise upward, the partner can gently lengthen the back leg to help release compression in the lumbar area.

Psychophysiological Benefits

Rājakapotāsana is a pose one can do to gain or regain confidence. There is a tendency for people to breathe in a shallow fashion using only the upper and smallest lobes of the lungs. In yoga, there is an emphasis upon breathing into the lower and middle lobes of the lungs, which corresponds to the abdominal and intercostal regions of the torso. It is important when learning the abdominal and intercostal breathing to bring the breath fully into the clavicle region, which fills the upper lobes of the lungs. This in known as the three-part yogic breath, the breath that moves from lower to upper parts of the torso affecting all parts of the lungs. Why limit our breath to only one area? It is okay to give ourselves permission to have it all.

The deeper reason for not breathing fully may be feelings of insecurity or unworthiness to deserve the fullness of what life has to offer. The inability to take in a complete and full breath may reflect one's early upbringing or a conditioning of lack. Limiting the breath may also reflect samskaras or deep psychic impressions that were created out of previous actions—such as vows of poverty, chastity, and humility.

These feelings or impressions may so deeply ingrained that it can be difficult at first to lengthen and extend the spine to create the upliftment that says, "I am worthy and can receive all that life has to give." As we quietly work through emotions and transcend past impressions, this pose reminds us that it's okay to give ourselves permission to "have it all," whatever "all" may mean to each of us.

In the full expression of Rājakapotāsana, the thoracic spine releases and offers itself into the front body, while the heart cakra lifts to the sky. It's as if we take flight, like the pigeon, transcending the old stuck patterns and contractive conditioning that had a gravitational pull on our bodies and our lives.

When bending the spine in Rājakapotāsana, it is important to remember the extension of the back leg to prevent lumbar compression and over-stimulation of the adrenals. As you lift to the light above, maintain awareness of the back leg, reaching it backward to balance the lift of the heart center. The lifting heart represents possibilities of future consciousness, while the back leg represents the past. We don't suppress or ignore the past but extend the leg as far back as possible, bringing the subconscious to the light of the conscious. Here, long-buried impressions can be transformed into a new confidence, filling those empty spaces with the prāṇa of a complete breath.

This pose can create positive changes in one's life. It's interesting to note that military recruits are trained to assume a posture of confidence and strength. Assuming a posture of confidence and strength, whether it's present or not, can create it. To paraphrase Shakespeare, "Assume an attitude, though you have it not, and it soon shall be yours."

Marīcyāsana II

Intermediate Seated Twist

Mārīca was the demon who was converted by fear in the Rāmāyana epic. Throughout the eastern scriptures, demons symbolize the ego, that element that sees and perpetuates separation rather than unification.

Philosophical Introduction

In the story of the Rāmāyana, Mārīca was the son of Tataka the demoness. Mārīca and his family were a threat to the society of holy men, creating havoc amongst the sages and saints by destroying peace in their forest. Together, Mārīca, his mother, and his brother Sabahu plotted to destroy the fire sacrifice that Rāma had planned. (Rāma was an avatar, an incarnation of Viṣṇu come to earth for the destruction of the demons and the protection of the pious.) The demons approached the fire ceremony and tried to pour blood and wine onto the sacrificial altar to make it unholy. They roared like thunder and appeared as different animals to drive away the assembly of sages.

Sabahu tried to kill Rāma, but Rāma's fire arrows reduced him to ashes. Mārīca grieved at the loss of his brother and wanted to retaliate. He showered thousands of arrows upon Rāma, like a swarm of humming bees, but Rāma's arrows covered all directions, dispelling the illusory power of the demon.

Rāma told his brother Lakshmaṇa, "Just a few hours ago, Sage Viśwāmitra taught me a secret mantra for this arrow. It will not kill the demon Mārīca but will toss him across the Seven Seas."

Rāma then launched the arrow, which hit Mārīca and carried him across the seas like a withered leaf on a tempestuous wind. Mārīca fell in a forest in the far of country of Lanka. Here, he built an ashram and meditated on Rāma out of fear. It is said that the fear of God is the beginning of knowledge. This was the beginning of Mārīca's conversion.

This twisting āsana symbolizes Mārīca's conversion or the metamorphosis of consciousness. The spine elongates and makes an evolutionary spiral, awakening consciousness from the egoistic, contracted mind to the expanded macrocosmic mind, where all thoughts are directed toward the Divine.

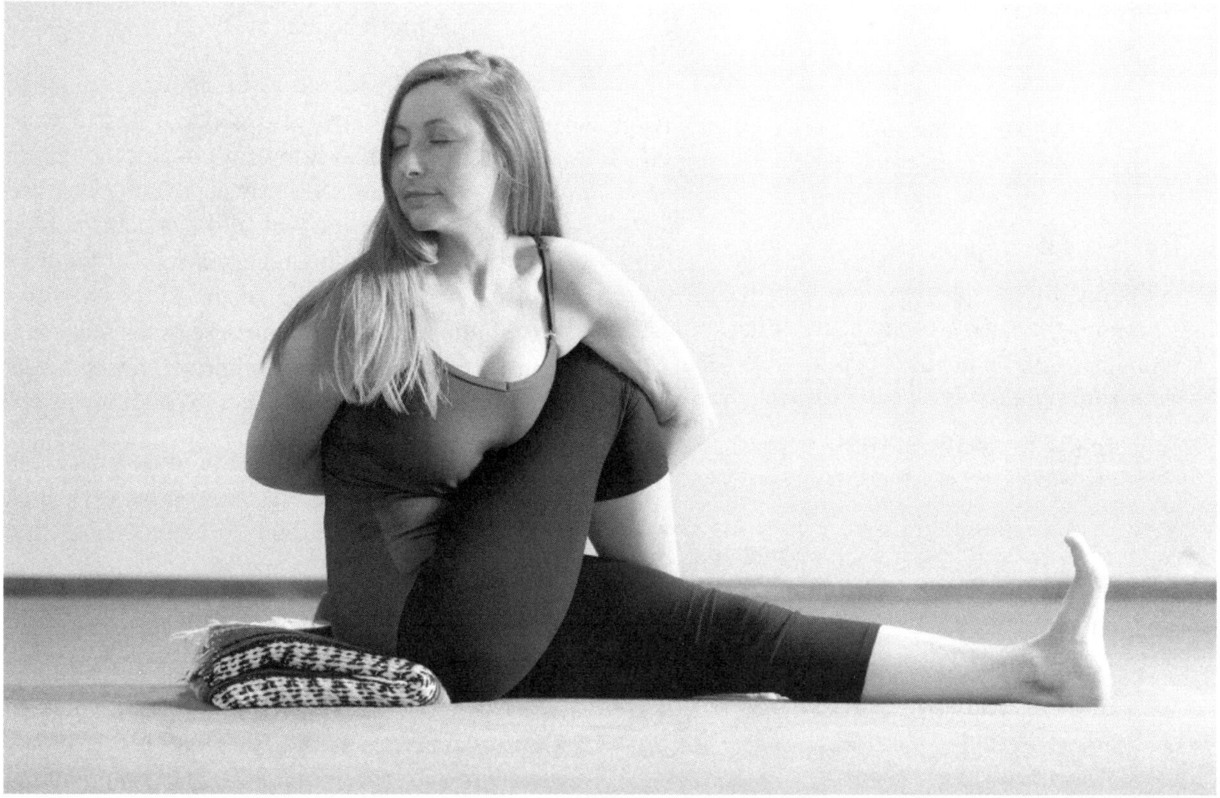

This twisting āsana symbolizes Mārīca's conversion or the metamorphosis of consciousness.

Guidance

1. Begin in Daṇḍāsana or from Marīcyāsana I (see page 129). If necessary, elevate the hips by sitting on a folded blanket. Bend the right knee, bringing the heel into the perineum and holding the hands around the front of the knee to give leverage. Keep the spine elongated and uplifted as much as possible.
2. Inhaling, allow the breath to round the back, lifting the base of the back ribs as much as possible.
3. Exhaling, keep the spine erect as you place the right hand on the floor behind the hips and bring the bent left elbow to the outside of the right (bent) knee. Don't rush into the pose.
4. Inhaling, let the breath round the back, finding new places where the lungs may not yet have experienced the breath.
5. Exhaling, bring the spine in like a backbend, moving the back of the body and the back of the left arm to the front. Press the right hand on the floor to give leverage for this rotation.
6. Inhaling, do nothing.
7. Exhaling, elongate the extended leg from the left side of the pubis all the way to the ankle. Keep the toes facing upward as the knee is lifted.
8. Inhale and allow the breath to round the back organically, moving the breath from the upper regions of the torso to the base.
9. Exhale and see if the body is ready to turn a little more to the right. Rotate the head only when the coccyx, the base of the spine, rotates. Draw the skin down the back and elongate the back of the neck without dropping the chin.
10. Inhale and do nothing.
11. Exhaling, lift the spinal vertebrae to give greater room for the intervertebral disks. If the spine is collapsing and compressing anteriorly, focus on elongation rather than continuing to twist.
12. Inhale and allow the breath to fill the back, rounding it to get more breath into the lungs.
13. Exhale and return to the center, pressing down with your hands upon the bone of the knee to lift the spine gently as you unwind.
14. When you're ready, outstretch the bent leg into Daṇḍāsana. Take time to breathe and elongate before bending the left knee and taking the pose to the other side.

Note: The most important aspect of this pose is to lift and elongate; after that the rotation of the spine will unfold in a gentle and profound way. The rotation comes out of the elongation. The neck does not turn on its own but simply receives the turn of the lower body.

Assist: A partner or teacher can stand behind the student and use the side of her leg to support the student's back. Draw the tops of the student's shoulders down on each exhalation (pausing on the inhalations). The focus of the assist is to help the student elongate the spine.

Psychophysiological Benefits

This pose has all the benefits of its beginning version, Marīcyāsana I (page 129). However, it is a more intense stretch, benefiting the pelvic as well as digestive organs. Done appropriately, with breath awareness and elongation of the spine, twists will strengthen the spinal ligaments, alleviate compression on the disks, and strengthen the nerve sheaths, giving greater emotional as well as physical stability. Marīcyāsana II helps to preserve strength and flexibility of the hips, and releases neck and shoulder tension. This pose is excellent for increasing the muscular peristaltic action of the large intension. When the breath corresponds with each movement and variation, this pose helps to activate and cleanse the liver and in turn benefit the heart.

Twistings are considered to be neutral poses and can be sequenced between backbends and forward bends. Twists are also excellent poses to take after inverted poses. All twists—seated, reclining, or taken as inversions—are excellent for balancing *samāna prāṇa,* the energy in the navel center that controls digestion and the digestive organs. If the twist can be felt all the way down to the base of the pubis and tailbone, it will also regulate *apāna prāṇa*, which is responsible for the elimination of bodily waste.

As the spine rises upward, it signifies the rise in consciousness. Spiraling from front to back, we look into the seat of the back body, which is equated to the subconscious mind. Thus, we fearlessly move from the known to the unknown. This pose is named after a demon who converted all his thoughts upon God. Even though he did so out of fear, he gained wisdom and knowledge and, as in this twist named for him, he made an evolutionary shift in consciousness. Marīchyāsana, like all poses, is a reminder not to destroy the ego but to transform it.

Matsyendrāsana

Lord of the Fishes Pose

Matsyendrāsana is the pose honoring the Lord of the Fish.

Philosophical Introduction

The fish is symbolic of the evolution of humankind. A wonderful story depicts this evolutionary process:

One day many *yugas* (ages) ago, the great Lord Śiva was dictating the Tantra Yoga Śāstras to his consort Pārvatī on the banks of a river. His teachings included a way that the householder—someone with a husband, wife, children, or job—could realize God. This was quite revolutionary at a time when only ascetics sought enlightenment. A fish that happened to be swimming by heard Śiva's profound discourses and became transfixed. (Pārvatī, it is said, fell fast asleep.) Śiva, who saw that the fish was becoming enlightened by these revolutionary scriptures, declared that anything that the fish desired would be his. The boon the fish requested was to become human. Śiva granted him his wish, and the fish moved through the entire evolutionary spectrum of creation. He became known as Matsyendra, or Lord *(indra)* of the Fishes.

Matsyendra is considered to be the first yogi to walk upon the face of the earth. The āsana named in his honor, Matsyendrāsana, is a seated twist. The bent knees and thighs resemble the tail of the fish, and the torso twists upward, symbolizing the evolutionary spiral from human to Godhead. Matsyendra's disciple Goraknatha continued the lineage of the masters of the Natha cult, who were considered to be the shining ones on earth, the Christ-like masters and the most powerful of all lineages. Yogis today speculate that their teachings are the origin of Svātmārāma's teachings, the *Haṭha Yoga Pradīpikā,* meaning a "little light" on Haṭha Yoga, which dates to the fourteenth century.

When sequencing a practice, it is good to do twists after the backbends. But then again, forward bends can help prepare for twisting poses too. Twists can be a bridge between backbends and forward bends or between forward bends and backbends. You can also end a practice with a twist because it's balancing and neutralizing.

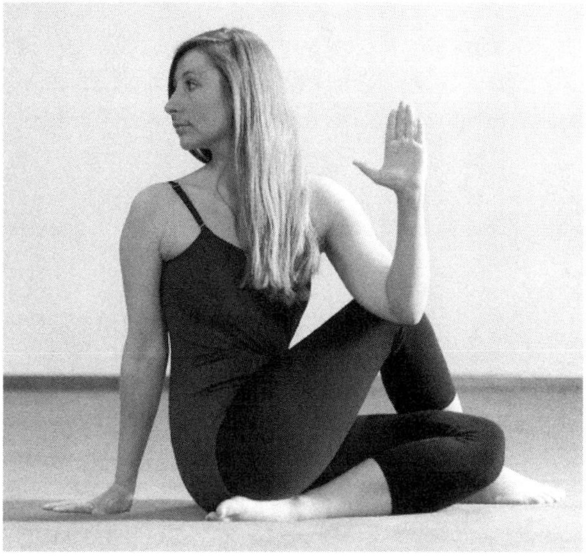

Twists can be a bridge between backbends and forward bends.

Guidance

1. Sit in Vīrāsana.
2. Shift the weight of the hips to the right side.
3. Cross the left leg over the right thigh, placing the foot on the floor.
4. Place both hands on each side of the hips.
5. Exhaling, press the fingertips against the floor to give leverage for each vertebrae of the spine to elongate upwards.
6. Inhale, round the back.
7. Exhale and clasp the hands together in front of the left knee. Use this resistance to elongate both sides of the spine.
8. Inhale into the back.
9. Exhale and bring the spine up and in tooward the front body like a backbend. To strengthen the abdominal muscles and spinal ligaments, stay here with several breaths, getting upliftment of the spine and elongation of the neck.

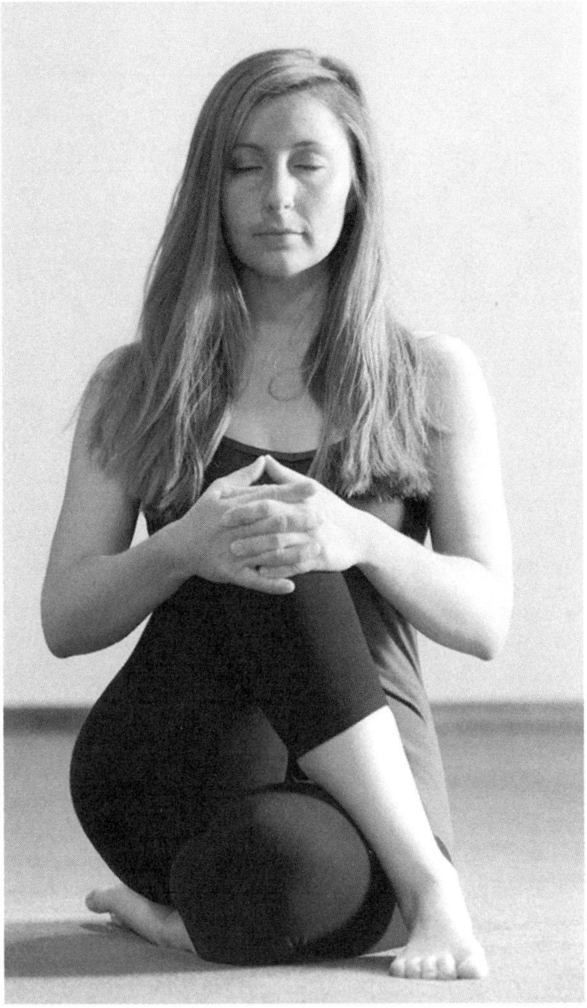

Press the hands into the knee to create leverage to lengthen both sides of the spine.

10. When ready to move forward, exhale and bend the right elbow, bringing it over the bent left knee. Bring the thumb and forefinger of the left hand into the crease of the left thigh; press down to give length between the left hip bone and the flesh of the thigh.
11. Exhale, lifting from the top of the pubic bone to allow the twist of the pose to begin in the pubis and the sacral region of the spine.
12. Inhale and expand horizontally across the back.
13. Exhaling, press the knee against the elbow as the elbow presses back against the outside of the knee.
14. Inhale, bringing the breath down from the upper shoulders to the thoracic and lumbar spine and down into the sacrum, if possible.
15. Exhale, growing down through the tailbone and rising up through the spine. Bring the skin of the back down towards the hips while elongating the neck.
16. On the inhalations, allow the breath to expand organically into the back, rounding it if possible.
17. On the exhalations, grow down through the buttocks as the spine soars upwards. Bring the spine into the front body like a backbend, lifting the heart center. Allow the head to turn, following the spiral movement that begins in the coccyx at the base of the spine. Do not *try* to turn the head, instead, allow it to receive the movement from the base of the spine.
18. Continue as long as the breath flows evenly and equally. When you are ready, come out of the pose the same way you went into it, remembering to breathe with every movement. Repeat on the opposite side.

Assists: Sit on a folded blanket to help elongate the spine. A partner can gently press down with the thumb and forefinger on the crease of the hip. This helps free the diaphragm and in turn the breath, and it helps prevent any compression of the intervertebral disks. A partner or teacher can stand behind the student's back and, on the exhalation, draw the shoulders down and back while gently pressing the side of the knee into the student's spine to draw it up and inward, like a backbend. When the head begins to rotate as a result of the rotation from the base of the spine, a partner can bring his or her hands to the base of the student's ears, drawing the neck and head upward while the shoulders move downward.

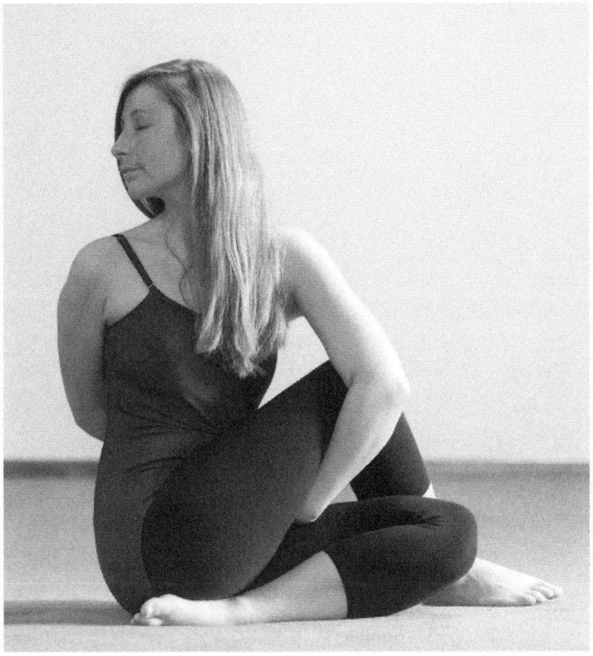

Clasping the hands together, another Matseyendrasana variation.

Psychophysiological Benefits

Whenever a pose twists or revolves—*parivṛtta*—I think of revolving the *vṛttis,* the mind waves. In all of the twisting āsanas, the front brain, or *manas* (the conscious thinking mind), turns around to look into the shadow side of one's self. It looks to the back body, the part that we cannot see with our physical eyes, representing the citta or subconscious mind, as well as the intuition. In any twist, we are taking the conscious mind and turning it to look into the seat of the subconscious.

In the twists, we bring the subconscious up to the conscious levels, and the conscious mind turns to look into the hidden depths of the subconscious. These poses may bring up long-buried memories and dreams as they stimulate Manipūra cakra (the navel center), which is the center of sight and insight. Twists also balance the samāna prāṇa, the flow of energy responsible for digestion, adrenal and kidney function, and the health of the eyes.

As we bring the shadow side to the light, this becomes a pose of transcendence, helping the practitioner to go beyond self-imposed limitations of body, mind, emotions, and spirit. We do this by creating immense space in the midline of the body, which opens neural pathways so that memories embedded at the cellular level can bubble up to the surface where we can transform them. It is best for beginning students to twist while lying on the back until the spinal ligaments and surrounding muscles are strong enough to transcend the gravitational compression of a seated twist.

Parivṛtta Jānu Śirṣāsana

Revolving Head-to-Knee Pose

Parivṛtta means "to revolve around." *Jānu* is knee, and *śirṣ* is the head.

Philosophical Introduction

This wonderful pose combines a forward bend, a backbend, and a twist. It gives all the benefits of Jānu Śirṣāsana, Head-to-Knee Pose, as well as the evolving spiral of the spine that turns the heart center and the face upward to receive the light.

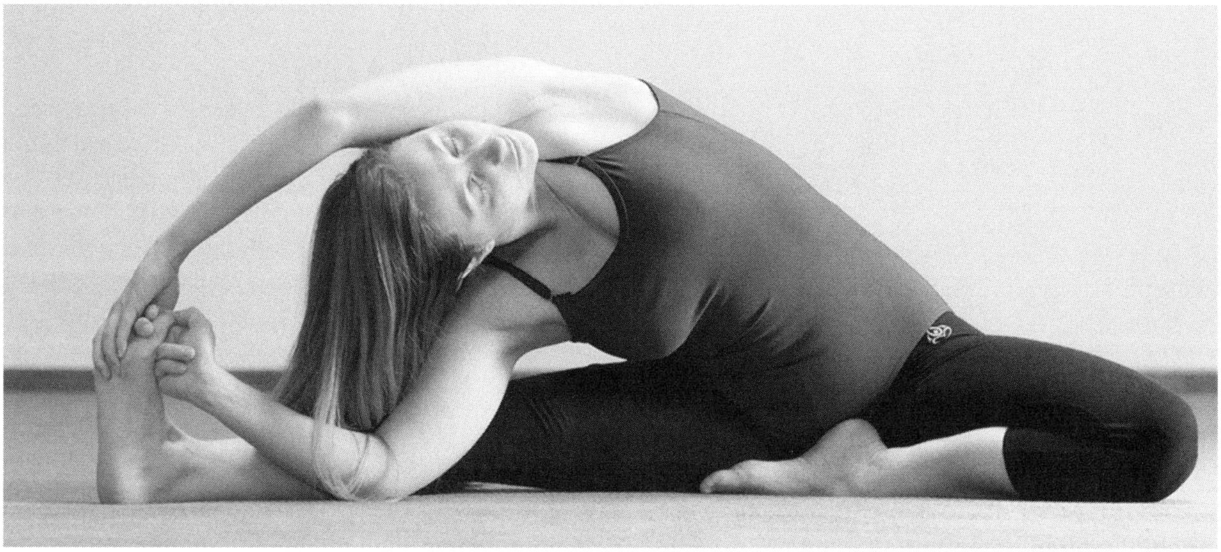

During twists, we turn to look into the hidden depths of the subconscious.

When we stretch and thin the midline and the pelvic plexus of the body, we activate the water element of the second cakra. The spine (like the great mountain that churned the ocean of milk) "stirs the waters" and brings up cellular memory and saṁskāras (deep psychic impressions) from the vaults of the subconscious. In the ancient story of the churning of the ocean of milk, the intent was to find *amṛta,* the nectar of immortality that lay at its bottom. Because this ocean is milky, not clear, one cannot see to its depth. Thus, the story is a metaphor of what lies within the unseen and hidden depths of what we refer to as the subconscious mind. As we clear the impressions embedded in the psyche, the celestial physician appears at last, holding the cup of the moon containing the coveted nectar of immortality. The moon represents the fullness of consciousness, the wholeness of our being. The nectar awakens our awareness to what already is; that we are immortal beings who have forgotten our connection to the Source.

Twists are powerful poses that reawaken our memory of immortality of the soul. They bring up the saṁskāras or latent impressions embedded in the memory vaults of the psyche. As it is said in Yoga, "The invisible must become visible before it can be eradicated" (or transformed).

Guidance

Standing poses help us prepare for the sitting poses by developing elongation of the spine. Otherwise, the tendency in a seated pose is to collapse. In this seated twist, the emphasis is on maintaining a Daṇḍāsana spine, which means to keep the spinal processes moving anteriorly, whether bending forward or twisting. When the spine moves into the center of the body, this prevents anterior compression of the vertebrae.

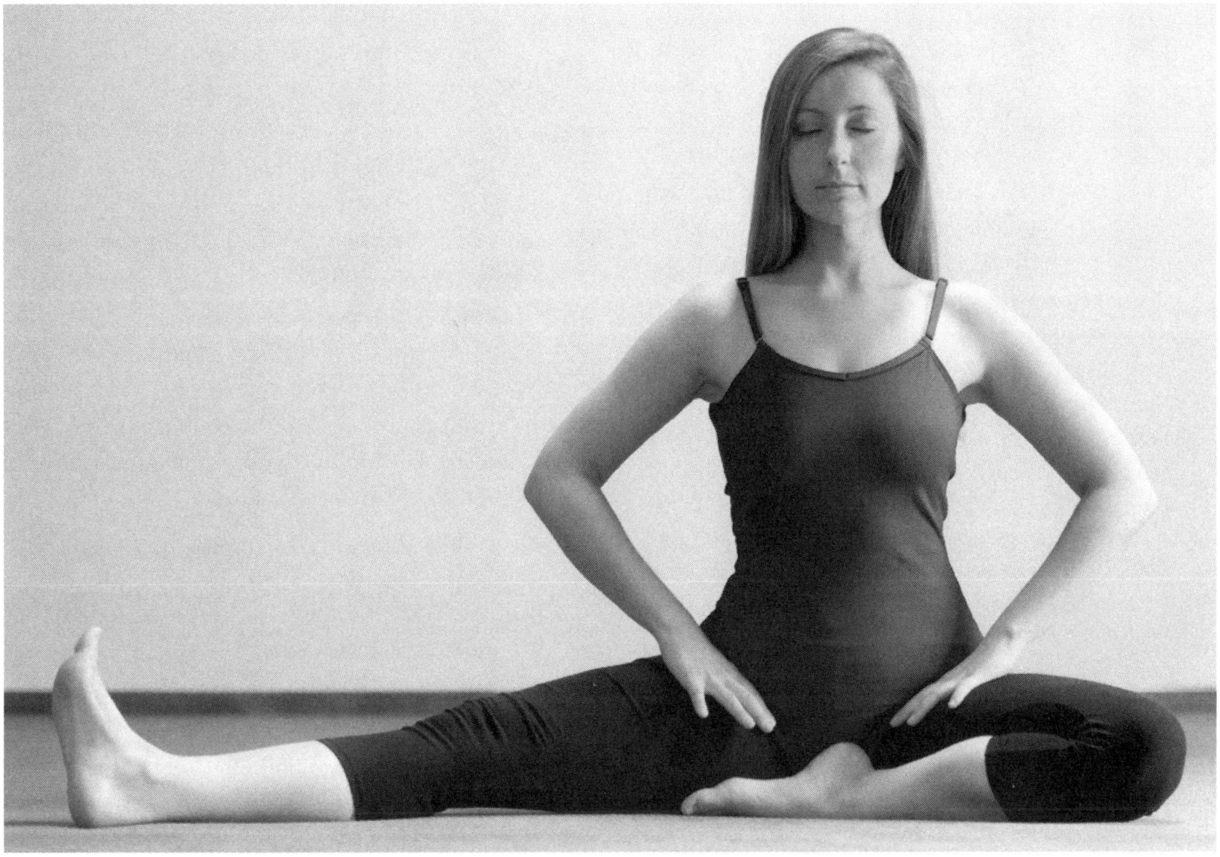

Lengthen from the inner thigh to the inner ankle.

1. Begin in Jānu Śirṣāsana with the right leg bent, bringing the foot as close to the right side of the pubic bone as possible. (Beginning on the right side activates the peristaltic flow of the large intestine, which moves up the ascending colon on the right side of the abdomen.) The left leg is outstretched, lengthening from the inner thigh on the left side of the pubic bone to the inner ankle.
2. Anchor the hip of the bent knee, rotating the thigh externally as the pelvic rim is lifted up and over the thigh of the straight leg. When moving into the pose, the thigh of the extended leg rotates inward as the bent knee thigh rotates outward.
3. Creating lift is essential in order to preserve the evenness of the spine. With every exhalation, as you move deeper into this pose, it's important to keep the front body as long (if not longer) than the back body, as if you are creating a backbend within the forward bend.
4. Emphasize the breath, pausing to inhale into the back. On the exhalations, elongate the spine, moving the navel and torso toward the thigh of the outstretched leg, bending from the hips (not from the waist).
5. Lift and widen the back of the rib cage on the inhalation.
6. Exhaling, continue to lift the lower back ribs, expanding them to the sides, and then lifting the front ribs, freeing the lumbar spine. Keep that lift as you exhale, preserving the opening in the ribcage as you bring the torso down toward the knee.
7. Inhale and continue to widen the back of the rib cage with the breath.
8. Exhaling, lift the tip of the sternum even higher. Imagine that the sternum is being offered to the knees and the diaphragm to the lower thigh. Try to lift the xyphoid process (the tip at the base of the sternum) over the knee as you extend from the top of the pubic bone.
9. Inhaling, expand the back.
10. Lower a little more, if possible, with each exhalation. Or stay on your edge and breathe.

11. We have a tendency to go slack in the inner thigh of the outstretched leg. The inner leg, like the inner arm, represents the subtle body. (The outer represents the physical body.) In this pose and in all others, we want to strengthen the subtle body (the prāṇamaya kośa) as much as the physical body (the annamaya kośa). On an exhalation, grow down from the back of the thighs as if into the earth, giving space for the pelvic rims to lift away from the flesh of the thighs. This lift creates a slight twist over the outstretched leg, freeing the diaphragm, which is attached to the lumbar spine. With the elongation in the lumbar area, the breath opens, and there may be a feeling of being able to stay in the pose comfortably. When the breath is compressed, there is an impatience to come out of the pose.

13. While you stay in the pose and breathe, keep the torso even on both sides. This balances the breath in the right and left nostrils and in turn equalizes the breath in the right and left lungs and balances the right and left hemispheres of the brain.

14. On each exhalation, the shoulder blades and skin of the back move gently down the back away from the ears to lengthen and relax the neck.

15. Keep one hand on the thigh of the bent knee, rolling the thigh back and down as you exhale and lift up out of that side, allowing the lung on the side of the bent knee to descend as the opposite lung ascends.

16. Align the pose so that there is no anterior compression of the spine. On the exhalations, elongate the spine, creating space between the disks of the anterior spine as well as the posterior spine. This increases the circulatory flow and helps preserve the health of the intervertebral disks.

17. Now that the body is in the "perfect" Jānu Śirṣāsana, stay in the depth of the pose as you begin to rotate the spine from the hips and sacrum around to the left, moving on the exhalations. Maintain the elongation of the spine on the bottom side of the torso.

18. On the inhalations, do nothing except breathe into the back and widen the ribs away from the spine.

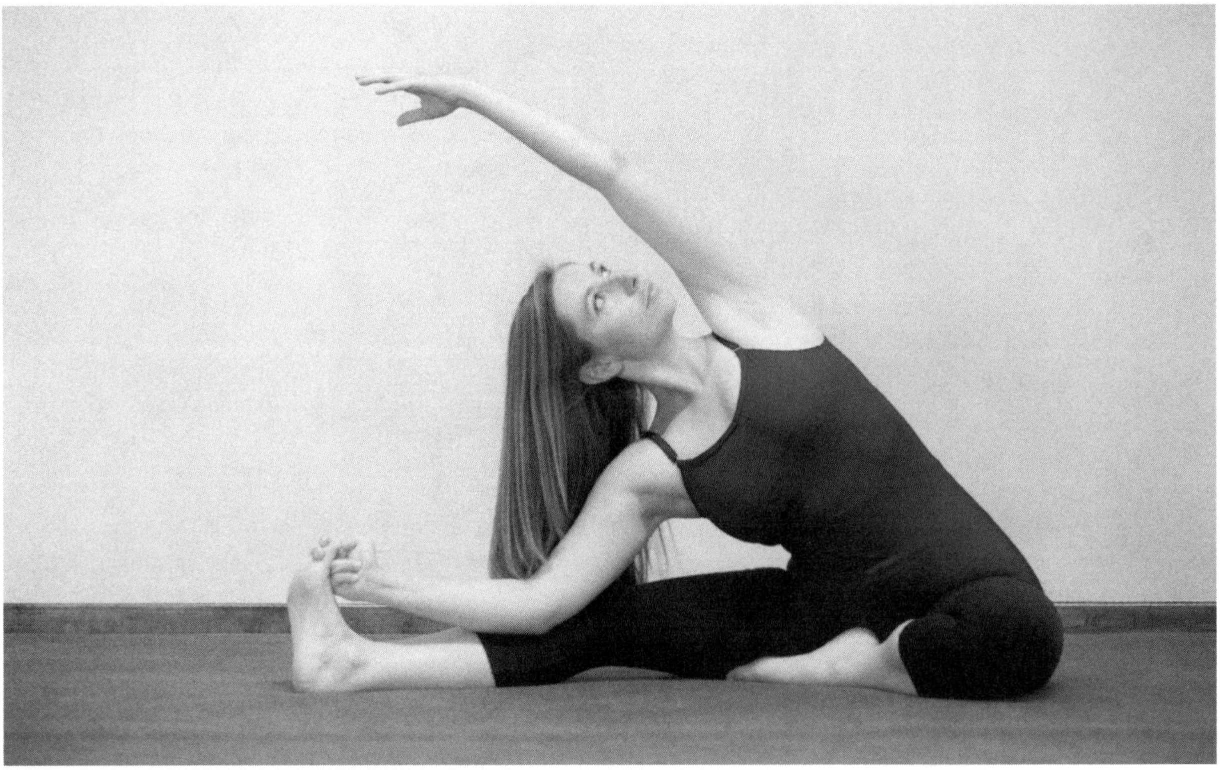

Focus on lengthening the sides of the torso equally as you reach for the foot.

19. Exhaling, continue lengthening the bottom side of the torso, eventually equalizing the extension of the top and bottom ribs, which equalizes the way the breath is processed in both lungs.
20. On the exhalations, bring the spine in like a backbend, moving the thoracic and lumbar spine into the front body while growing down through the backs of both thighs.
21. Do not intentionally turn the head but allow the rotation of the cervical spine to grow organically from the rotation at the base of the spine.
22. On an exhalation, lengthen the neck and move the skin of the upper shoulder down toward the buttocks as you bring the arm to the side of the head. Keep the elbow bent if you notice a tendency to bring the top of the shoulder to the ear (which produces neck tension). Even if the arm does not touch the side of the head, the bent elbow alleviates any neck tension.

Note: The idea is not to "get somewhere" in this pose but to be and to breathe, allowing the breath to rotate the navel, heart center, and face to receive the light of illumination from the solar regions of the universe while you remain deeply connected to the earth.

Assist: Students may use a folded blanket under the buttocks (not the thighs) to help create the lift of the spine. The knee of the bent leg should be lower than the pelvic rim in order to prevent compression of the spine. If the bent knee doesn't reach the floor, it can be supported with blankets. The bottom elbow can rest on the lower thigh just above the kneecap, with the hand facing upward to support the side of the head and allow that side of the neck to elongate. When the neck is relaxed, the lumbar spine and sacrum can more easily release and lengthen.

Psychophysiological Benefits

Parivṛtta Jānu Śīrṣāsana lengthens the hamstring muscles and adductor muscles of the inner thigh. Like Jānu Śīrṣāsana, this āsana releases neck tension if it is entered with the breath. The spine is stretched, increasing the intervertebral circulatory flow, which helps prevent disk degeneration.

This pose helps release excessive fluid buildup in the sacrum and pelvis. The lymph system in the pelvic area can become coagulated because of excessive sitting and compression. When the circulation is sluggish, stagnant blood can build up in the pelvic region or in the uterine area in women.

Parivṛtta Jānu Śīrṣāsana aids elimination by stimulating peristalsis through the natural massage to the abdominal organs: the ascending, descending, and transverse colon, the appendix, the procreative and reproductive organs, including the ovaries and prostate gland.

When it is practiced by focusing on breathing and elongating the spine, Parivṛtta Jānu Śīrṣāsana helps alleviate many back conditions. Through its particular stretch to the side and back of the body, it benefits the liver, spleen, gallbladder, and stomach, as well as the kidneys and adrenals that perch on top like little nightcaps. This is a wonderful pose for releasing neck tension, while preserving the flexibility of the hips and youthfulness of the spine. It impacts the subtle as well as physical body through its potential to relax the solar plexus and open the heart cakra.

In sequencing a practice, twists are a bridge between backbends and forward bends or between forward bends and backbends. You can also end a practice with a twist because it's balancing and neutralizing. Parivṛtta Jānu Śīrṣāsana activates the autonomic nervous system through the parasympathetic nerves that come off the sacral and cervical spine. And when bringing the spine into the front body on the exhalations, the pose becomes a backbend, and the bend in the thoracic and lumbar spine stimulate the sympathetic nervous system. As the spine moves in an evolutionary spiral, it can at times feel as if the life force of prāṇa is spiraling upward from the lower to upper cakras.

Parivṛtta Jānu Śīrṣāsana is a graceful reminder of Patañjali's Sūtra on āsana (II:47): "It is through relaxation of effort and meditation on the infinite that āsana is perfected."

Vīrāsana

Hero's Pose

Supta Vīrāsana

Reclining Hero's Pose

Supta means "to recline." *Vīra* is loosely defined as "hero." In the Warrior Pose (Vīrabhadrāsana), vira is energy, fortitude, and stamina, the qualities equated with a hero. However, this Sanskrit root implies much more. *Vīra* is also known as enthusiasm leading to sustained effort (*tapas*). In the Yoga Sūtra commentaries, it has been said "where there is Śraddhā (faith) there is Vīrya. Both relate to the attainment of Kaivalya, the state of liberation. When the mind in meditation is tired and wants to drift to a different subject, the power which one has to bring it back to devotional practice is Vīrya."

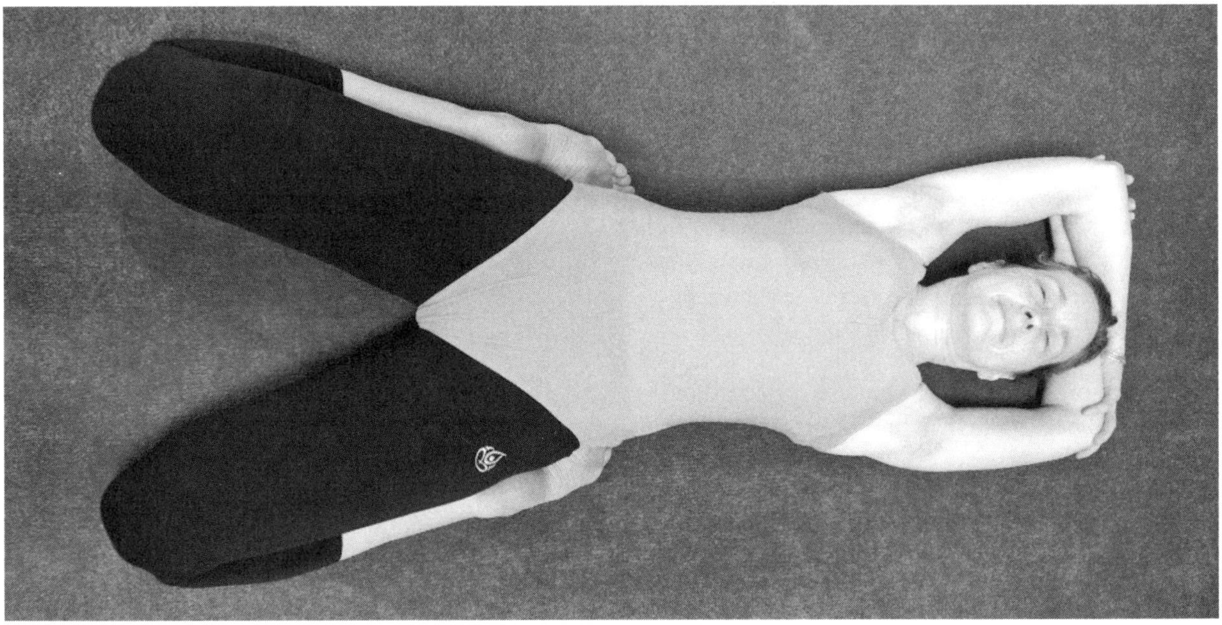

Supta Vīrāsana impacts the parasympathetic nerves, making it an excellent pose for hypertension and sleep disorders.

Philosophical Introduction

Vīrāsana is related to Vīrabhadrāsana, the pose of the warrior. Both poses symbolize unwavering faith, stability, and steadfast concentration. They also give bravery. Bravery in this sense does not mean fearlessness, but having the courage to face one's fears. Instead of turning away from fears, one develops the courage to face them, humbly facing into the wind and the storms of life rather than recoiling or retreating. Like Vīrabhadrāsana, Vīrāsana creates balance and steadiness with alertness and a 360-degree of peripheral vision of whatever situations may arise within life. In Vīrāsana, as a peaceful warrior, we learn not to react but to act with dispassion, compassion, and equanimity in all of life's situations.

In yoga, it is believed that if we have no reverential faith in our objectives, we cannot apply any energy to attain them. When the mind gets fixed repeatedly on a subject, it leads to concentration, which brings forth wisdom and knowledge. In the DhammaPāda, Lord Buddha said that all sorrows can be cured through good conduct, reverential faith, enthusiasm, concentration, and correct knowledge.

Yogis who adopt the tranquility of mind that is experienced through reverential faith are sustained and supported like a child in the arms of a loving mother. This kind of faith gives the seeker an energy that makes the mind undisturbed and conducive to concentration. In such a mind dawns the light of discriminative knowledge, where the Yogin begins to understand the real nature of things. We sit in Vīrāsana to steady the body as a vehicle for steadying the mind.

Guidance

1. To sit in Vīrāsana, bend the knees; the shins are at the sides of the hips, the thighs internally rotated. Relax the buttocks (the gluteous maximus muscles) and elongate the spine, offering the heart center up towards the light of the heavens. Use a blanket under the hips if necessary. Balance the weight under both right and left hips to balance the twin hemispheres of the brain.
2. Place the fingertips on the floor, bend the elbows back, and press down to create leverage to lengthen the spine on each exhalation.
3. If you can keep the length of the spine and the openness of the heart, then turn the palms up, resting the backs of the hands on the thighs. Join the thumbs and forefingers as a way of recycling the pranic energy that flows through the fingertips back into the body.
4. Inhaling, spread the awareness of the breath across the back body from shoulder to hips.
5. Exhaling, elongate the spine, lifting the base and top of the sternum toward the head while keeping the length of the lumbar spine.
6. Continue breathing slowly and deeply on the inhalations and exhalations.

Supta Vīrāsana

1. When you feel ready to progress from Vīrāsana to Supta Vīrāsana, exhale and lean back, bringing the elbows and forearms to the floor behind you.

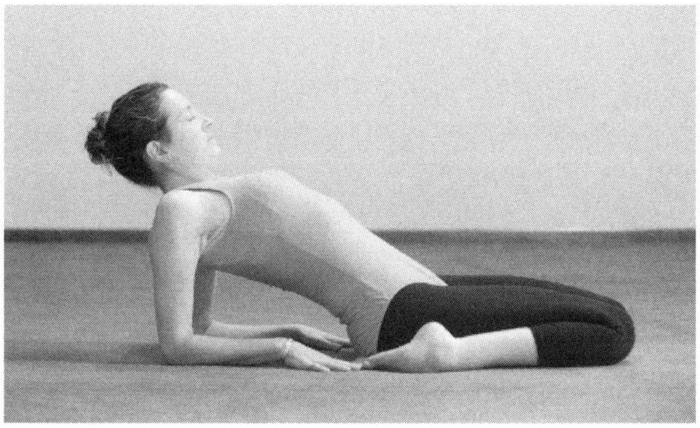

2. Inhale and do nothing except breathe into the back, focusing especially on the sacrum and lumbar area.
3. Exhaling, lift the hips gently from the floor, offering up from the base of the pubis without dropping the vīrya of the heart center. Lengthen the lumbar by bringing the muscles of the right and left buttocks together, which lifts and lengthens the psoas muscles.
4. Inhale and stay in this position while organically rounding the back with the breath.
5. Exhaling, bring the spine into the heart center like a backbend, lengthening the back of the neck.

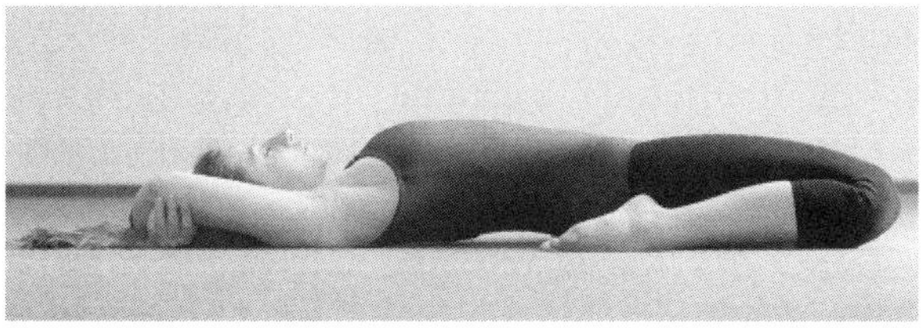

6. Continue proceeding in this way, inhaling as a way to re-center the mind in the pose, and exhaling to lift and offer the heart, as well as the base of the pelvis, to the heavens. Bringing the heart and pelvis up simultaneously preserves the length of the lumbar.
7. If it is right for you, use the exhalation to lower yourself more deeply into the pose. Are you in svadharma? Go only to the point that is right for you, letting the breath be your gauge. As long as the breath is slow, powerful, and deep, see if the body will allow you to move more deeply into the pose. If the breath changes, becomes rapid, shallow, or erratic, stop and evaluate. Is the breath telling you to wait at this point and not proceed further? If you have gone a little too far, back off your edge, find your calm and easy breath, and then, on the next exhalation, see if there is space within you to ease a little more deeply into the pose.
8. Using your breath, come out of the pose the same way you went in.

Assists: Place a blanket under the hips to prevent strain on the knees. Build the blanket up until any medial pressure is relieved. In Supta Vīrāsana, place a bolster or a stack of blankets for the shoulders and back of the head to rest upon. When the upper body is at rest, excessive contraction of the thigh muscles can release.

Partners can assist students in the reclining position. As the student exhales, the partner can place both hands at the back of the hips to give greater length to the lumbar area and release the psoas muscles. A partner can also lengthen the back of the neck, which helps to release the lower back and gives greater stimulation to the parasympathetic nerves, which dilate, cool, calm, and relaxe the system.

Psychophysiological Benefits

As one proceeds cautiously in Vīrāsana and Supta Vīrāsana, and the thighs rotate internally, the nerve plexus in the sacrum is activated. The plexus of nerves that come off the five fused vertebra of the sacrum and the four fused vertebra of the coccyx (tailbone) is part of the parasympathetic nervous system. The parasympathetic nerves stimulate digestive fluids and the eliminative functions of the body. Supta Vīrāsana in particular impacts the parasympathetic nerves that stem from the sacrum and coccyx as well as the neck, making it an excellent pose for hypertension and sleep disorders. Both Vīrāsana and Supta Vīrāsana are excellent preparation for backbends. They alleviate neck tension and can be used after the Headstand.

Practicing Vīrāsana helps to balance the cross-legged sitting poses, in which the external rotation of the thighs can tighten the gluteus maximus (buttock) muscles. Vīrāsana requires the opening and expanding of the buttock muscles. When the buttocks are squeezed together briefly during Supta Vīrāsana, there is an opening of the psoas muscles and the base (not the top) of the pubis rises to the light of the heavens. When the floor of the pelvis is "offered up," the heart center is also offered to the heavens. This creates greater length in the lumbar area, which in turn lengthens the psoas muscles and the quadriceps of the thighs.

The gradual opening and lengthening of the psoas muscles can bring up long-stored emotions, which helps to free the mind and the emotions stored in this area. This helps open the channels for spiritual remembrance or for the awakening of the psycho-nuclear energy within the human system that is a microcosm of the Universal macrocosm.

Practicing the Hero Poses also gives the steadiness of mind to face situations we have avoided in the past. All poses with the root *vīra* or *vīrya* in their names represent the inner peaceful warrior. We may not be fearless, but like the warrior, we have the courage to face our fears.

Triang Mukha Eka Pāda Paścimottānāsana

The Three-Limbed Forward Bend

The name of this pose tells us how to assume it. *Tri* is three and *ang* is limb. *Eka* is one and *Pāda* is piece or little part, like the foot. Pāda also refers to a chapter—as in the Pādas of the Yoga Sūtras. Paścimottānāsana is the pose of the stretch of the backside of the body, which refers to the setting sun, one of the eight directions that is portrayed by yantra. Triang Mukha Eka Pāda Paścimottānāsana is a derivation of Paścimottānāsana, with an intense stretch of the back body and the face moving to one limb. Triang (three limbs) are showing: the first limb is the thigh of the leg that is folded back, and the other two are the upper and lower parts of the extended leg. Mukha, the face, extends over the eka Pāda (one foot or piece), which is the extended leg.

Philosophical Introduction

In Indian mythology, there is a presiding deity for each direction. This side of the setting sun is where darkness falls and we cannot see. We cannot visibly perceive our back body without a reflection. Therefore, as Mr. B.K.S. Iyengar would say, "We have to retire within ourselves and there we will 'feel' the back body." It is the intuitive side of our being and is said to be one of the directions that is ruled by the gods and goddesses of the ten-sided Universe, the direction known as *paścima.* The pose invokes the Lord of the West, the light or agni of the setting sun.

In this pose, we are humbling the head, the symbol of ego, to the lower limb. As the back is exposed to the light of the heaven, we receive knowledge directly through the back brain or cerebellum as a holographic intuitive feeling. When we are in this state, we don't have to sift through sequential concepts or ideas trying to deduce them logically. Instead, knowledge may arise holistically as a symbol, a vision, a feeling, or a sense of knowing.

This back brain stimulation can also be felt in Paścimottānāsana, in which both legs are extended, and in Jānu Śirṣāsana, in which one leg is bent out to the side and the other is straight.

The Triang Mukha Eka Pāda forward bend may be more difficult for some, and it requires a little more "letting go" with self observation. Again, it is important not to go beyond your Sva Dharma, but to move, breathe, and stay on your edge, and at times, even back off your edge.

Like all forward bends, Triang Mukha Eka Pāda Paścimottānāsana is a humbling pose in that we offer the self. This is the fifth niyama, Īśvara Praṇidhāna, surrender to Self or to the Lord of the Universe. Forward bends are wonderful poses to practice breathing and letting go even when you may reach an obstacle of pain. Do not plunge through the obstacle but honor it, breathe into it, and circumambulate the nucleus of the pain, releasing any tension or armoring that has

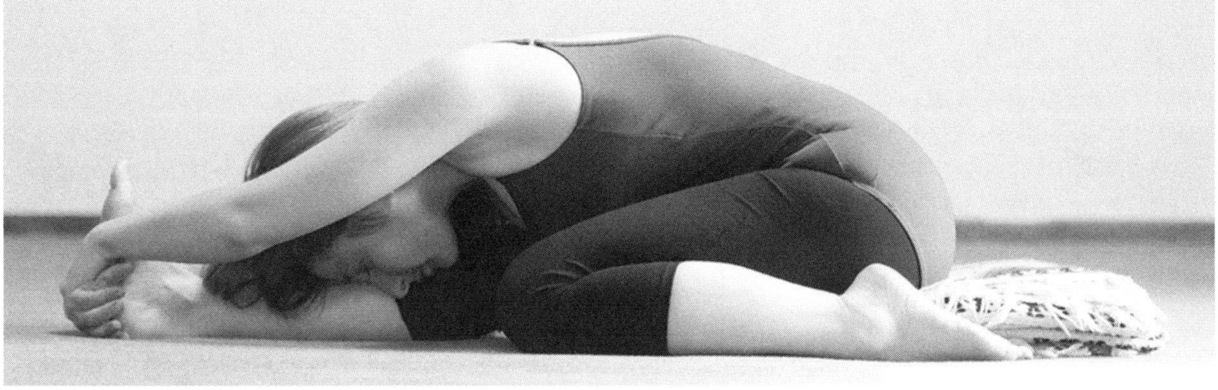

In forward bends, we practice breathing and letting go, not plunging through an obstacle but honoring the body's ability.

been used to protect its tender center. Slowly move in this way, honoring your body's ability.

Close your eyes to alleviate any goal orientation. There is nowhere to go; you are already there. There is no goal in this pose, only to be and to breathe and to become one with the Eternal Cosmic Vibration. This is the definition of āsana.

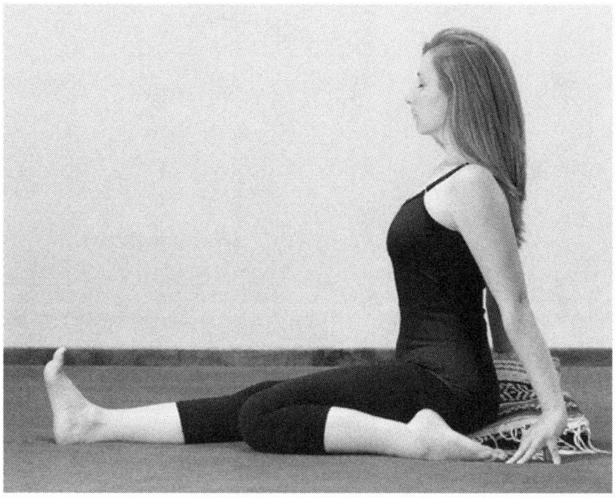

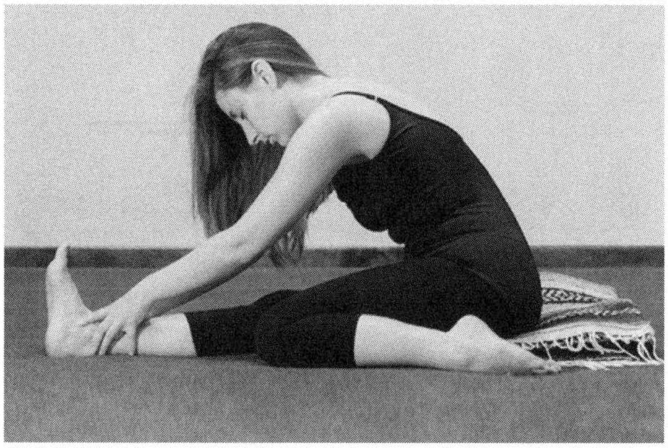

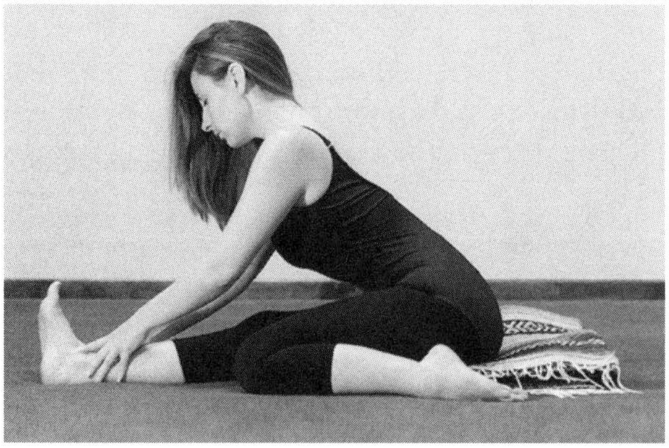

From a strong foundation with the thigh internally rotated, move breath by breath, expanding on the inhalations, lengthening on the exhalations.

Guidance

1. Begin in Daṇḍāsana. Fold one leg back, rotating the thigh internally.
2. Place the hands on the floor beside the hips.
3. Inhaling, breathe into the back, allowing the breath to round the back organically.
4. Exhaling, press down with the hands, and draw the skin of the shoulders down as the neck elongates upward to the base of the skull. (Do not compress the neck.) As the exhalation continues, elongate the spine upwards toward the head, moving it slightly in as if in a backbend.
5. Inhaling, keep the lift and elongation while breathing into the back, rounding it again.
6. Exhaling, lift even higher, pressing down with the hands, bending the elbows back, and opening the chest.
7. It may be enough for some to inhale and exhale in this seated position, without taking the pose deeper.
8. Exhale and lift out of the hips, elongate the spine, and offer the navel over the extended leg.
9. Inhaling, stay where you are and breathe into the back, rounding it. (Remember to relax the neck.)
10. Exhaling, see if it is possible to press down with the hands and lift, elongating the spine and opening the heart center a little more as the navel center comes closer to the thigh of the extended leg.
11. Inhale, allowing the breath to round the back from shoulders to hips.
12. Continue exploring the pose with each outgoing breath, moving only to your edge. See if you can bring the torso close to the leg and place the hands on the calf, ankle, or sides of the foot. Bend and raise the elbows up to release any tension in the neck.
13. Inhaling, offer the spine to the heavens and to the Lord of the West.
14. Exhale and allow the spine and upper torso to surrender to the lower limb. Closing the eyes helps draw the prāṇa of the eyes backward. This stimulates the cerebellum, the back brain, which is activated by the "setting sun."
15. When you are ready, inhale, rounding the back to lift up and come out of the pose.
16. Exhaling, elongate the spine and slowly straighten the bent leg, returning to Daṇḍāsana.

Note: This pose transitions well with Krauñcāsana (page 208). After returning to Daṇḍāsana, you may continue on the same side with Krauñcāsana. When lowering out of Krauñcāsana, go back to Triang Mukha Eka Pāda Paścimottānāsana. Usually, it is possible go a little deeper into this pose on the second repetition. Return to Daṇḍāsana before practicing Triang Mukha Eka Pāda Paścimottānāsana and Krauñcāsana on the opposite side.

Psychophysiological Benefits

This pose is similar to Jānu Śirṣāsana, but instead of bending the knee out to the side with the foot near the perineum, this time the bent leg is in a Vīrāsana position. Through the internal rotation of the thigh, this position stimulates the parasympathetic nervous system and has a cooling and calming effect as it aids in digestion and elimination. The pose affects the ascending, transverse, and descending colon. Because of its effect upon the back brain and the pineal gland, the gland that stores melatonin, this pose helps alleviate insomnia as well as what is now called "restless leg syndrome."

It is important to keep both sides of the torso as equal as possible, for this balances the breath in both lungs. This is experienced when the breath flows through both nostrils equally, and this in turn balances the twin hemispheres of the brain.

Whether the name of this pose can be pronounced or not, it doesn't matter. Eventually the pose becomes more comfortable, and we begin to feel it as a surrender beyond whatever has held us back in the past. The root *tan* in Paścimottānāsana means "to stretch and go beyond past limitations." These self-imposed limitations will show up as discomfort when trying to move more deeply in the pose. Go only to your edge, breathe, and see if there is space to release a little more.

Often, this pose brings up psychic imprints more often than the other forward bend poses do. It teaches us to allow repressed emotions to bubble to the surface, and to know our momentary edge. This edge becomes the Guru or teacher that gives gentle reminders not to plunge through the pain that arises, but to allow it to reveal the source of the self-imposed limitation. Yoga does not create anything but only reveals what is already there.

Krauñcāsana

Heron Pose

Krauñca, according to the Indian scriptures known as the Purāṇa, is the fifth of the seven Dvīpas. A dvīpa is a continent, island, place, or plane of existence.

Philosophical Introduction

Krauñca, a mountain, has vistas that spread like wild mustard seeds and is surrounded by seven seas. One is of salt water, while the others taste of sugar cane juice, wine, butter, curds, cream, and milk. It is said that in this Dvīpa dwell the virtuous devas or heavenly beings and humans after their death.

In this Dvīpa, there was once an asura (a contractive force) named Krauñca. He was aimlessly wandering the world when Sage Agastya began praying to Lord Śiva. Śiva appeared and granted him a boon. The sage wanted help in creating a holy place in Bhuloka, a plane of existence between heaven and earth. Śiva agreed but upon the sage's return, Krauñca mischievously blocked his way by assuming the form of a mountain and making it rain heavily.

The sage lost his way and roamed the forests for a very long while. Eventually, he understood what had happened, and he cursed Krauñca to remain forever in the form of a mountain. This legendary mountain may be the one the Mahābhārata refers to as Mahā (great) Krauñca. This mountain in the Himalayas was said to be a mine of all kinds of gems, which are symbolic of gems of wisdom and insight into things that cannot be seen with the physical eye.

A unique feature of Mahā Krauñca is its elliptical shape with a diametric narrow pass. According to legend, this gap was created by Kartikeya (also known as SubRāmaniyam), who was the son of Śiva and the brother of the elephant god Gaṇeśa. It is said that Kartikeya pierced the mountain with his mighty sphere in a battle with the Demoness Tharaka, who was hiding inside. In Krauñcāsana, the body assumes the shape of the two sides of the mountain. The mountain's central gap can be seen as the space between the upward leg and the torso and head.

According to ancient scripture, swans, vultures, cranes, and herons would fly out of Krauñca on their journey to Meru, the central axis of the planetary mountains. Krauñca is also the Sanskrit name for the heron. Herons are birds of the marshlands and shallow waters. They have long thin legs, long necks, and sharp bills. In the Mahābhārata, the Kauravas used a military formation based on a pattern resembling a heron's flight. When the heron flies, its head is folded back in a flat S-shaped loop, which is symbolic of an internalization of consciousness, even in action.

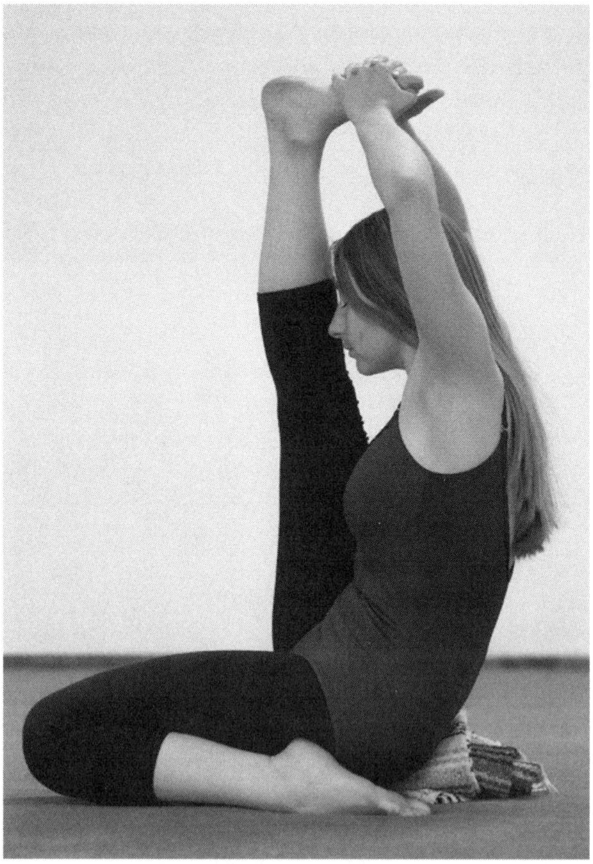

Krauñcāsana lengthens the hamstrings and calf muscles, where we have a tendency to hold knots of emotion.

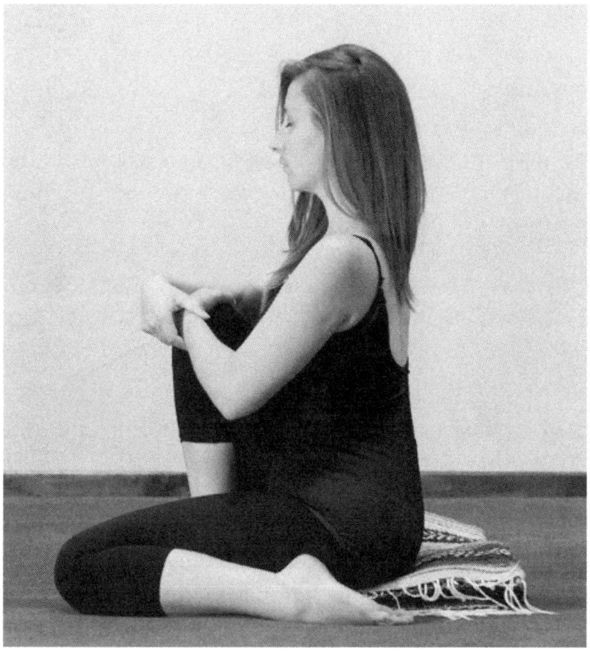

Krauñcāsana is naturally sequenced after Vīrāsana and Triang Mukha Eka Pāda Paśchimottānāsana.

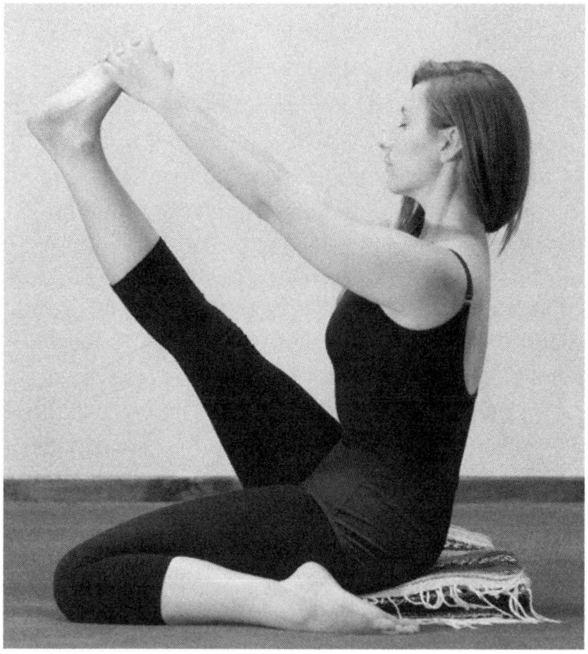

If the hamstrings are tight, you might hold the ankles or calf, or use a strap.

Guidance

1. Begin in Triang Mukha Eka Pāda Paścimottānāsana, one leg folded back (as in Vīrāsana) and the other leg outstretched. Inhaling, allow the breath to expand over as much surface area of the back as possible, rounding the back to feel the breath even more deeply.
2. Exhale and elongate the spine, bringing the spine into the front body like a backbend. Keeping the spine elongated and perpendicular to the floor, bend the knee of the outstretched leg, bringing the thigh as close to the torso as possible and holding each side of the foot with the hands. If the hamstrings are tight, you might hold the ankles or even the calf.
3. Inhaling, enjoy rounding the back to gain even greater fullness of breath in the lungs
4. Exhaling, elongate the spine, trying to bring it into the front of the torso as in a backbend.
5. Inhaling, allow the breath to widen and round the back.
6. Exhale as you straighten the knee, continuing to hold the foot, ankle, or calf.
7. Inhale, allow the breath to round the back.
8. Exhaling, bring the spine in, opening the chest, which allows the head and neck to move back as if in an S formation.
9. Inhale and do nothing.
10. Exhaling, bring the leg toward (not to) the torso as the torso lengthens, bringing the spine in like a backbend.
11. Inhaling, feel the breath in the back
12. Exhaling, lift out of yourself majestically, elongating the spine toward the heavenly planes. Bend the elbows out to the side and see if the upper body and the lower leg can close the gap of separation.
13. Inhaling, remain in this position while bringing the breath into the back.
14. Exhale and bend the upper knee, bringing the foot to the floor. Straighten the leg and bring the torso once more to the leg as in Triang Mukha Eka Pāda Paścimottānāsana. (You may now find it a little easier to bring the upper to the lower body for this forward bend.)
15. Come out of the pose very slowly on the exhalation, the same way you went into it.

Psychophysiological Benefits

The heron is a marsh bird; its long, thin, delicate legs symbolize balance and being able to wade deeper into the waters of life while connected to the earth. Long legs also symbolize the ability to transcend what others would find insurmountable. The longer the legs, the deeper the waters the heron can wade in.

Even though the heron's legs are thin and fragile looking, they are strong, symbolizing that we don't need massive pillars for support to remain stable; rather, we can stand on our own and yet explore other dimensions above the earth. Some varieties of herons are lone hunters, like some individuals who do not need a lot of people in their life. They are not pressured by opinions of others but seek their own uniqueness.

The pose can lengthen the hamstrings as well as elongate the gastrocnemius and soleus muscles of the calf, where we have a tendency to hold knots of emotions. The pose strengthens the hip area and increases its flexibility, if we keep lengthening the spine and torso without compression of the hip joint.

The heron is as graceful in flight as it is in water and on land. When the heron flies with the head pulled back, this reflects the internalization of awareness and the innate wisdom of being able to maneuver through life and control life's circumstances by adjusting to any situation. The long beak of the heron reflects an assertive movement towards opportunities that present themselves. The birds that fly out of the mountain Krauñca are moving toward Meru, the central axis of all mountains. In Yoga, the spine is known as the Meru Daṇḍa, the central axis of creation out of which all things arise and all things return.

The form of Krauñcāsana creates diagonal angles, which represent the activation of Śakti or dynamic energy. The triangular apex of this pose is in the buttock bones. The pose brings the prāṇa into the lower cakras, which when honored draw energy and offer it up to the higher cakras. It is the lower that feeds the upper in this pose.

The splitting of the mountain to release the demoness is symbolic of opening that place within ourselves to free the dark, restricted corners of the psyche. The mighty spear of Kartikaya pierces past contracted conditions to open a space and free the light so it can shine through. This pose, an upward surrendering, brings the two sides of the mountain together, bridging the gap and reuniting the upper and lower polarities that give the illusion of separation. Krauñcāsana reminds us not to get caught up in this illusion, but to remember, even in what appears to be a gap or separation, that we are united with Divine Source.

Urdhva Mukha Paścimottānāsana

Upward-Facing Forward Bend

Urdhva means "upward" and *Paschim* is the name for the god who rules the western direction. The west relates to the backside of the body, the side of the setting sun. *Tan* means "to go beyond self-imposed limitations." In short, this pose is the upward-facing stretch of the backside of the body, or Upward-Facing Forward Bend.

Philosophical Introduction

The Sanskrit name of this pose tells us what we are to do in the pose. We activate the back brain and the pineal gland that stimulates the parasympathetic nervous system. Doing this helps us retire within ourselves and find space between the thoughts and a quietness of mind.

In this pose named for the western direction, we also stretch with equal intensity the *Pūrvā,* which means east, the side of the rising sun. When the sun rises we can see. We can see the front of the body with the physical eyes. Paścima, however, is the side of the setting sun, the backside of our body, the part we cannot see. Mr. B.K.S. Iyengar once asked his students if we could see our back body. "No," we replied. "The back body is like God," he said. "You cannot see it. Therefore, you must retire within yourself, and there you will feel and come to know it."

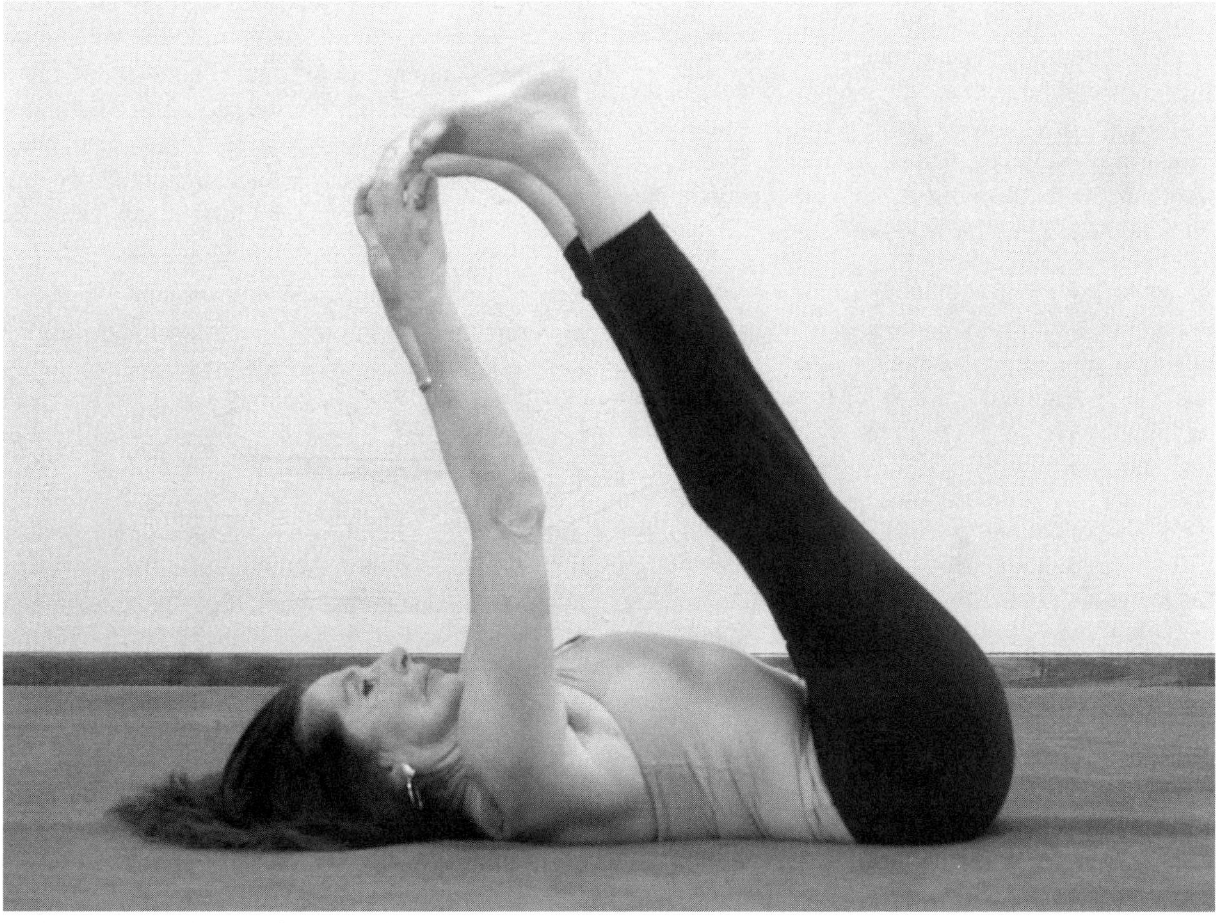

In this pose, the front and back of the spine are equal to one another, as the pose and counterpose are done simultaneously.

The posterior nerves of the spine activate the cerebellum at the base of the brain. In yoga, this correlates with the subconscious seat of mind. Like the back body, the hidden part of the mind is a part we cannot see and voluntarily access. This is why Sri Aurobindo Gosh called yoga "compressed evolution." The practices of āsana, prāṇāyāma, meditation, and chanting open channels to reach deep into the hidden parts of the psyche. These practices can help to bring past imprints, known as saṁskāras, to the surface of the conscious mind, which is represented by the front of the body and the anterior spinal nerve roots. The saṁskāras come up for healing and releasing.

In this pose, the posterior spine and anterior spine have an opportunity to be equal to one another as the pose (Paścimottānāsana) and counterpose (Pūrvottanāsana) are done simultaneously. Urdhva Mukha Paścimottānāsana honors the Lord of the east (Pūrvā), the rising sun, as it opens the east or front side of the body. It simultaneously stretches and opens the side of the setting sun or Paschima, the God of the west.

Reclining in Urdhva Mukha Paścimottānāsana helps to release the hamstring muscles without effort, while keeping the spine extended equally in front and back. It is a form of Śavāsana, which helps to release the "efforting" that tightens rather than lengthens the hamstrings. When the hamstring muscles are tight, they cause restrictions throughout other parts of the body as well within the mind and emotions.

As the legs are gradually brought closer to the torso, the base of the buttocks should move in the opposite direction. The spine does not round but moves from the back to front body as if doing a backbend while holding the feet. This preserves equal length of the east and west.

As the skin of the back of the thighs move toward the earth with the buttock muscles, the legs move toward the face and torso. This is a pose of neutrality. The spine is dynamic, as the head, face, and mind are practicing the second Sūtra: *Yogaḥ cittavṛtti nirodhaḥ.* It is a wonderful pose to learn what is described in the Bhagavad Gita as "relaxation within the action."

Guidance

1. Begin in Śavāsana. Exhaling, bend the knees and bring the soles of the feet to the heavens.
2. Inhale and allow the breath to spread across the back from buttock to shoulders.
3. Exhale and, without raising the shoulder blades or neck from the floor, reach for the outer edge of the feet, holding the big toe or behind the knees.
4. Inhaling, spread the breath across the back while keeping the navel passive.
5. Exhaling, gently elongate the spine, bringing the spine into the front body and offering the heart center toward the head.
6. Inhale and relax as the breath horizontally expands across the back from hips to shoulder blades.
7. Exhale and stay relaxed as you explore the possibility of bringing the legs closer to the torso while drawing the base of the buttocks lower to the floor. This gives a backbend effect to the spine as it is brought deeper into the front of the body.
8. Inhale and exhale, repeating the previous movements as long as feels comfortable. Preserve the relaxation within the action and the stillness of the waves of the mind as you exit the pose. Without shortening the front of the torso, bend the knees into the chest, and then bring the feet to the floor, sliding (not lifting) them out to the Śavāsana position. Relax and let go.

Note: Bending the knees into the chest helps to prevent lumbar strain. If the abdominal muscles are weak, this begins to strain the spine, eventually weakening the lumbar area. As we strengthen and lengthen the abdominals, we strengthen the lumbar and all parts of the spine.

Assist: If the hamstrings are tight, and the practitioner tries to reach the toes, this will pull the body out of alignment and disturb the quiet state of the mind. Using a belt around the bottoms of the feet can be helpful as long as there is no tension in the arms, neck, and shoulders. It is important to keep the outer shoulder blades and the back of the head—even better, the base of the skull—on the floor. Doing so allows the body to keep the heart center open and gives equal length to the front and back body. If the hamstrings are tight, it is also helpful to hold the back of the knees and the thighs, but only if the torso and head do not lift from the floor. If the chin or shoulder blades lift from the floor, this will produce a restless mind.

The most important thing in this pose is not to round the lower back. Urdhva Mukha Paścimottānāsana is not about trying to get the legs to the upper torso but to preserve equal length of the east and west sides of the body. Do this by bringing the buttocks and even the backs of the upper thighs toward the floor as the calf skin moves upward toward the heels. This is a subtle movement but one that can bring the practitioner into the fullness and intent of the pose.

Psychophysiological Benefits

Urdhva Mukha Paścimottānāsana is a wonderful pose to precede Śavāsana when coming out of Halāsana. This pose is a great teacher for learning how to relax within the actions of our lives. It teaches us to be centered in everything we do and not be thrown off or imbalanced when faced with difficult situations.

The second Sūtra in Chapter I of Patañjali's Yoga Sūtras is the most important; it tells us why we are practicing yoga. "Yoga is to still and quiet the waves that arise in the field of the mind." To do this in Urdhva Mukha Paścimottānāsana, we equally honor two of the ten directions of our planet, which are associated with the gods and goddesses of the Universe. We offer to the east, the side of the rising sun, and to the west, the side of the setting sun. These directions relate to the masculine (the frontal lobes of the brain) and the feminine, the intuitive part of one's being (associated with the back body and brain).

As we attempt to equalize these two polarities, the shoulders remain on the earth and the heart center lifts to receive the light. When space is created between the earlobes and the top of the shoulders, it creates space and equanimity within the mind.

Baddha Koṇāsana

Bound Angle Pose

Baddha means "bound," and *koṇa* is angle.

Philosophical Introduction

Though commonly thought of as a "hip opener," Baddha Koṇāsana is much more. In this pose, we not only create and preserve hip flexibility, we also create the yantra of two triangles meeting at their base to form the shape of a diamond. The angles of the legs and the joining of the feet can be seen as a modified tetrahedron, which gives Baddha Koṇāsana its own particular energetic effect. The tetrahedron symbolizes harmony and equilibrium. Its corner points, the apex of the triangles, are equal distance from one another, creating geometric equilibrium. (When the distances between the points of the angles differ, the result is stress.) Thus, this pose gives rest with no strain or tension, as long as one does not try to go beyond "the edge" or svadharma—what is right for that individual.

The equilibrium of Baddha Koṇāsana brings the mind into a state of balance and equanimity. When the feet are brought together with equal pressure, the pose expresses "Namaste," saluting the divinity in another as we acknowledge it also within ourselves. This mudrā of prayer is also a way of balancing the left and right hemispheres of the brain. Mudrā (Sanskrit for "seal") brings the electrical current of prāṇa back into the system, not allowing it to be dispersed through the bottoms of the feet or through the fingertips and palm of the hands.

As the feet and hands come into alignment, Baddha Koṇāsana creates one-pointedness of mind and evokes the star tetrahedron known as Merkaba. (In the language of ancient Egypt, *Mer* means light, *Ka* is spirit and *Ba* is the body.) This sacred geometric form is also familiar as the Judaic Star of David. In Hinduism, the upward- and downward-facing triangles represent Śiva and Śakti, the Divine masculine and the Divine feminine, which join at the heart center to create the perfect equilibrium of the Sri Yantra. The tetrahedron incorporates the Divine patterns used in the design of everything in creation, including the cellular formation of the human body, all aspects of nature, and the sacred geometry of architecture. Our third-dimensional world is built up in cubic form that is hidden within itself.

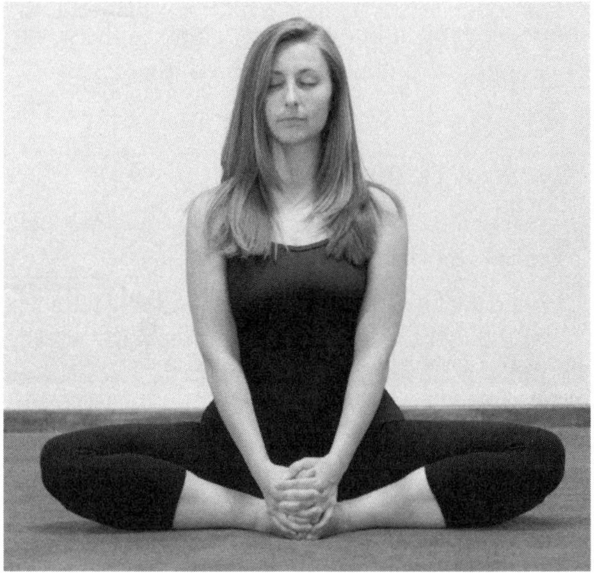

As the feet and hands align, Baddha Koṇāsana creates one-pointedness of mind.

Two tetrahedrons rotating in opposite directions become a vortex or yantra that transports spirit and body from one light dimension into the next. The Merkaba is a geometric electro-magnetic field that extends through all possible dimensions and parallel universes. It is a living dynamic field of energy. It is the spirit/body which is surrounded by counter rotating fields of light and is a vehicle to transcend the space-time continuum.

When we bend forward in this āsana, we enter into that perfect order that the star tetrahedron symbolizes. As we offer the upper to the lower body, the senses internalize. Instead of darting outward to the external world, the senses turn inward in pratyāhāra to explore the universes within. Baddha Koṇāsana is a reminder that we can only connect with our center of Divinity within ourselves rather than directing our attention to the outer world.

While bending forward in Baddha Koṇāsana, it is important to tilt the pelvis so the tailbone can lift, bringing the top of the pubis into the center of the base of the triangles. In this point of the body there is an opening, a portal that reaches from the base of the spine to the crown cakra. As we offer from here and then from the navel center into this geometrical pattern that pervades all of creation, we are drawn into the center of the universal equations duplicated within the cellular structure of our own body.

Guidance

1. Begin in Daṇḍāsana with the legs equally outstretched. If the pelvis has a tendency to drop back, and the spinous processes become prominent (indicating anterior compression), sit on the edge of a folded blanket. Build the blanket up to the point where the spine moves anteriorly in order to protect the vertebra and give space to the disks. It is important for the knees to be lower than the iliac crest of the hips.
2. Bend the knees out to the sides, bringing the soles of the feet together. Bring the heels toward the pubic bone an arm's length away.
3. Inhale, allowing the breath to expand horizontally across the back.
4. Exhale and elongate the spine, rising up out of the hip joints. Clasp the toes of both feet together with the left hand, and then bring the right hand over that. This binds the energy of the angle to energize the system through its own circuitry.
5. Inhale across the back from shoulders to hips.
6. Exhale, bending the elbows out to the sides. Bring the skin down the back as the neck elongates in the opposite direction.
7. Inhale, rounding the back to expand the breath into all lobes of the lungs.
8. Exhale and elongate the spine upward as the skin moves down the back. Tilt the top of the pelvis forward.
9. Inhale into the back and do nothing; take no movement or adjustment. Just breathe, allowing the back to round and expand horizontally.
10. Exhaling, lift up out of the hip joints and offer the top of the perineum to the center of the angle. Bend the elbows out to the side as the torso offers itself to the lower body. It is important to bring the spine in like a backbend when lowering the torso. For some, it may be enough to sit in this position, making sure the spinal vertebrae are not moving posteriorly but anteriorly—toward the front of the body. Offer the thoracic spine into the heart and lift the heart center toward the heavens. Instead of lifting the chin, continue to lengthen the back of the neck and the base of the skull to prevent neck compression.

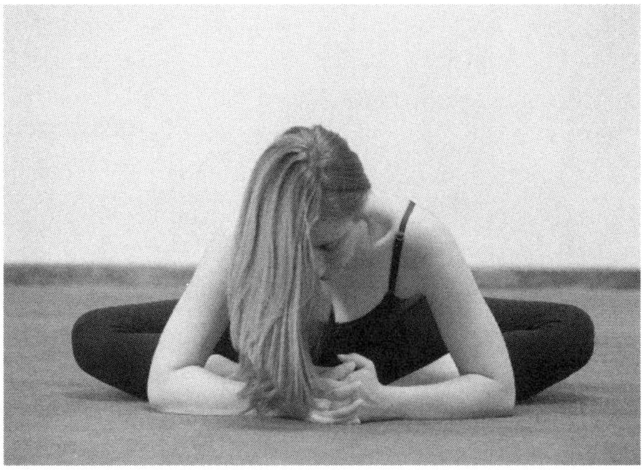

Baddha Koṇāsana is an excellent hip-opener, useful for preparing for other sitting poses.

11. Inhale the breath slowly, allowing it to horizontally expand the back
12. Exhale and, wherever you are in the pose, slowly rise up out of the hip joints, elongating the spine and bringing it into the front body.
13. Inhale across the back from shoulders to hips.
14. Exhaling, continue to lengthen the spine, rising up from the base of the pubis and bringing the spine in like a backbend.
15. Inhale, expanding your breath across the spectrum of the back from shoulders to buttocks. Stop at your threshold of discomfort, breathing into any painful areas and releasing the tension around the painful area on the exhalation.
16. Exhaling, continue lengthening the spine, including the neck. Relax the head and face as you move into the center of the geometrical form of the bound angle.
17. Inhaling, remain unmoving, simply allowing the breath to fill as many areas of the back as possible, correlating to the upper, middle, and lower lobes of the lungs.
18. Exhale deeper into the center of the tetrahedron of the pose. If you are able to explore the full expression of the pose, with the heart center offering itself into the center of the angles, bring the head to the altar of the feet. This completes and recycles a circle of energy emanating from the head and the feet.

Assists: To help a student gain leverage for elongating the spine, a partner or teacher can assist from behind, bringing the thumbs and forefingers to the crease where the hip meets the thigh, applying gentle pressure. At the same time, the student can press down with the fingertips on the outside of the thighs. To help the student expand the breath, a partner can assist from the front by reaching to gently guide the neck forward on the exhalations, then placing the hands on the shoulder blades to guide the skin up the back on the inhalation and down the back on the exhalation. From behind, a partner can guide the breath down into the lower part of the middle lobes of the lungs by placing his or her hands on the student's lower rib cage, and then the sacrum, using gentle pressure on the exhalation to help guide breath into the lowest, deepest, and most unused parts of the lungs.

Psychophysiological Benefits

Baddha Koṇāsana elongates the adductor muscles of the inner thighs and externally rotates the hip joint. This preserves youthfulness in the hips, giving space for the flow of synovial fluids responsible for joint mobility and flexibility. The pose strengthens the gluteus maximus, preserving the stability of the sacroiliac joint (where the pelvis meets the sacrum), and elongates any contracted attachments to the pubic bone. Even though Baddha Koṇāsana can be an end in itself, it is also a wonderful preparation for other sitting poses such as Padmāsana, Siddhāsana, and Samāsana.

As the base of the spine moves back and the iliac crests (the tops of the anterior pelvis) tilt forward into the geometric space of the pose, the movement of the pelvis allows the navel center, the seat of personal will, to surrender into the central adjoining bases of the triangles. The heart center offers itself into the powerful energy field that this pose creates. Last but not least, the head, the symbol of ego, humbles itself toward the altar of the arches of the feet.

The center of the star tetrahedron of Baddha Koṇāsana is slightly above the perineum, where there is an energetic opening in the subtle body. The energy from this point runs through the central canal of the spine, all the way to the crown cakra at the top of the head, and beyond. The perineum is important in our yoga practices, a powerful center of stored prāṇa that rises upward to awaken the heart center and release the granthis or knots at the throat cakra. The subtle opening at the top of the perineum can awaken the two lower cakras, the dwelling place of Kundalini Śakti, creating a counter-rotational field of light and prāṇa. If unimpeded, this energy can rotate up the spine to awaken the crown cakra where the inter-dimensional secrets of the cosmos reveal themselves. It is important to extend and not compress the back of the neck in this pose so the prāṇa can flow freely from just above the perineum to the crown of the head.

The physical perineum is located between the vaginal and rectal area in a woman and between the testicles and rectum in the male body. There is an energetic triangular connection between the coccyx, the pubic bone, the perineum, and the sacrum. In some methods of Chi Gong training, attention is placed on the perineum as the center of gravity, strength, and empowerment. Even the power of the voice is said to come from the peritoneal area rather than the throat or the solar or pelvic plexus.

As we honor this deepest part of our body, we honor the deepest part of the authentic self. When we reach down into this place of origin, there is no repression, no hiding or protecting an image we have of ourselves. When we face and become familiar with the base and essence of Being, there is no psychological sleep or tuning out when something appears uncomfortable. When we reach down into this place of the origin of Self, we awaken that dormant storehouse of energy that helps transcend the ultimate fear of the unknown. Awakenings in this pose can bring us into a Divine encounter and a symmetrical alignment with the collective unconsciousness of the planetary field and the collective psyche of humankind.

The primordial form of matter, Prakṛti, is built around the divine tetrahedron. The star tetrahedron is a replica of the subtle body and is a connecting link between spirit and matter, heaven and earth. Thus, Baddha Koṇāsana is a reminder that the geometrical patterns of universal life are a manifestation of the Divine Self and dwell within each one of us.

Upaviṣṭha Koṇāsana

Upa means to "approach," "go near," or "come down near." *Kona* is an angle. *Viṣṭha* is from *vesha* or *esha* meaning "life" or "to live." The name of this āsana tells us to sit or come down near, enter in, and live within the angle.

Philosophical Introduction

The angle in this pose is the yantra (universal energy field) of a triangle, with the pubis at its apex. Practiced as a reverential offering, Upaviṣṭha Koṇāsana can reveal the inner secret of itself. We practice the pose as if we are entering into a cosmic constellation or a Kendra, an angular house, the most auspicious houses in Vedic astrology.

Every āsana has a *bindu,* a seed point within the center of the yantra or angles of the pose. Bindu is the seed of the entire Universe beyond time and space. When finding the bindu or point of stillness within a posture, our consciousness can soar beyond time and space, bringing us into the true meaning of āsana. The perfection of Upaviṣṭha Koṇāsana lies within its bindu, the center of the pelvis between the pubic bone and the navel.

This āsana is an opportunity to offer the ego, represented by the head and the solar plexus (as self will), to the Iṣṭa Devatā or personal deity within the angle of the pose. In Upaviṣṭha Koṇāsana, when we focus on offering from the base of the pelvis and the seed point above the pubis, we give from the fullness of our Being. When we move from the strength and power of this base, eventually we can offer the heart center to the earth, and then the forehead can touch the earth in final surrender to the Lord of the Angle. The point bindu of the third eye center, *Ājñā cakra*, awakens to the teacher and teachings within. As the forehead offers itself to the earth, it simultaneously receives, for the bindu is the beginning and end point of Universal creation.

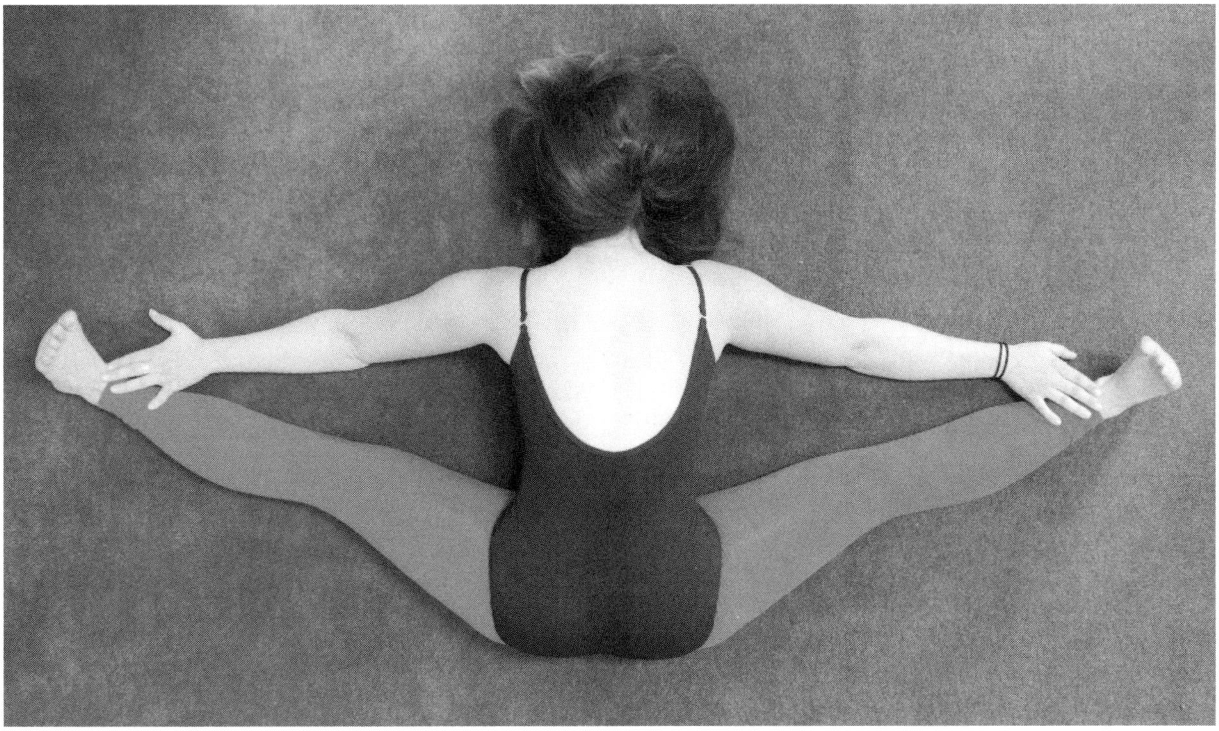

The yantra of Upaviṣṭha Koṇāsana is a triangle known as Kendra or angular house of Vedic astrology.

This pose, like many poses, expresses the unfolding of the fourth niyama, *svādhyāyāt iṣṭadevatā saṁprayogaḥ,* which is given in Sūtra (II:44):

Svādhyāya = one's own meditation
Iṣṭa Devatā = on that which they wish to shine like
Saṁprayogaḥ = brings forth and becomes one with
Yoga = Union or Oneness with All Creation

Upaviṣṭha Koṇāsana is a pose of Bhakti, a devotional offering of one's self into the triangular field or yantra of the pose. It is an opportunity to center one's self, to breathe, and to begin the offering not from the upper body (which is only a pretense of giving) but from the pelvic procreative force within. This is a full offering of every part of self, a full-hearted prostration from the base of Being. It is a form of giving our all, so to speak. As one enters into the yantra in the spirit of this giving, the pose gives back, and we become the sūtra, as we become one with the deity or energy field of the yantra.

3. Exhaling, press down with the fingertips to extend the spine upward and inward like a backbend. It is not as important to go down as it is to go up.
4. Inhale and allow the breath to round the back, relaxing the neck and bringing the breath from the shoulders to the buttocks.
5. Exhaling, elongate the spine upward and tilt the top of the pelvis forward, bringing the top of the pubic bone toward the earth. Continue moving and breathing in this way, taking your time, pausing on the inhale and lengthening on the exhale.
6. Inhaling, round the back to let the breath flow in.
7. Exhaling, lift the tops of the kneecaps toward the thighs and press down with the fingertips or palms to give leverage to elongate the spine.
8. Inhale and stay wherever you are in the pose, breathing into the back.
9. Exhale and extend the inner thighs out from the sides of the pubis, offering the back spine to the front of the body and the body toward the earth. Continue in this way, only moving as far as a calm, deep, and easy exhalation will allow.

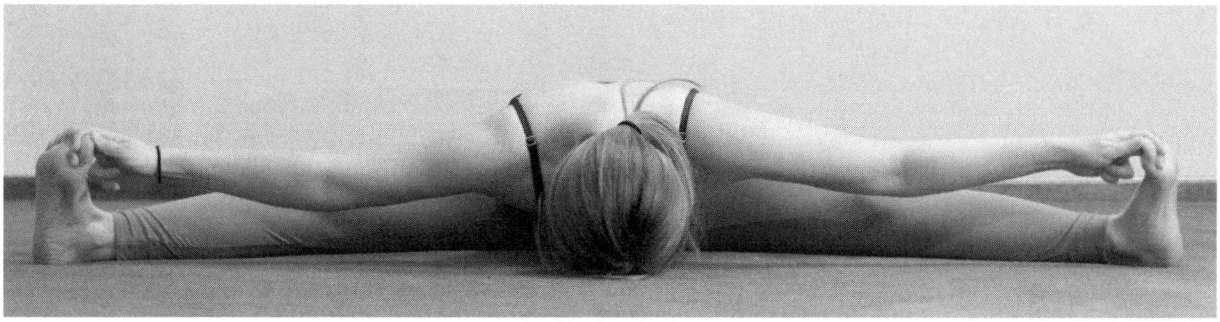

Deepen the pose only if the breath will allow.

Guidance

1. Begin in Daṇḍāsana. Bring the legs equal distance apart, as far as possible without discomfort. If the lower back is rounding, elevate the hips, sitting on a blanket or cushion high enough for the pelvic rim to be able to move forward. (Sit on the back of the thighs, not on the base of the spine.) Draw the flesh of the buttocks backward and diagonally, coming to rest more on the base of the pubic bone. Extend from the inner thighs to the inner ankle without dropping the feet out. Without shortening the Achilles tendon, extend to the ball of the big toe to relax the spinal reflex in the sole of the foot.
2. Inhaling, place the fingertips on the floor between the thighs, shoulder width apart.

10. Slowly come out of the pose breath by breath, the same way you went into it.

Assists: A teacher or partner can sit behind the student and use thumbs and forefingers to press down on the tops of the thighs at the hip joints, rolling the skin of the upper thigh externally while the student turns the bottom legs internally. A partner can hold and support the student's arms (without pulling) to allow the spine to lengthen and not bend prematurely. Alternatively, the practitioner can place her arms and hands on a chair to help lengthen the spine.

Psychophysiological Benefits

Emotional constrictions manifest in a variety of ways in our body. In Upaviṣṭha Koṇāsana, we may confront long-held tightness within the point where the inner thighs meet the butterfly shape of the pubic bone. Restrictions in the procreative plexus fan out, preventing the psoas and adductor muscles from opening into the full expression of this forward bend. It is important not to push or strain within the pose but to move only to the point of svadharma—one's own truth—and hold as long as the breath is calm and fluid. Whatever the āsana, wherever we are is the sacredness of the moment and the perfection of the pose. In this āsana, it is far more important to bring the top of the pubic bone to the earth than to over-effort, straining and rounding the back, which causes anterior compression of the spine.

Upaviṣṭha Koṇāsana helps maintain the flexibility of the hips, as well as the strength of the knees and spine. As we attempt to do a backbend with every exhalation, the spine and nervous system are strengthened. The external rotation of the thighs tones the gluteus maximus muscles and stabilizes the sacroiliac joint. It is an excellent pose for opening space to bring the circulatory currents to the male and female reproductive organs. The stretch and opening to the inner thighs and legs increases awareness of the subtle and intuitive body, represented by the inner legs and arms.

When the forehead touches the earth in the yantra of this pose, it is a form of *trātaka* or steady gazing. Trātaka is a method for establishing concentration of mind as a prelude to meditation. It is one of the *ṣaṭ kriyās,* but rather than being a cleansing of the body, trātaka steadies the mind. Trātaka can be internal or external. When the student finds the internal seed bindu within this (or any) āsana, then breathes into and moves from this center, the mind becomes one-pointed. If that concentrated state is held for twelve breaths or twelve seconds, the subject and object merge as one: This is dhyāna or meditation.

Meditation is the mergence of subject and object, where consciousness is compared to an uninterrupted stream of oil being poured from one vessel into the next. It is possible to enter into concentrative and meditative states in āsana, as well as the first stages of Samādhi. Trātaka is often practiced using a particular deity or yantra as a way of transcending normal experiences to become one with the object of one's focus. In this āsana, we enter in and become one with the formless energy field of the yantra as an expression of the Divine.

Siddhāsana

Adept's Pose

Siddhis are the yogic powers outlined in the third part of Patañjali's Yoga Sūtras, and Siddhas are the great ones, the perfected beings who have developed through many years or lifetimes of spiritual practices and realizations. They are able to access yoga's hidden powers.

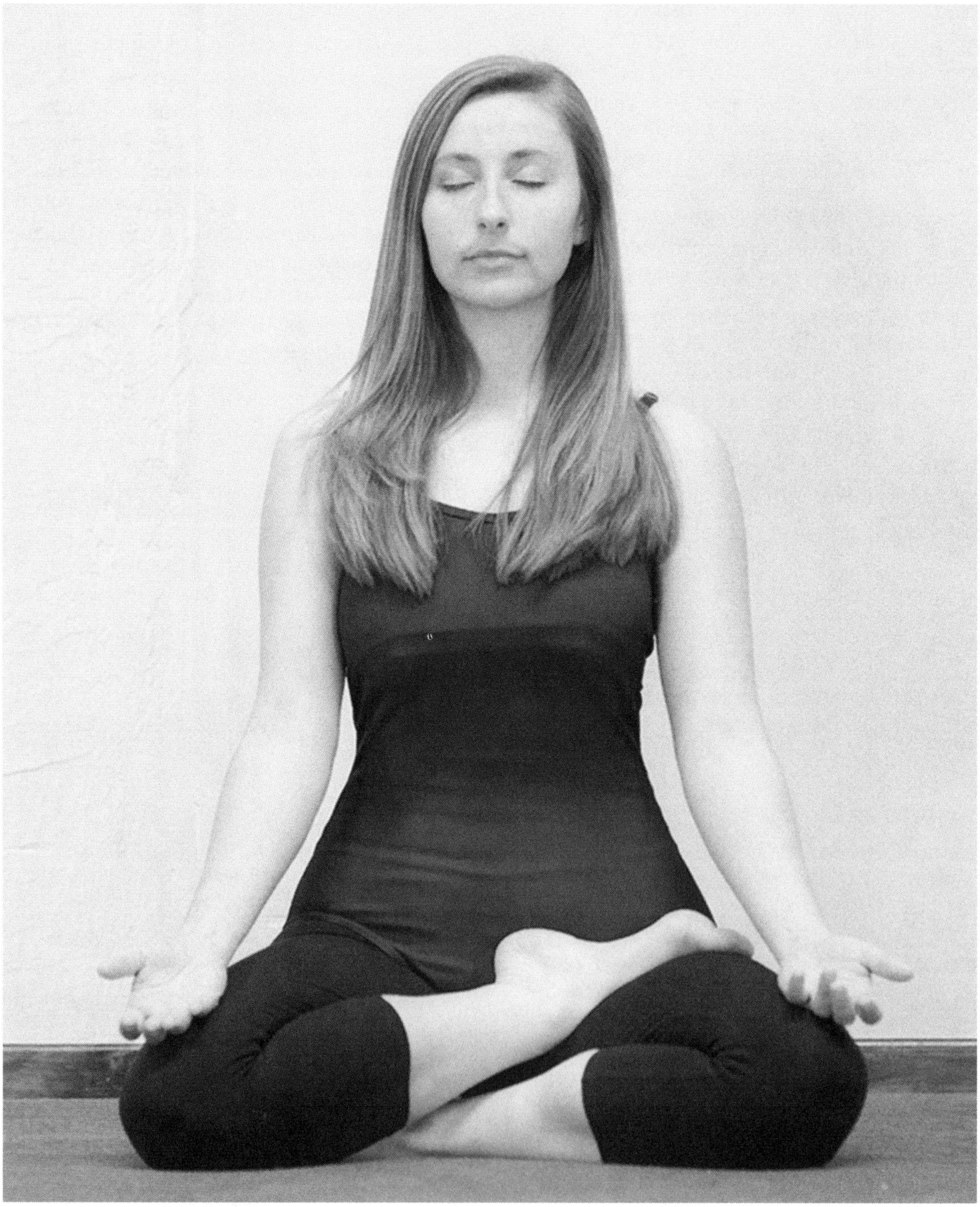

In Siddhasana, the heel is pressed into the root cakra, sublimating that cakra's energy and bringing it up to the higher centers.

Philosophical Introduction

Siddhas may sit long hours in meditation, and thus they are usually celibate. Siddhas live monastic lives, although householders can be Siddhas as well.

The traditional way to sit in Siddhāsana is with the heel pressed into the root cakra. This sublimates the energy and brings it up to the higher centers, rather than allowing energy to build up in the reproductive glands. The right heel would be placed on the left side of the pubic bone. The left foot is then crossed over the right thigh, placing the foot between the right ankle and thigh. Siddhāsana does not require as much elongation of the adductor muscles as in Padmāsana, the Lotus Pose, but it does require flexibility of the external rotators in the joints of the hips.

Classically, the right foot comes in first, and then the left foot, whether one sits in Samāsana, Siddhāsana, Sukhāsana, or Padmāsana. The right side of the body is associated with the sympathetic nervous system, which is more activating. This division of the autonomic nervous system stimulates the adrenal glands, which prepare us for fight or flight, and in turn activate the prefrontal cortex of the left brain, which is logical and sequential and does not always perceive the bigger picture.

When you prepare to sit for meditation, however, it's time to curb the restlessness of the sympathetic nervous system or, in terms of the guṇas, the rajasic part of one's nature. When we sit, if the right foot is brought in first and then the left, the left foot becomes dominant over the right. This position creates a little more stimulation of the parasympathetic nervous system. The parasympathetic division is associated with the receptive, calming, and cooling nature of the right brain, and it dilates and opens the physical and subtle nerve channels. This helps our body to become an open receptacle for the Divine.

Mr. Iyengar taught that if we practice a meditative pose one way, we should practice it the other way at times in order to preserve the balance of right and left hemispheres of the brain, the sympathetic and parasympathetic. In his teaching, Mr. Iyengar was considering the hip joints because after a while, a meditator can develop tremendous tension in one hip. He was addressing the structural aspects of the sitting poses and, in terms of structure, it is helpful to alternate sides.

Throughout the years, I have alternated the placement of the legs at times in the sitting poses. However, when placing the left foot first, making the right foot dominant, I found more frontal brain stimulation, which seemed to make the mind more outgoing and sensitive to the external world. For meditation, I prefer the classical pose, with the right foot in first and then the left foot crossed over onto the right. This creates more of a right brain dominance, which is related to spatial and holographic awareness. In this placement, you will notice that the erector spinae muscles on the left side of the spinal vertebrae are more active. This reveals more activity in the parasympathetic division of the nervous system. This side of the nervous system quiets and calms the mind, bringing it into a more receptive state. I have found fewer thoughts enter the mind when the left foot is crossed over the right.

Through Padmāsana and Siddhāsana, we learn to sit in continual silence, stillness, and deep meditation. It is in this profound stillness that we contribute to the equilibrium of the planet and all life forms dwelling within this dimension.

Padmāsana

Lotus Pose

Padma is one of the names for a lotus flower. The lotus is a phenomenal symbol, not just of sitting but also how we can live our life.

Philosophical Introduction

The beauty and purity of the lotus grows out of mud and murk. Its root system goes beneath the waters, deep into the mud and earth. The stalk of the lotus represents our spine. It's thick at the bottom and it grows thinner as it comes up to the top. The lotus flower blossoms above, but it is still deeply connected to the earth beneath the waters. As the prāṇa of the spine rises, it is still connected to the earth plane through the Mūlādhāra cakra at the base of the spine. The Śakti rises like the flower to reunite with the energies in the crown cakra, the Sahasrāra, depicted as the thousand-petalled lotus. (In the East, a thousand means infinite.) The human neck, like the pad of the lotus, floats lightly upon the waters of life, and our head rests upon its axis. When the energy is awakened, the petals of the crown cakra unfold like the lotus flower that opens with the light of the rising sun.

Although the lotus flower appears to float effortlessly on the water, a sinewy stalk keeps it connected to the earth. If the spine is strong and powerful, we have the same rooted connection to the earth. We can feel it through the hips, through the buttocks, and through the back of the thighs. From here, we can lift and extend while the mind can be in a calm and peaceful state. When the light dawns within us, it feels as if there are petals unfolding from the top of the brain stem, like the lotus opening to the dawn of the new day. This unfoldment, when the effulgent light dawns within our own Being, seems infinite, without end.

The Bhagavad Gītā emphasizes how we should cultivate an attitude of nonattachment. Sri Kṛṣṇa urges that one should live in the world like the lotus leaf, which is unaffected by water. When the yogin places all actions in the Eternal, abandoning attachment to the results, he or she can live in the world—upon the waters of life. Yet, like the lotus leaf that grows from the mud beneath, the yogin is not affected by the mud or by the water. In other words, the yogin is in the world, but is not of it.

In the beginning stages of the Lotus Pose, students usually practice a loose variation in which the ankles are bent, overarching the outer ankle and compressing the inner ankle. As the body accustoms itself to the pose, the knees may come closer together, helping the feet to be more relaxed upon the thighs. Eventually, the inner and outer ankles become equal to one another without ankle compression. In the "tighter," more advanced version of this pose, energy is not restricted or blocked in any way. The feet become dynamically alive and the coccyx (tailbone) is automatically lifted off the earth away from the downward pull of gravity. Certain materials, such as animal skins, were once used to insulate the base cakra from the downward pull of the earth's energy. But when practicing a "tighter" Lotus pose, the tailbone is automatically lifted away from the downward magnetic pull of the earth.

The full Lotus Pose is like *abhyāsa* (the first instruction that Patañjali gives in the Yoga Sūtras), a way to still the turbulence of the waves of the mind. *Abhyāsa,* commonly translated as "continual practice," means "checking the downward pull" of both body and mind. Lotus Pose helps lift descending energies upward to the higher cakras and eventually to the crown cakra, the center of the thousand-petalled lotus.

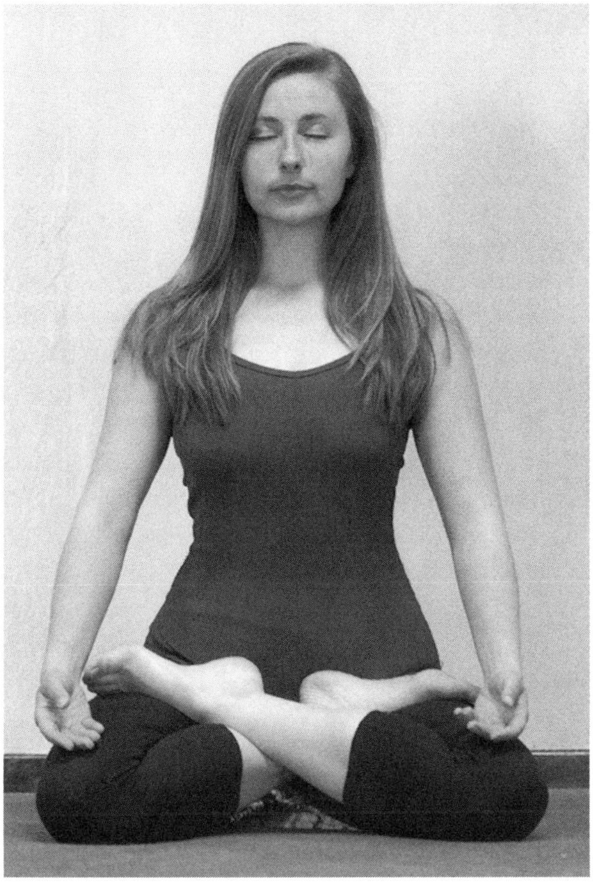

When the feet are dynamic in Padmāsana, this helps to keep the mind alert for meditation

In Padmāsana, when the feet become dynamic, they create a mudrā that keeps the mind alert. The essence of the full lotus is also to keep the spine locked into the position so that we don't compress or tense the spinal nerve roots to hold the pose. Padmāsana recycles prāṇa or energy that flows out through the bottom of the feet, bringing it back into the spine to renew the pranic currents of the subtle body and the nerves system of the physical body. The spine and torso are locked into a vertical position so that prāṇa can flow unimpeded through Suṣumna, the subtle spinal center. Yogis believed that if one were to enter the state of Samādhi (altered state of consciousness) while meditating in Padmāsana, the body could not fall over. The torso and spine would remain erect and the body would not fall. Throughout years of meditative experiences, however, I have learned this is not true. When in a trancelike state, one's legs can remain folded in Lotus Pose even when toppling backward.

The seated poses are conducive to a meditative state when the erect alignment of the spine brings the crown of the head over the base of the spine. This brings the mind into a "thoughtless" state of awareness. It cannot be emphasized enough: The sacro-occipital alignment is important to meditation. As Mr. Iyengar said, "When the heart is an extrovert, the mind is an introvert."

Padmāsana is the most desirable sitting pose because it helps the spine, breast, neck, and head to come into this natural alignment. (If one cannot do the Lotus Pose, however, this does not preclude practicing meditation from any position.) In Padmāsana, the head and mind are not leaning forward into the future or pulling back into the past—they come into the moment. We don't have to wrestle with the mind to banish thoughts. Instead, the space is opened to receive Divine grace. The meditative seat becomes, according to Sri Aurobindo, a self-offering or dedication of self to the Divine. This pose is Īśvara Praṇidhāna, surrender or devotion to Īśvara, the lord of this world, the teacher of even the most ancients.

The Lotus Pose is our reminder to float upon the waters of life, lifting and unfolding with the effulgent light that is always shining. Even though the lotus grows from the earth beneath the waters, the mud cannot cling to it, and droplets of water cannot penetrate it. Just as we may have grown out of the darkness of the past, we rise up into the light of the new day and open ourselves into the infinite and unending unfoldment to Spirit. The mud of past hurts can no longer penetrate the purity and openness of our soul. Nothing can cling to us as we continue to open with the Divine light that shines from within.

The Yoga Sūtras (III:35) tell us: "By practicing Saṁyama on the lotus of the heart, knowledge of the mind is acquired." Commentaries on the sūtras explain this in more detail. One commentator says, "The Citadel of Brahma is the heart center which is shaped like a lotus. There is a small aperture in it that is the seat of knowledge. By concentration and meditation on this point, perception of citta (mind) arises. It is from the heart that one can watch the action of the mind."

Śavāsana

Corpse Pose

Sava means "corpse."

The Deeper Levels of Śavāsana

The practitioner can experience four different layers of consciousness in Śavāsana, which is why it is considered the hardest pose. With foundational teacher training and general yoga classes, it is helpful to open with Śavāsana to engage deeper breathing. This occurs as we stretch the neck to release the cervical vertebrae and nerve roots because the C3, C4, and C5 nerves fuse together to create the phrenic nerve, which innervates the diaphragm. When the practitioner releases the sternocleidomastoid (SCM) muscles that run along the sides the neck, this relaxes the diaphragm and, in turn, the breath. The SCM and the diaphragm are two of the four breathing muscles. Next, by elongating the neck and moving the legs in the opposite direction, we also the free the other two breathing muscles, the rectus abdominus and the inner and outer intercostal muscles. The elongation and alignment of Śavāsana that occurs with the relaxation allows the breath to open spontaneously.

When Śavāsana is experienced on the surface level, the upper eyelids pull away from the lower eyelids and the eyes will turn up to the frontal lobes of the brain. When the front brain is active, the mind is restless. To calm the mind, place something under the back of the head to bring the hairline higher than the chin. Then the eyes and eyelids drop down while the eyes recede into the back of the skull. If the head is positioned correctly, the energy of the eyes will descend downward to the back of the heart. This helps the senses to turn inward (pratyāhāra) and the whole body comes to a deep state for rest.

Avoid arching the lumbar spine. When the lumbar is elongated, coming as close to the earth as possible, this also helps to quiet a restless mind. The teacher or student may place a pillow underneath the knees to bring the lumbar and sacrum to the floor, which helps relax the sympathetic nerves that come off the lumbar spine and, in turn, the adrenals. Eventually, however, we want the whole leg to extend and relax so the prāṇa can move freely through any blocks in the knees to pass through the soles of the feet without impediment. This relaxes and creates cellular space within the spine and internal organs.

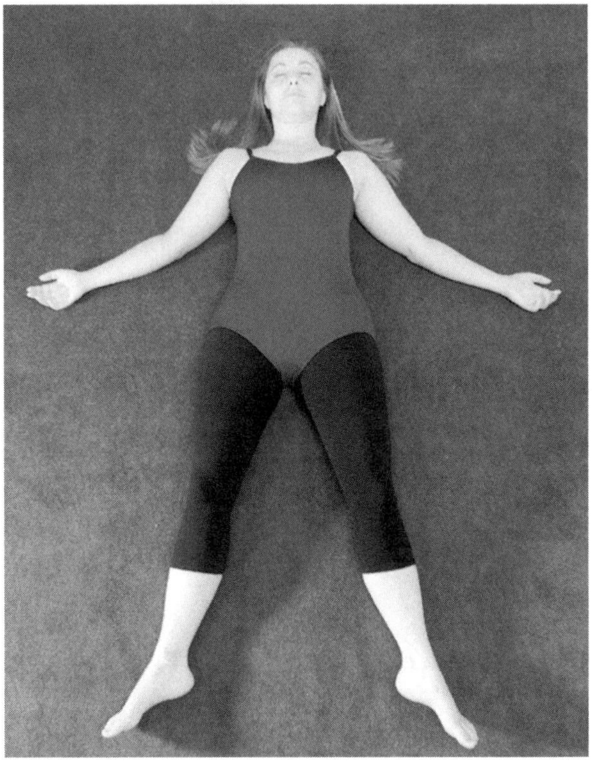

Śavāsana

The next phase of Śavāsana is when the student's consciousness is not on the surface but moving toward the mid-plane of the body. At this level, there may be only a partial release; if the practitioner lacks trust in various aspects of life, she may subconsciously believe that the earth may not support her. This lack of trust keeps students from total release. Also, there may be a fear of giving too much of oneself because the floor, like people or situations in life, may not always be there to give total support.

In the next phase of the pose, as trust develops, the practitioner eventually lets go. The front body drops into the back body, and the energies of the front brain come to rest upon the back brain. The cerebellum, the seat of the subconscious, is where the akāśic records are stored individually and collectively. In this state, we can access the latent impressions (saṁskāras) stored in the psyche, where they may surface to conscious awareness to be transformed or released. This is the state where the hypnogogic images emerge out of the subconscious to the conscious mind. Here, in the theta mind wave state, one learns to dwell between the conscious and subconscious.

At the surface level of Śavāsana, we experience beta brainwaves. Alpha waves are present at the midline level, and at the third level is the theta wave. At the fourth level, the body relaxes so deeply that the organs, glands, and soft and hardened tissues release whatever it is they have been holding onto, and the awareness of the body drops away. In this state, it feels as if the earth's contours begin to mold to the shape of the body. Initially, it may feel as if the arms are higher than the torso as the body sinks into the softness of the earth. Finally, one comes into the thoughtless state of awareness where thought cannot even take form. There is no bodily awareness. It is like returning to the source and substratum of the Puruṣa that lies like a seed within one's self. It is the bindu from where we have sprung and where we will return.

APPENDICES

Creative Sequencing

The idea of practicing āsana is to create internal space. We also need to create space and inspiration in the way we sequence our poses. Like the choreography of dance, in yoga āsana one movement flows into the next. Composing a class is like composing music, with augmentations and resolutions that morph into the next pose with grace and ease.

When I began training yoga teachers in the 1960s, the new teachers wanted to outline prescribed pose sequences for their classes. Many would put the outline on a note card and hide it during class. Some would write a class sequence on their hands for easy referral. One teacher was so nervous when teaching her first class that her hands perspired, erasing her carefully planned sequence.

When I was asked for my thoughts on writing a class outline, I would say that it was fine to do this, as long as they forgot it when they entered the classroom. The reason: When there is too much preplanning, we are not open to the creative impulse that is attempting to move through and guide us. There may be times when we veer from the planned poses, not knowing why, until one or more students say, "That was just what I needed."

More than once, I raced to an evening class planning to do vigorous standing poses. When I arrived, the students were in Śavāsana on the floor, obviously fatigued by the day's activities. All my best-laid plans flew out the window as I gauged the energy in the room, attuned to it, and let go of my carefully structured sequence along with my expectations. Times like this reminded me to be sensitive to the moment and to adapt to the students' needs.

While teaching an unchanging set of postures may satisfy the need for structure and security, it does not always allow us to be present to the changing needs of the moment, or to exercise one's own creativity and responsiveness. Teachers who have taught the same set of poses for a few years have said that after a time, they felt "dry" and uninspired. If we parrot the words and teachings of our mentors without finding the depth of those teachings, it is difficult to stay inspired.

I learned the art of sequencing in the Sivānanda method, as taught by Swami Satchidananda, Vishnu Devananda, and Walt and Magana Baptiste. I have also been inspired by T. K. V. Desikachar, and I was strongly influenced by Mr. B. K. S. Iyengar's alignment-based methodology. Mr. Iyengar worked with me on sequencing many years ago, when I established a yoga teacher training school in San Francisco. The presentation of Āsana I and II in this book is a combination of different methodologies that have been inspired by my personal teachers, based upon a sequence that can be altered and adapted to one's own practice or teaching.

Whether you are a teacher or a student, remember that the practice or teaching does not come from us; it comes through us. Creative sequencing helps us continue to feel inspired, fulfilled, and attuned to the Divine essence that teaches through us. By allowing creativity to direct our teachings, we become instruments of Divine grace. We don't just lead people through poses; we help them experience the eternal cosmic vibration through each pose.

Creative sequencing draws on knowledge of how āsana realigns, balances, and regulates the physical and subtle body. It is based on the biological understanding of āsana in relation to the autonomic nervous system, the endocrine system, and the body's subtle energies. This understanding increases self-awareness and self-observation through āsana practice. Through sequencing poses and adapting them for our own (or our students') personal needs, we develop greater awareness of the efficacy of āsana. We learn to adapt, adjust, and balance emotional needs and energetic patterns. For teachers, creative sequencing expands consciousness to embrace and invoke the presence of the masters who have gone before.

Creative sequencing teaches flexibility—not just of the body but in all areas of life. We learn to trust in our intuitive impulses and allow guidance to enter into our teaching. When we create a sequence, we create a mood—a mantle for the presence of the Divine to enter the room and our hearts. When this happens, we benefit in both body and spirit.

Sequencing and the Autonomic Nervous System

Whether sequencing one's own practice or teaching a class, it is important to understand the function of the autonomic nervous system (ANS), which consists of the sympathetic and parasympathetic nerve ganglia that run laterally along the spinal column. (The chart on page 232 illustrates the ANS.) The sympathetic and parasympathetic nerve ganglia also relate to the left and right hemispheres of the brain. All sequencing is based upon balancing the ANS through forward bends, backbends, inversions, and twists.

The sympathetic division of the ANS correlates to what was known in ancient times as Ha. The syllable Ha, in Sanskrit, refers to the sun, the projective energy that heats, constricts, and activates. Ha is associated with the masculine universal energy. The parasympathetic division was known as Tha, one of the Sanskrit words for moon. The moon is known for its cooling influence, balancing the heating and constricting effects of the sun. Like the moon, the parasympathetic aspect dilates; it is a receptive energy associated with the universal feminine.

The essence of āsana practice is to balance Ha and Tha, sun and moon, heat and cold, day and night, masculine and feminine, and all polarities that comprise life's existence. General sequencing is based on the bilateral integration of the autonomic nervous system. When these two opposite forces are brought into balance, prāṇa is automatically brought into the central canal of the spinal cord, awakening the universal intelligence that lies dormant within.

The Sympathetic Nervous System and Backbends

The sympathetic ganglia arise from the spinal nerves of the thoracic and lumbar vertebrae. The sympathetic nerves have a stimulating impact upon the heart, thymus, and adrenal glands, preparing us for fight or flight. The adrenals are sometimes known as the body's brain. It is logical to assume that backbends affecting the thoraco-lumbar spine would impact the sympathetic nervous system. This is why backbends have a stimulating affect, speeding up the general metabolic rhythms and functions of the body. Backbends and other postures that influence the sympathetic nervous system are excellent for conditions such as chronic fatigue, depression, hypothyroidism, and low blood pressure.

If backbends or other āsanas related to sympathetic stimulation (Headstand, for example) are taken at or near or the end of an āsana sequence, the constrictive effects make it difficult to relax in Śavāsana, and feelings of anxiety, anger, and agitation may arise after the practice.

The Parasympathetic Nervous System and Forward Bends

The parasympathetic ganglia radiate out from the cervical spine and the sacrum. When the parasympathetic nerve plexuses are activated through āsana, blood vessels dilate, which reduces excessive heat and inflammation and balances sympathetic stimulation. It is the parasympathetic nervous system that helps the mind to become more focused and calm. Its activation is helpful for reducing anxiety, hyperactivity, and high blood pressure.

It is logical to assume that the main āsanas impacting the parasympathetic nervous system are forward bends, shoulderstand, and plow pose. Therefore, it is highly advisable to end an āsana sequence with poses that engage the parasympathetic response, such as a forward bend variation. Forward bends and other parasympathetic poses have a calming and relaxing influence on both body and mind, preparing the body for final relaxation in Śavāsana.

Twists

Twists are neutral. It is important to extend the spine before twisting; the movement must start at the coccyx (tailbone) at the base of the spine before proceeding upward through the sacrum, lumbar, thorax, and cervical vertebrae of the neck. Twisting that involves the whole spinal spectrum in this way creates a marvelous combination of a backbend in a forward bend. As a result, twists impact both the parasympathetic and sympathetic ganglia. This is true for both supine and seated twists.

In twists, the bottom half of the body is in a modified forward bend. The spinal elongation and rotation creates a backbending affect by stimulating the sympathetic nerves that emanate from the thoraco-lumbar spine. The cervical spine (neck) mirrors the alignment of the base of the spine, and the movement of the sacrum and neck activates the parasympathetic nerves.

In sequencing, twists can be taken between backbends and forward bends or between forward bends and backbends. Along with forward bends, twists are recommended for evening practices. These poses affect the cervical and sacral plexuses—the parasympathetic nervous system—and help the practitioner to relax and prepare for sleep.

Standing Poses

It is suggested that morning classes start with standing poses, while evening classes can begin with relaxing poses before introducing more vigorous poses. Standing poses also impact the parasympathetic nerves and in turn influence apāna, the pranic flow that carries waste matter and energy downward. Standing poses develop strength, balance, and trust in one's own strength.

Since standing poses and forward bends have a dilating impact upon the parasympathetic nervous system, they can have the effect of reducing high blood pressure. This is one of the reasons that standing poses are usually sequenced before the Headstand. It is recommended that students with high blood pressure practice forward bends for at least twenty minutes before attempting to invert the body. Students with low blood pressure should avoid excessive practices of standing poses, as they can cause fatigue.

For a basic practice, one would begin with standing poses: The body isn't as tired at the start of practice, and the standing poses will help stabilize high blood pressure before taking inverted poses. Or, a practice session may begin with Downward-Facing Dog, followed by a preparation for Headstand, with standing poses taken afterward to help regulate blood pressure and release any neck tension. People with low blood pressure and/or chronic fatigue would need more inversions and fewer standing poses. Students with high blood pressure will benefit from standing poses when they are practiced before inversions or backbends.

Inverted Poses

Inverted poses are a good choice in the afternoon when one's energy level drops. Low blood pressure and chronic fatigue are brought into balance through inverted poses. The main inverted poses are Headstand, Handstand, Peacock Pose, and the most important of all inverted poses, the Shoulderstand.

The Headstand stimulates the sympathetic nervous system. If the Headstand is done appropriately, the thoracic spinal nerves are stimulated, while the elongation of the nerve roots of the neck, lumbar spine, and sacrum creates a balance between sympathetic and parasympathetic stimulation and, in turn, a balance between the polarities of Ha and Tha associated with the crown of the head and base of the spine.

Shoulderstand is known as Sarvāṅgāsana, which translates roughly as "the pose of the whole or entire body." The name of the pose reflects the fact that Sarvāṅgāsana affects all parts and systems of the body. It is important to include Shoulderstand (or its modified variations using a wall or chair to support the feet and legs) in every practice session. Shoulderstand activates the parasympathetic nervous system through the angle of the neck and cervical nerves. When taking variations such as Halāsana (the Plow), the nerves in the sacrum are also stimulated, creating major impact on the nerve plexuses associated with the parasympathetic response. Halāsana has a calming and balancing effect upon the mind, and helps to bring the entire endocrine system into balance.

After practicing Headstand, Handstand, Peacock Pose, or their preparations, it is recommended to follow with Shoulderstand or one of its variations. If Shoulderstand is not taken immediately, it can be sequenced toward the end of the session, then followed with forward bends and final relaxation. Though it is usually recommended to end an āsana session with forward bends or twists, which have a calming and soothing effect through the activation of the parasympathetic nervous system, the Shoulderstand can also be sequenced at the end of a practice session.

When practicing inverted poses or even just their preparatory positions, if the Shoulderstand is not taken immediately after them or near the end of the session, one might later feel heat and constriction and a weakness in the nervous system. This could be expressed as impatience, frustration, and anger, reflecting too much sympathetic stimulation.

The Autonomic Nervous System and the Subtle Body

All āsana is based upon balancing the sympathetic (masculine) nerves and the parasympathetic (feminine) nerves, the anterior and posterior spine, and the left and right hemispheres of the brain. Sequencing based on these polarities would include standing poses, which stimulate the apāna prāṇa (downward flow), and then inverted poses that stimulate the prāṇa

prāṇa, the flow that brings the descending energies upward and helps prevent depression and fatigue.

It is important to note that when we balance the sympathetic and parasympathetic responses, we are also balancing the subtle energy channels known as the nāḍīs. The central channel, which correlates to the physical spinal cord, is known as *suṣumnā.* The channel that runs along the left side of the suṣumnā, which correlates to the parasympathetic nervous system, is known as *iḍā.* The channel that runs along the right side of the spine, correlating to the sympathetic nervous system, is known as *piṅgalā.* Every āsana is based on bilateral extension, and so is the way we design a sequence for a class or practice session.

In the classical traditions of yoga, the physical nerves and subtle channels are brought into balance by taking a pose and then the counter-pose. However, in the methodology of this book, we practice the counter-pose within the pose. In this manner, we can maintain continual balance of the autonomic nervous system and the subtle energy channels (iḍā nāḍī and piṅgalā nāḍī) in each āsana. This has the effect of quieting the waves of the mind, which is the very essence of yoga, according to Patañjali's second sūtra. Instead of doing the poses in order to curb restlessness so that one can meditate, by doing the counter-pose in the pose, the mind can find that stillpoint of meditation in the pose.

The Endocrine System and the Subtle Body

The endocrine system and its relationship to the cakras (shown in the chart on page 247) is another major aspect in designing an āsana sequence. The endocrine glands are internally secreting; that is, they secrete their hormones directly into the bloodstream. Also known as ductless glands, the endocrine glands include the hypothalamus, pituitary, pineal, thyroid, parathyroids, thymus, adrenals, and reproductive organs.

The endocrine system is the physical correlate of the body's subtle energy centers, or cakras. A *cakra* is a wheel. *Ca* means "to go" (as in the word "chariot"). *Kra* is from *kri,* meaning "to do" or "to act." Cakras are commonly thought of as vortices of energy. The seven major cakras relate to the endocrine glands, but there are also minor cakras located throughout the subtle body—between the seven major cakras, at the physical body's moving joints, in the palms of the hands, the soles of the feet, and the backs of the knees. I call these sub-cakras.

Cakras cannot be seen with the physical eye but are experienced in the subtle sheath that is known as *prāṇāmāya kośa.* (For more about the kośas and the subtle body, see page 245.) The health and balance of the endocrine system is considered to be an important component in opening the subtle channels of each gland's corresponding cakra. The classical sequencing is brilliantly designed to insure the balance and health of each endocrine gland in turn. After beginning with sun salutations or a few standing poses, the Headstand or inverted poses would come next.

Once, the pituitary was thought to be the "master gland" that controlled and regulated the entire endocrine system. Now, however, the hypothalamus is recognized as the master endocrine gland. The prefix *hypo-* means "under," and this gland is located under the thalamus, in the topmost center of the brain. Within subtle anatomy, this area correlates to sahasrāra cakra, the thousand-petaled lotus.

Śīrṣāsana , the Headstand, directly affects the thalamus and hypothalamus located at the top of the head. Śīrṣāsana is called the king of all āsana because it regulates and balances the entire endocrine system through these master centers. The Headstand is meant to bring balance to the endocrine system through the activation of the thalamus, which in turn affects the master gland of the hypothalamus. The Headstand creates a pranic current that can activate a portal opening of the crown cakra.

Next, the Shoulderstand would be taken, which brings the pressure to the base of the skull, influencing the pineal and pituitary glands. Shoulderstand draws the masculine energy of the pituitary backward and slightly upward in the brain, where it unites with the receptive feminine energies of the pineal gland. When these two pranic currents come together in a unified field of consciousness, ājñā cakra opens. Ājñā, located at the forehead centerpoint, is the command center where the inner guru may appear. It is from this center that intuitive guidance arises.

Practicing Shoulderstand also benefits the next endocrine glands further down in the chain of command. Located at the throat center, the thyroid stabilizes metabolic processes of body, mind, and emotions. The parathyroids, which are embedded within the butterfly-shaped thyroid gland, regulate the metabolism of calcium. Shoulderstand is the very best pose for balancing the thyroid and parathyroid glands. Due to its direct impact upon the thyroid, the Shoulderstand stabilizes a hyperactive or hypoactive thyroid and in turn regulates the heart rhythm.

Following Shoulderstand, the next posture that is usually taken is the Plow, which is a variation of Shoulderstand. When the legs drop behind the head in Halāsana, the balancing effects on the thyroid are even greater, moving downward to the center of the chest to include the thymus gland. The thymus, named for the thyme flower, is the body's immune center until puberty, when it shrivels. The thymus relates to the cardiac nerve plexus and the heart cakra, known as anāhata, which means "unstruck sound," or sound produced without friction. When the subtle nerve channels open within us, we hear the Divine sound that is ever existent and is produced without friction.

In classical sequencing, Fish Pose is usually taken after Shoulderstand and Plow. Matsyāsana is intended to balance and preserve the C-curve of the cervical spine. It stimulates the immune system through its direct affect upon the thymus gland. It is an excellent pose for balancing an underactive thyroid. Students throughout the years have also found Matsyāsana helpful in bringing balance to hypoglycemic conditions.

Fish Pose elongates the solar plexus, helping to release built up anxiety and tension, and also releasing toxins in the liver, gallbladder, pancreas, and spleen. It is a good preparation for more complex backbends. All backbending poses stimulate the sympathetic nervous system through their impact on the thoracic and lumbar nerves. They temporarily speed up the cardiac rhythm, giving an aerobic effect to the heart.

After backbending, the forward bends are taken to balance the autonomic nervous system. Forward bends benefit the endocrine system through the procreative organs, influencing the healthy balance of the ovaries in women and the testes and prostate in men. For this reason, it is important that the movement of forward bends originates in the hips rather than the waist. This also preserves a healthy alignment of the spinal vertebra.

Breath and Sequencing

One day in India, I asked Mr. Iyengar why he did not mention the breath in coordination with the alignment of the poses. He emphatically said, "First you get the pose, then you get the breath."

"Sir," I timidly asked, "Will we ever get the pose?"

Over the years, sometimes practicing up to twelve hours a day, I found that I would never "get" the pose and that āsana was infinite. It was the exploration of the internal universe. Each time we think we reach the boundaries of the fullness of the pose with the breath, a new portal can open, expanding consciousness into ever-new galaxies of self-discovery.

It is difficult to teach or write about sequencing without mentioning the importance of the breath. Originally, many of us were taught to take a pose and then a counter-pose. Now, I teach students to use the breath to find the counter-pose within the pose. In so doing, we create a balance between the sympathetic and parasympathetic divisions of the autonomic nervous system in every pose.

If we enter into a pose without using the propulsion of the breath, inner space can close down, creating compression and repression of deep cellular memories, known in yoga as saṁskāras. If we allow the pose to follow the breath, we open the inner space for these deep psychic impressions to be released. A commentary on Patañjali's Yoga Sūtras says, "The invisible must become visible in order for it to be eradicated." If the pose follows the breath, we allow the embedded subconscious imprints (saṁskāras) to emerge to the surface of the conscious mind. When these saṁskāras arise, the invisible becomes visible, making healing and transformation possible.

If there is no conscious breathing when entering, exiting, or staying in the pose, it is difficult to direct the currents of prāṇa into the subtle nerve channels. This is why I emphasize bringing the breath into āsana, allowing each pose to emerge and unfurl from the center of each breath.

I believe that breath is the most important essence, whether we are practicing āsana or spontaneously choreographing a sequence. I found that if I allowed the alignment of the pose to organically unfold from the breath, it would open consciousness to the vast unexplored spaces within. Through this organic unfoldment from the inside out, one movement would determine the next, allowing for a spontaneous choreography of sequencing to occur.

With breath, I felt that the pose could be held for an indefinite period of time. The breath would also indicate when it was time to come out or to stay in the pose and continue to explore the infinite space of the universe within.

AUTONOMIC NERVOUS SYSTEM
Sympathetic and Parasympathetic

SYMPATHETIC
(Thoracic and Lumbar)

- Assists in dilating pupils
- Inhibits excessive saliva
- Inhibits digestive fluids
- Accelerates heart rate
- Increases thyroid and parathyroid metabolism
- Increases blood pressure
- Speeds up metabolism
- Controls vasoconstriction

PARASYMPATHETIC
(Cranial and Sacral)

Parasympathetic Divisions*

- Stimulates juices, fluids and pranas that govern peristalsis of intestines
- Digestion
- Bladder and kidney function
- Lowers blood pressure
- Slows metabolism
- Helps lower an overactive thyroid

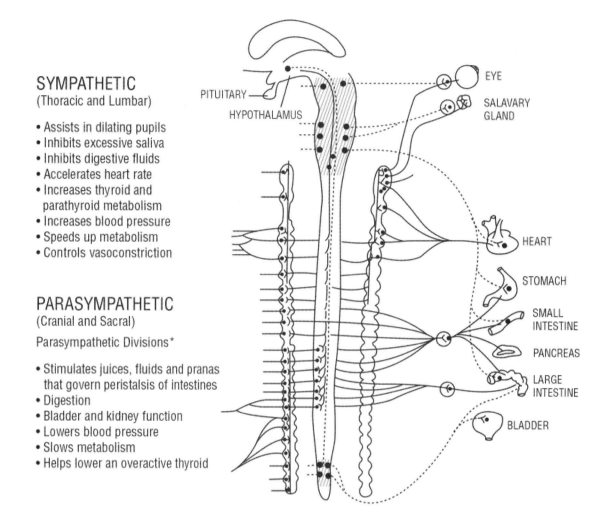

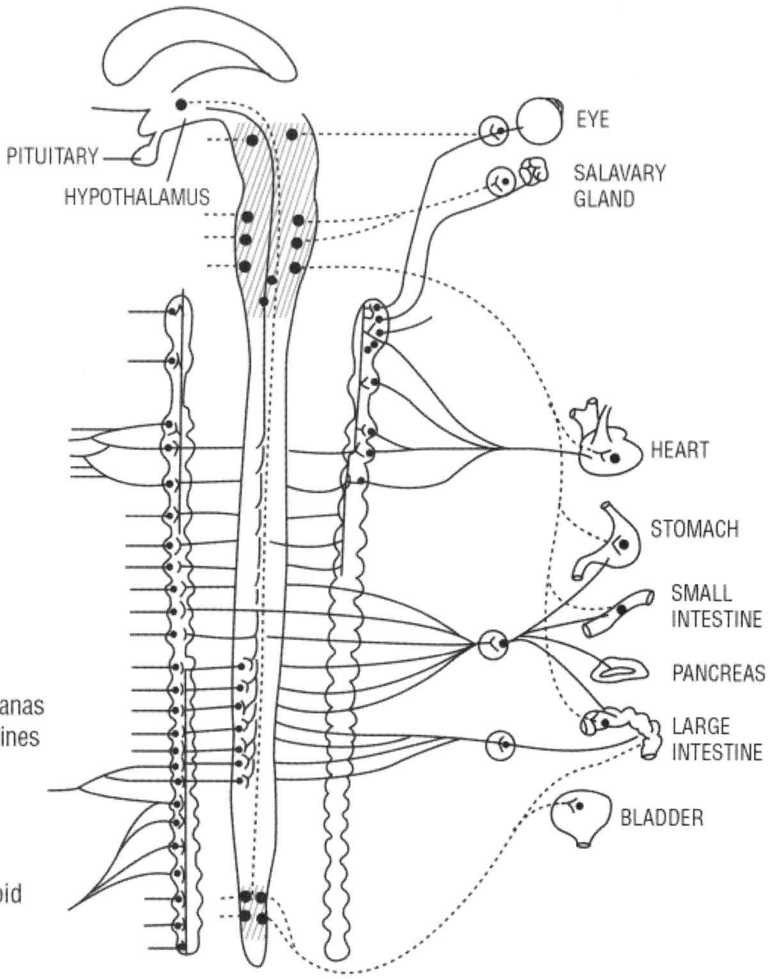

The ANS acts as protagonist and antagonist, and it is desirable for the parasympathetic to be more dominant. It relaxes, digests, and repairs. The body heals with deep sleep and relaxation.

* The sympathetic is illustrated by the solid lines. The parasympathetic connections are shown by the broken lines. Notice the two parasympathetic divisions; cranial and sacral.

Aṣṭāṅga: The Eight Limbs of Yoga

The eight limbs of yoga, according to Patañjali's teachings in the Yoga Sūtras, are the steps to transcend the painful afflictions in our life known as kleśas. Once the seeds of the kleśas are scorched, never to germinate again, we can reach full spiritual potential. Though I will describe all eight limbs separately, my experience over the years is that they are not sequential and that they can be simultaneously experienced in āsana. The eight limbs (*aṣta* = eight, *aṅga* = limb) are:

1. Yama (the five restraints or ethical disciplines)

Ahiṁsā (non-violence) is practiced in thought, word, and deed as inoffensiveness, non-destruction, and non-injury. Violence is a state of mind, not only a state of diet. To be in ahiṁsā is to be free of fear and anger.

Satya (truthfulness) is not limited to speech alone, although there are four sins of speech: abuse, obscenity, gossip, and ridicule of the beliefs of others. What appears as truth in one man's eyes can be an error in another. Since the definition of truth is illusory and colored through the lens of the ego, we must all be motivated from the absolute resources of inner truthfulness.

Asteya (non-stealing) negates the desire for the possession of another's property, also misappropriation or the gathering of more than one's needs.

Aparigraha (non-covetousness) means to be free from the desire to possess or steal. Poverty of spirit is taking things that one does not require immediately. Detached from loss or gain, the yogi finds his needs provided at the right time. "To those who worship me alone with single-minded devotion, who are in harmony with me every moment, I bring full security. I shall supply all their wants and shall protect them forever" (Bhagavad Gita, IX:22).

Brahmacarya (abstinence) is commonly interpreted as celibacy or sexual abstinence. The ancient teachings seem to consider the manifestations of sexual impulses to be gross obstacles on the spiritual path. To the brahmacari, however, sexual abstinence does not mean a forced negation and repression of the sexual impulse. The sexual impulse in the form of energy is sublimated, transformed, and used as an instrument for God-realization. Also, a brahmacari is one established in Brahman, one who sees divinity in all things or who studies the sacred Vedic lore.

2. Niyama (the five devotional observances)

Śauca (purity) is cleanliness, both internal and external. By purging the darkened recesses of the body through sattvic diet, āsana, kriya, and prāṇāyāma, and burning the impurities and confusion of the intellect with the fires of svādhyāya (study of the self), the mind and emotions are freed from disturbing emotional influences. When freed from obstacles of debris, the temple of mind, body, and emotions emanates radiance and joy.

Santoṣa (contentment) is to be without desire—content, tranquil, and serene. If the mind is filled with movements of cravings (either conscious or unconscious) it is not content and therefore is not concentrated. Santoṣa is a state of mind that must be cultivated so that the seeds of one-pointedness can grow into unwavering steadiness of thought. It is through this steadiness that the flame of spirit cannot be snuffed or even disturbed by the winds of desire.

Tapas (self-training) is from *tap,* meaning "to burn," "to illuminate," or "to be consumed by heat." The austerities of tapas burn all desires that block divine aspirations. Without the archer's arrow of tapas, there is no aim, no value in ritual or prayers. Life without tapas is like a heart without love. The three disciplines of tapas relate to the body (action, postures, breathing), to speech (japa, prayer), and to meditation. Whether the choice is one or many forms of disciplines, the chosen methods are tapas.

Svādhyāya (study of the scriptures) dispels ignorance through the study of one subject, which is the foundationless fulcrum from which all other subjects have formed their base. As the bee draws nectar from many flowers, so too does the spiritual aspirant savor the nectar in other faiths that enables greater appreciation of his own. Yoga is the science of religions, not a religion by itself. As we study sacred writings, we gain greater understanding of the faith of others as well as our own faith. As we write, so we revise our own book of life.

Īśvara Praṇidhāna (love of God) is the giving of one's smaller self (aham) to the larger self (Brahman) as the instrument of divine action and love (Karma Bhakti). All life's actions then become the love offering to the divine. Mere adoration and devotion without strength of character is an inert, trance-like stupor. Physical strength and the attainment of siddhis (powers) without bhakti is deadly. The gratification of the senses, whether in worldly pursuits or in meditative pursuits, creates attachment and a desire to repeat the experience. Only when the mind is emptied of desires and gratifications can it be filled with thoughts of absolute divinity. As we become open to higher ideals through love and devotion, illumination will penetrate the darkened corridors of our travels with the light of divine direction.

3. Āsana

The third limb of yoga is āsana, a word that means much more than "pose." *As* means "to be" or "to breathe"; *san* is from *sam,* meaning "to become one with"; and *na* means "the eternal cosmic vibration." Āsana brings steadiness, flexibility, health, and levity of limb. A steady, unwavering posture produces mental equilibrium and prevents unsteady and fluctuating thought. Āsana strengthens the physical nerves and subtle channels for the body to withstand the light of illumination.

One of my teachers once said, "A soul without the body is like a bird who has lost the power to fly." The yogi believes that his body is not for the enjoyment of the senses alone but is for the service of his fellow men. He does not consider it "his property" and therefore is respectful and does not abuse it. Care is taken to oversee the health of the body but not to the exclusion of mind. Āsanas are named after all aspects of creation and are called "prayers" as each position is a position of humble reverence for life and its creative force. Their names are significant and symbolize the principle of evolution. They have assumed the names of vegetation, insects, birds, reptiles, warm-blooded animals, and legendary heroes.

The body is not an impediment to spiritual liberation, but it is an instrument or vehicle or realization. It must be fit to serve and not to burden. The body is the temple of the divine spark (or spirit). The yogi does not turn his gaze outwards toward the heavens but toward the kingdom within, knowing and experiencing them to be one and the same.

The body is the basis for all longings and spiritual aspirations of the mind. Āsanas are performed by the body but are considered a reflection of the mind. Where does one begin and the other leave off? The inter-relation of the body and mind are part of this same all-pervading universal consciousness subservient only to change, with no beginnings and no endings.

4. Prāṇāyāma

Let your life be measured not by the number of days but by the number of breaths. Prāṇāyāma harnesses the life force by converting breath into prāṇa.

The meaning of the word *prāṇa* is as vast as the word *yoga*. Prāṇa is breath, respiration, the vital life force, wind, or strength. It also corresponds with and is related to "soul" more than it is the body. It is used in reference to the vital breaths or winds of the body. (For more information about the five prāṇas, see the chart on page 254). *Ayāma* means length, expansion, stretching, restraint, control, or retention. Hence, *prāṇāyāma* would be the control of the vital winds, breaths or forces of the body through all three respiratory functions—inhalation (pūraka), exhalation (rechaka), and retention (kumbhaka).

A kumbha is a pitcher, water pot, jar or chalice. Just as a container may be emptied of all air and filled only with water, it may also be emptied of all water and filled only with air. This pertains to the lungs and the three states of kumbhaka: 1) *aṅtara* refers to suspended breath on the inhalation, 2) *bāhya* is suspended breath on the exhalation, and 3) *kevala* is the spontaneous fusion of inhalation and exhalation, where the mind is void of thought waves. Kevala means "isolated and absolutely pure."

Prāṇāyāma, the science of breath, is a defined and regulated procedure where the patterns and waves of rhythmic breath correspond to the patterns and waves of the mind. Cessation of one brings stillness to the other. The out-breath is symbolic of emptying the mind of its illusions, and the in-breath symbolizes the realization of the Ātmā (I am) or existence of the individual soul. Steadiness and concentration on the Ātmā or "I am" then becomes the kumbhaka only when it is retained and held firm within memory.

Each breath is the unconscious prayer *So Ham. Sah,* meaning "he" or "that," is taken in on the in-breath.

Aham, meaning "I am," is expelled on the out-breath. In reverse, *hamsah* would mean "I am that," like the mantra *Tat tvam asi,* meaning "Thou art that," and "That is thou." This unconscious repetitive prayer is automatically breathed by all living creatures.

The word prāṇāyāma can also be understood another way. *Pra* means to bring forth; *na* is the eternal cosmic vibration; *ya* means "yeah" or "yes," referring to the Śakti that moves it forward; and *ma,* meaning to measure, represents third-dimensional awareness where we experience polarity and separation. This is known as maya, the illusory world. Prāṇāyāma, therefore, is to bring forth the eternal cosmic vibration into this world of maya.

The calming and soothing effects of prāṇāyāma upon the nervous system diminish cravings and desires and prepare the mind for the fifth limb of the eightfold path.

5. Pratyāhāra (sense withdrawal)

Pratyāhāra is often translated as "withdrawal," not to be confused with escapism. Contrary to escape, pratyāhāra is the sublimation of the less intense states of consciousness that are identified with the worldly five senses that consistently dart outward. With these senses circumvented and brought to one point through the previous limbs of yoga, the mind is freed from external desires. The mind of the aspirant then turns inward toward contentment and joy that rise from the internal wellspring of "self."

Pratyāhāra is also referred to as non-attachment in the sense of renunciation from externals—for example, leaving one's home, family, position, money, possessions, etc. The integrated man, however, withdraws daily for meditative moments or hours, depending upon his schedule, believing that true renunciation comes from the heart, not from the pocketbook. He is *in* the world but not *of* the world. He shares the joys of physical, mental, and spiritual well-being with all who are eager to learn.

When there is true detachment, there is no need to push away or physically divorce oneself from sense objects. The desire for sense objects automatically vanishes, and these objects are observed with dispassion and detachment (vairāgya). It is only when doubt and difficulty arise due to inner conflicts that the aspirant may feel the need to divorce from society and remain in silence and seclusion, helping humanity from afar through vibrations of strength and peace.

6. Dhāraṇā (concentration)

When the body is freed from the pains of opposition, the mind cleared and refined through the fires of breath (prāṇāyāma), and the senses circumvented by pratyāhāra, the aspirant reaches the sixth limb of dhāraṇā. Concentration is defined as bringing together to a common center or point of union, or to intensify by removing non-essential matters. The mind of the aspirant must become one-pointed to engage in meditation. Mental states have five groupings, described in the Introduction and illustrated on page 30: mūḍha, kṣipta, vikṣipta, ekāgratā, and nirodha.

The mental state of concentration is ekāgratā, which means "one and foremost." In this state, the mind is closely attentive, with concentrative ability for a single object. An ekāgratā personality knows just what he wants and uses his powers to achieve it and has superior intellectual powers. Ruthlessness can happen in this state. If the senses roam unbridled, the mind follows. Mental equilibrium can be kept through the anchor of bhakti and concentration on divinity. The guṇa of sattva predominates in this state.

From ekāgratā, the aspirate approaches the mental state of nirodha and the next two limbs on the eight-limbed path. In the state of nirodha, the mind (manas), intellect (buddhi), and ego (ahaṁkāra) are all harnessed, controlled, unified, and offered to the Divine to be moved and used as an instrumentation of clarity and divinity. This is sometimes referred to as "self-offering to the divine." No longer is there the separation of "I" and "Thine." Without the previous state of mind (ekāgratā), nothing can be mastered. Without nirodha—concentration on the divinity that defines and shapes the universe—one cannot experience or unveil the divinity within to become a universal man or woman.

7. Dhyāna (meditation)

Dhyāna occurs when there is uninterrupted flow of concentration (dhāraṇā), and the subject has merged with the object of meditation into the blissful state of unity and higher perception. Just as the bulb of electricity is illumined and lighted by the uninterrupted flow of electrical currents, the yogi's mind becomes illumined by dhyāna. Body, breath, senses, mind, reason, and ego integrally harmonize and merge into oneness with the object of his contemplations. The universal spirit pervades within this state of consciousness, which transcends all forms.

The outward manifestations of one who is experiencing dhyāna include physical lightness, steadiness, clarity of countenance, a beautiful voice, and freedom from cravings. There is humility and subservience to Divinity. The mind is balanced, serene, and tranquil, taking up and giving up actions only for the sake of the work and not for the reward. Free from the bonds of karma, the meditator becomes a *jīvāmukti,* or liberated soul. Even within this blissful state of consciousness, the meditator is still aware of separation between himself (the lover) and the Divine (the beloved). The mind within the state of dhyāna still perceives.

8. Samādhi

During samādhi, mind and intellect stop, as if in a deep state of sleep. Even though appearing to be unconscious and oblivious to the world, the realized soul is fully conscious and alert. As if in a deep sleep, he experiences only the consciousness of truth and unspeakable joy and the attainments of true yoga (union). This is "the peace that passeth all understanding." *Sam* means "to bring together," and *adhi* means "adhere" or "stick to." No longer of the material world, the yogi is merged in the eternal, free from duality or separation between the knower and the known.

Practicing Yama and Niyama in Āsana and Life

Yama

Ahiṁsā (Nonviolence)

"As the yogin becomes established in non-injury, all beings coming near him cease to be hostile." (Yoga Sūtras, II:35)

Ahiṁsā In Life

To be truly nonviolent—physically, mentally, and verbally—it is necessary to cultivate a spirit of nonjudgment and forgiveness. Nonviolence requires a continual refinement and awareness of one's own inner process. It also requires the reduction and eventual elimination of judgment, criticism, and projections onto others. Not merely an attitude of negating harm to others, true nonviolence is the development of a positive dynamic quality of universal love. Mahatma Gandhi once said, "Nonviolence is the finest quality of the soul, but it is developed by practice. Almost everything you do will seem insignificant but it is important that you do it."

Ahiṁsā In Āsana

To practice ahiṁsā in āsana, it is important to allow the breath to be taken in and given out in such a way that it does not produce friction, either on the membranes of the internal region of the body or the external region around the body. If the breath is so refined that it does not disturb the waves of the mind or even move a hair within the nostrils, it is a breath of ahiṁsā.

When one moves into āsana with this refinement of breath, the pose becomes sattvic—serene with a sense of lightness. As āsana unfolds from the center of the breath, it is possible to move through space without creating a ripple of disturbance in the atmosphere, both within and without. A refined breath calms the turbulence of the mind in the poses of yoga and of life. When we are in this state, we don't even disturb the earth beneath our feet or head. This is the essence of yoga.

A gentle, frictionless breath is the protection against moving too fast and too far, which can cause strain and even injury. Breath brings us into an attitude of nonviolence within ourselves and with others. If we use the breath to unfold organically into the pose, we preserve the inner space and the continuity of breath, which calms the mind. If we move without breath, it produces more restlessness of mind, which is opposite of the essence of yoga, and we close the inner space and compress organs and muscles. As the second sūtra tells us, Yoga citta vṛtti nirodhaḥ, or "Yoga is to quiet or calm the waves that arise within the field of the mind."

Satya (Truthfulness)

"When truthfulness is achieved, the words [of the yogin] acquire the power of making them fruitful." (II:36)

Satya In Life

Throughout the years, I've heard it said that satya meant being truthful to others and staying truthful to oneself. But how is that possible if we don't know the Self?

Satya is keeping one's word, following through with the simplest things such as saying we will do dishes or take the dog for a walk. It is following through with self-commitments or vows. Satya precludes procrastination. In keeping one's word, the mind and concentrative powers become stronger. If we say one thing to someone while saying something else to another, it is considered to be speaking with a forked tongue. The energy of our words is scattered in two or more directions, and they lose their power of manifestation. Satya is being "seamless" in all situations, being as authentic in front of a thousand people as we would be with one.

This yama is purity of speech, which means not speaking about what we perceive as negative qualities of another and especially not speaking ill of one person to the next, negatively influencing one against the other. Gossip, even though tempting, is not satya. Denigrating another is more likely to occur when we feel insecure about ourselves and have low self-esteem. Truthfulness is the gift of non-criticism. It expresses the thoughts and words that heal rather than wound the hearts of others. There is great power in truthfulness. When truthfulness is achieved, words acquire the power of fruition and manifestation.

Satya In Āsana

We observe satya internally and externally in āsana, by setting an intention to practice, by practicing without distractions, and by going deep within to observe the pose from one's own experience rather than having to rely on the perception of another. In satya, we observe sensations that arise in āsana with equanimity, without identifying sensations as pain or pleasure. If the breath becomes shallow, back off the edge of the pose until the breath can flow easily and calmly, and then, when the time is right, see if there is an opening to proceed further. Honor your own abilities, not seeing them as limitation but simple as what is. Stay in the moment without psychologically tuning out. Keep the mind present to what is, not what you would like it to be.

Asteya (Not Coveting or Stealing)

"When non-stealing is established, all jewels present themselves." (Yoga Sūtras, II:37)

Asteya In Life

Non-covetousness creates a feeling of nonattachment. We only want or covet what we feel we lack, whether it is material possessions or qualities we admire in others. If we envy the possessions and qualities of others that we feel we lack within ourselves, it can create territorialism, competition, envy, and in turn, the "downplaying" of others in order to boost our low self-esteem. When we are fulfilled, there is no need to compete, criticize, or gossip about others to make ourselves feel superior. When there is no envy or wanting what others may have whether it is possessions or qualities, we can delight in their joys and successes as we would our own. When we give up wanting, many things will be given unto us and manifest in a variety of unexpected ways.

Asteya In Āsana

When we don't feel confident or satisfied with who we are, there is a tendency to compete with others. Sometimes we even compete with ourselves, attempting more even if the body is not ready. In this phase, we always are seeking a new goal, a new horizon to conquer. Asteya is to refrain from coveting the gifts, talents, and abilities of others. If we compete with others in yoga, it propels us beyond svadharma, what is right for us. By consciously or subconsciously competing with another in a yoga class, we may prematurely stretch beyond our edge to "get" the pose.

To remain in asteya during āsana, close your eyes, draw within, find your own center, and allow the āsana's unfoldment, like a flower blossoming out of the breath from the inside out. When the eyes are closed, it prevents competition, even with oneself. This helps us find what is right for ourselves, rather than trying to accomplish what is right for another. To practice asteya, it helps to let go of the past, even yesterday's practice, and approach each pose as if coming to it for the first time.

We can never do the same pose twice. If we can let go of trying to recapture a pleasant sensation previously experienced in an āsana, the mind will be in the power of Now. When we experience being in the moment, we are able to cooperate rather than compete, remembering that there are no "others."

Aparigraha (Non-Possessiveness or Non-Acceptance)

"On attaining perfection in non-acceptance, knowledge of past and future existences arises."
(Yoga Sūtras, II:39)

Aparigraha In Life

Another scholar gives us this translation: "Questions regarding the past, present, and future states of one's body, in the form of 'Who was I and what was I? What is this body? How did it come about? What shall I be in the future? How shall it be?' get properly resolved in a yogin."

Aparigraha, physical and emotional, is a natural sequential step from asteya, even though Patañjali doesn't order it this way in the Yoga Sūtras. The prefix *a* negates; *par* is "to fill" and *graha* is "dwelling." Therefore, aparigraha means "not filling one's own dwelling." Aparigraha could be interpreted as avoiding the over-accumulation of possessions that leads us to protect and defend. This also refers to the emotional storehouse of memories of anger, resentment, projections, and aggressive thoughts toward others.

As we develop a feeling of giving in all areas of our

lives, we experience a growing sense of trust and non-defensiveness. When we are bound by the ordinary desire of a variety of needs for security, the walls we build to keep something in are also the walls that keep something out. We become possessed by our possessions and our need for security, which can also take the form of attachment to personal, ideological, socio-political, religious, and spiritual beliefs. When the desire to possess and accumulate is absent, we seek nothing for our separated and individual self. Non-possessiveness is the stage when one learns that "more is not always better," and unlearns "if only things could be different, then I would be happy." It is the realization that little is required for love and the true experience of happiness.

Aparigraha In Āsana

To practice aparigraha in āsana, we focus on the exhalation and releasing into the pose with the outgoing breath. It requires courage to "let go" and ride the wave of the out-going breath. But if we can see the body as the dwelling place of spirit, we can then clear unnecessary emotional hoarding to create space for the light of spirit to shine forth. Then we allow the out-breath to carry us deeper into the newly created space within each āsana.

According to one commentary on the Yoga Sūtras, "It is on the outgoing breath that the ego unravels itself." Aparigraha aids in the growing awareness that we are not this body, not this mind, not this passing personality. Aparigraha in āsana is the ability to release into the spiritual center of one's own being, as if diving into a sea of infinity through each pose.

Brahmacarya (Regulation of the Senses)

"When continence is established, vīrya is acquired." (Yoga Sūtras, II:38)

Brahmacarya In Life

Brahm is "to wander," and *acarya,* refers to a teacher or conduct. Or the word can be translated as *Brahma,* the creator, and *carya,* meaning "to go." Brahmacarya can be one who goes or travels and teaches of God, or one who wanders and teaches. In ancient times, designated teachers traveled from village to village and were fed and given shelter in return for spreading teachings of the scriptures, the word of God. To prevent attachments, these acaryas stayed no more than three days in one place. Because it took time for relationships to develop, they could not foster a relationship that would lead to marriage. They were celibates whose dharma was to travel and teach, and they put their teachings first, before their own needs.

One commentator on this sūtra stated, "Incontinence deprives the nerves of vital powers. Practice of continence prevents loss of vitality and increases vīrya or energy." It is believed that the words of wisdom of an incontinent person do not go deep into the mind of a student because of the loss of vitality. However, one who is established in self-regulation has the vital power or vīrya to instill wisdom into the minds and hearts of students far beyond the spoken word.

In our world today, brahmacarya could be interpreted as avoiding physical and emotional self-indulgence. Sensual regulation is not the repression of sensual needs, but the sublimation of desire into the sacred act of giving oneself. For instance, it is meeting one's sexual partner as a manifestation of the Divine. It is moving from self-gratification to understanding the roots of the needs of the human soul. Brahmacarya is regulating the senses not only in reference to food, drink, and the sexual drive but also to self-pity. When our eyes are filled with our own tears, we cannot see the suffering of others. When we indulge in our own emotional pains, we cannot extend our hands to another. Self-pity is ego turned in on itself. It creates separation rather than unification. One absorbed with the self does not have the energy to serve the greater good.

The word vīrya in this sūtra means far more than energy. It implies śraddhā, or faith and tranquility, a feeling of reverence. Vīrya is also enthusiasm that leads to sustained effort. When the mind is tired and drifts away from a focal point of concentration, the power that can bring it back to devotional practices is called vīrya. Śraddhā or faith leads to vīrya. If we have reverential faith in our objectives, we then have the enthusiasm and energy to pursue them.

Brahmacarya In Āsana

Brahmacarya is associated with an ascetic or one who practices celibacy, sublimating the śakti by bringing it from lower to higher centers of awareness. In true celibacy, one raises the bindu from the procreative plexus, transforming it to ojas within the ājñā cakra, the center of wisdom.

As a householder or as an ascetic, we can practice āsana as a brahmacarya by bringing the primal instinctual nature (propelled by nature's need for procreation) up from the procreative plexus to the co-creative center within the upper cakras. This is done not through forced bandhas, which may cause prāṇa to coagulate in the maṇipūra cakra, the center of self-will, and increase the ego's assertions. Instead, we allow bandhas to develop naturally while keeping the navel plexus passive as the spine is elongated. This allows the prāṇa to move upward from the coccygeal and sacral plexuses to the heart, throat, and forehead cakras. For bandhas to occur organically, it is important to take the pose on the exhalation when the ego unravels itself. This is the Vedic form of prāṇāyāma, where we empty ourselves of form in order to transcend duality.

In forward bending poses, if we lift the buttocks and tailbone to receive the light from above, this inversion creates a polar shift, leading to a natural ascension of śakti that creates sublimation and self-regulation. If the navel is kept passive, without effort or muscular contraction, this organic or natural mūla bandha becomes uḍḍīyāna bandha, the great bird whose energy flies upward. Unimpeded by the contraction of the navel center, śakti can rise from the base of the spine to the heart cakra and even beyond. In this organic sublimation, the energy centers of the lower cakras energize the upper centers, creating an integration of śakti in which prāṇa can flow freely between all the energy vortices within the sphere of the physical and subtle body.

Master Sivānanda used to say, "One desire fulfilled leaves room for ten more unfilled." Sri Aurobindo Gosh, however, felt that one should give unto life what is called for in life, rationing one's desires so they are not repressed. He believed that as one grows older, a natural sequential sublimation can occur, and that premature celibacy can be psychologically detrimental, creating a backlash in one's being, one's life, and one's practice. There is a thin line between repression and sublimation. He emphasized the importance of self-regulation.

Niyama

Śauca (Purity)

"Purification of the mind, pleasantness of feeling, one-pointedness, subjugation of the senses, and the ability for self-realization are acquired." (Yoga Sūtras, I:41)

Śauca In Life

According to one commentary on this sūtra, "The yogin practicing cleanliness gets purification of the heart, which leads to mental bliss, or spontaneous feelings of joy. From mental bliss develops the power of realizing the Self. All these are attained by establishment in purification." But this sūtra is extremely difficult to translate into today's world. In a positive framework, it can be interpreted as "purity of motives." As we release arrogance, attachments, and the motive of power and recognition, we learn to take up each action for the sake of the action alone, letting go of the need or attachment to a particular outcome. As we purify our motives, we become spontaneous channels for the outpouring of love, with no self-reference or need for self-recognition.

Purifying one's motives requires continual observation of all desires and hidden agendas that cross our mental horizons. This means endeavoring to take an action while at the same time, letting go of the desire for a specific result. Without purity of motives or intentions, there may be desire for achievement or an attachment to the result, and pride may be the outcome. Pride breeds separation and is a hindrance to our sense of oneness with all humanity.

Śauca In Āsana

Why have we been drawn to the practice of Yoga? Whatever the motive, it is likely that the motive will change over time. We may begin āsana for physiological relief from a condition. That may lead to a deeper understanding of the mind and a desire for more peace. We may want to relax, to experience better health, or simply to work out, while others may desire to "work in." One day, however, we may forget why we are practicing. And that is considered the time when the true practice of yoga begins, when practice no longer has a motive behind it.

The purity of śauca occurs when we practice āsana for its sake alone, without a motive or desire to get something from it. We know we have reached the state of śauca in āsana when the pose spontaneously comes through us and not from us. This is what the Bhagavad Gita refers to as detachment from the fruit of the action. This is the true Karma Yoga, when we practice an āsana without trying to reach a goal or overreaching beyond oneself.

Santoṣa (Contentment and Serenity)

"From contentment, unsurpassed happiness is gained." (Yoga Sūtras, II:42)

Santoṣa In Life

Dr. Andrew Weil was once asked about being happy all the time, and why people are miserable trying to achieve happiness. He answered, "Negative and positive moods like bliss and despondency mark the edge of our emotional spectrum. They can help us discover a neutral midpoint of emotional health. That midpoint is contentment, which is an internal state of well-being." Dr. Weil went on to say that this state of well-being is independent of what we have or don't have, of "getting a raise, a new car, a new lover. Contentment . . . is an inner feeling of calm. It's not dependent on external circumstances, possessions, or a period of good fortune."

Santoṣa is the spirit of nonattachment, experienced as the witness or onlooker who sees all people and happenings through the light of Universal love. Contentment is not a state of repression but a state of serenity that transforms the negative into the positive, recognizing that every thought we have is contagious and the time is coming when every thought will become public property. Santoṣa can be seen as purification of mind, pleasantness of feelings, one-pointedness, internalization of the senses, and opening to the possibilities of self-recognition or self-realization.

In santoṣa, inner contentment radiates out and creates an atmosphere of serenity and peace. Contentment is the deep, calm peace of a soul devoid of emotional disturbances. It is seamlessness, where we are the same in all life's situations, whether at home, in the workplace, or on the battlefield. We cannot always avoid situations of stress or conflict, but we can help heal them by contributing our own calmness, serenity, peace of mind, and compassion. Contentment and serenity are the way of the peaceful warrior.

Santoṣa In Āsana

Happiness often depends on getting something in order to fulfill a desire. Santoṣa is the happiness that exists for itself alone, not based on getting or acquiring. This is as true in āsana as it is in life. In the first sūtra on āsana, in Patañjali says, "Establish steadiness and comfort in any pose" (Yoga Sūtras, II:46). This could be translated as "Take any pose and be comfortable." Often, however, it is interpreted as "Take any comfortable pose." Big difference. To practice santoṣa in āsana, one finds a level of equal comfort in every pose, not preferring one pose over the other. This would be reflected in the pose by a calm and easy breath.

Santoṣa can be seen as the act of serenely moving from the known to the unknown. In āsana and its variations we move from the familiar—that which is comfortable or known—into a more expanded perimeter of the unknown. Eventually the new spatial relationship of the unknown becomes the known. Santoṣa is being the same, holding to one's center in all situations, in all āsanas, even while exploring new variations that represent unknown or unfamiliar situations. In this way, we expand the perimeters of our consciousness instead of staying in old stuck patterns, which can contract consciousness. We calmly explore the unknown areas of āsana without attachment or aversion, accepting each variation equally without fear of the unknown.

Santoṣa requires discernment. Are we content within a pose, or stuck in the familiarity of the past? Discernment is needed to see if we are overreaching, going beyond the svadharma of what is right for us in that moment. Are we trying to achieve conscious or unconscious ambitions? Is it possible to find contentment, happiness, and serenity where we are, rather than trying to get somewhere or something out of the pose? In practicing santoṣa, a calm breath will reveal contentment and an abrasive breath will reveal aversion within an āsana. If we can create a calm, even inhalation and exhalation it helps us to be able to accept all poses with equal serenity, not attaching to one while avoiding another.

Tapas (To Burn)

"Through the destruction [transformation] of impurities, practice of austerities brings about perfection of the body and the organs." (Yoga Sūtras, II:43)

Tapas In Life

Tapas help the human psyche to transcend pain, like gold that does not fear the flame because it cannot be destroyed. This is adamantine hardness, or hardness like a diamond. Hanuman, the great monkey god of the Ramayana, was known as the "diamond-bodied one." A diamond is incorruptible; it can be changed only through the purity of another diamond. It has many facets and dimensions as it reflects the Universal Light upon earth. It represents not just adamantine hardness of body but also of spirit—a spirit that cannot be tempted, corrupted, or lured away from the ultimate goal of self-realization.

Rather than trying to get rid of life's difficulties, be thankful that they are there to smooth the ragged edges of the personality and to teach greater compassion for others. Find a point of inner peace in the midst of any or all conditions of life. Achieve equanimity both in praise and blame, success or failure, where the opinions of others have no hold over your mind or emotions.

Tapas In Āsana

Tap is "to burn," symbolizing the fires of the blacksmith who forges and shapes and reshapes molten metal giving new form, new life. The practice of tapas in āsana is a metamorphosis that changes every cell and atomic particle of one's being. It refines the body, the emotions, the thoughts, and even the quality and gentility of one's words. The practice of āsana is tapas, moving us from rigidity and contraction into the fires of expansion and self-transformation. It brings our consciousness from the darkness into the light.

When my young children were in school, I would immerse myself in yoga practices for six hours or more a day. For me, āsana was like a deep meditation, pulling me deeper into its secret chambers. I felt restful, peaceful, and even blissful as I let go of resistance and went deeper than ever before. As I tasted the fragrance within and between the poses, I didn't want to stop, but it was time to greet the children as they came home from school and to prepare the dinner. As I've said to students a thousand times: "When we put the practice mat in the closet, the yoga begins."

I continued to explore how it was possible to take the *bh⊠va,* that feeling or mood from my yoga practice, into every action and interaction of life. I was torn between immersion in āsana, which became a meditation, and fulfilling my duties as a mother and householder. As I pondered the meaning of tapas as discipline, I realized the practice of yoga had become like tasting the sweet nectar of ambrosia, and that for me, the true tapas was to stop the practice and cook dinner (with love).

A friend once said, "We seem to spend our time doing all the things we think we should be doing to avoid the things we know we should be doing." What is it you've been avoiding? What is your tapas? Doing that which we've avoided relates to the fourth kleṣa, *dveṣa* (aversion). *Dukḥa anu⊠ay⊠ dveṣa* (Yoga Sūtras, II:8) means, "To go along with that which is hard or painful leads to aversion or avoidance." In this instance, tapas is to face into the wind and move toward rather than away from that which is hard.

We usually attach to (raga = attachment) and overdo the poses that come more easily, āsanas that do not produce pain or fear and that are comfortable. You may avoid poses you are afraid of because of where they might lead, or poses where there is weakness and hence, a lack of trust in your own support, such as arm balances or inverted poses. To practice tapas in āsana, take time for the poses you've avoided. Using the breath as your guide, proceed slowly and cautiously, until you have transcended aversion and fear, and these poses become comfortable and familiar.

Is tapas stopping life's "busyness" to take a few moments to internalize our consciousness through yoga practice? Or does tapas mean stopping our practice to attend to the poses of life? Perhaps one day the two will find their balance, like raga and dveṣa, attachment and aversion, in a unified field of opposites.

Svādhyāya (One's Own Meditation)

"Through one's own meditation on that which one wishes to shine like [chosen deity or role model] become one with and bring forth yoga." (Yoga Sūtras, II:44)

Svādhyāya In Life

Svādhyāya is usually translated as "self-study" or the study of the scriptures, which is associated with Jñana Yoga. However, this is erroneous. *Sva* means "one's own," and *dhy⊠ya* refers to meditation. Viewed from the perspective of Bhakti Yoga, the meaning of this sūtra, *Svādhyāya iṣṭa devatā saṁprayogaḥ,* is "From study and repetition of the mantras, communion with the desired deity is established." Bhakti Yoga commentaries say, "The heavenly beings, sages, and the siddhas (celestials) become visible to the yogin who practices svādhyāya and the yogin's wishes are fulfilled by them."

During dhāraṇā, the state of concentration, as the subject and object come closer, concentration merges into meditation or dhyāna. This sūtra reminds me of the nightingale who serenades the rose as her iṣṭa devatā (desired deity). Tears of sorrow stream from the inner corridors of her eyes, tears of joy from the outer corridors. Her love of the beatific and fragrant rose is so great that she chooses to be separate rather than merge with her beloved. In the separation, she can worship on the precipice between agony and ecstasy, experiencing the pangs of separation and the joy of offering fully of herself. Her ardor is so great it is like a magnet invoking the Divine into manifestation. There is a saying, "If we take one step toward the Divine, the Divine takes a thousand steps toward us."

To practice svādhyāya, contemplate the lives and teachings of inspirational role models, both living and non-living, who have incorporated principles of nonviolence, love, compassion, and forgiveness into their daily lives. During life's difficulties, the dark nights of the soul, remember those who have shed light on the darkened corners of mind and heart. Role models help us to aspire to courageous heights and unimagined vision that transcends the human mind. Whatever or whoever your iṣṭa devatā might be, hold it in the heart as a symbol of transcendental awareness that will lift you above any spiritual and material obstacles that may appear on your path to the "pathless land."

Svādhyāya In Āsana

This sūtra is a form of puja, an offering of oneself onto the altar of Spirit. In āsana, one part of the body can be an offering. In Uttānāsana, the head, the symbol of ego, is brought toward the floor. The tailbone, that which lies in darkness, is brought to the light. This puja is a reversal of the polarities of heaven and earth. In Jānu Śīrṣāsana, the upper body is like the nightingale and the extended leg is like the rose, a symbol of the Divine. If we were to practice this forward bending pose as a Bhakti Yogi, we would honor the separation between subject (the upper body) and object (the lower body). As the two come closer and closer, the magnetic force would fuse into a sense of Oneness. Then we would be in Īśvara Praṇidhāna, total surrender and offering to the Universal Source through our body, the Temple of spirit.

As we devotionally offer one body part to the other, we create an altar that awakens the life force within every cell of our being. When an object of divinity, the iṣṭa devatā, is invoked with intensity and faith, it is said to appear before the devotee. If this practice is done half-heartedly and mechanically, it will not produce the same results. The mental state during the practice will determine the outcome of the practice. If the mind of the practitioner is not focused during the practice, it can produce a more restless mind rather than a quiet mind.

During āsana, the breath produces a strong nervous system and a concentrated mind. In svādhyāya, when the one-pointed concentration from subject to object is held, the yogin enters dhyāna, the state of meditation where subject and object merge as one. This prepares the practitioner for Īśvara Praṇidhāna.

Īśvara Praṇidhāna (Surrender or Devotion)

"Devotion to God, samādhi is attained." (Yoga Sūtras, II:45)

Īśvara Praṇidhāna In Life

⊠⊠ is "to wish"; *war* is from *var,* meaning "to fill"; *pra* is "to bring forth"; and *dh⊠na* is "wealth." Īśvara Praṇidhāna is the bringing forth or filling with wealth, where the knowledge of everything that is known or wanted is fulfilled. Īśvara is the lord of this world and the teacher of the most ancients. The sūtra says that by the attainment of samādhi, the yogin knows all that is desired to be known—whatever happened in another life, in another place, at another time, or even that which is happening at present. As one commentator says, "This enlightenment reveals things as they are."

Whatever our beliefs (or non-beliefs), when we remember God or higher self in all life's actions and interactions, life takes on a sense of centeredness and fulfillment. In Īśvara Praṇidhāna, one develops growing sensitivity to the inner voice that leads to the defenseless endeavor to dwell in the Higher Self. By devotion to God, one can more easily hold the "remembrance" as perfect steadiness of inner poise. This means holding onto the inner vision while performing the outer work on the physical plane. It is doing the work of the world with one hand, while holding the remembrance of God or higher self with the other.

Īśvara Praṇidhāna In Āsana

As in Svādhyāya, the previous niyama, we are offering to our iṣṭa devatā, the symbol of Divine Consciousness. When the subject and object of devotion come together and merge, it is like the moth that professes his love of the eternal by encircling and then entering into and becoming consumed by the flame. This is Īśvara Praṇidhāna. When we surrender all thoughts and actions to Īśvara or God, it means mentally merging oneself into God.

This can be practiced in āsana by releasing the separation in a pose. "The distance between the upper and lower body," Mr. B. K. S. Iyengar once said, "is the distance between you and God." This does not mean we have to effort, strain, and overreach to close the gap of separation, but simply to breathe and release into the pose. In Īśvara Praṇidhāna, we realize that we are already filled with the fullness of God Consciousness, and as we move into a pose, we carry that remembrance and devotion with us, aware that we have never been separated from the Source. Like the moth that merges with the flame, we mentally merge into the bliss of this God Consciousness within each pose.

Sometimes, like the nightingale serenading its beloved rose, we may feel separation between ourselves and the Universal. Other times, we may take a deep breath and let go of fears, attachments, aversions, and forgetfulness of the Divine or the higher self to delve deeper into a pose. As we release past self-imposed limitations and remember that there is a power greater than ourselves, we discover the true āsana, which means to breathe and become one with the eternal cosmic vibration.

The Pañca Kośas or Five Sheaths

Ancient yogis recognized subtle fields of energy, called kośas in Sanskrit, radiating from within and around the human body. The physical (or gross) body is visible and palpable. It is the part of our being that we take to a doctor or health practitioner for diagnosis and treatment. The kośas are also associated with the body's energetic or subtle body, invisible and impalpable. These five energy fields, commonly described as sheaths or layers, are interconnected. They can be thought of as an ethereal egg-shaped membrane that allows spirit to interact in the environment of matter.

Yoga āsana uses the body to transcend the body in order to connect with the subtler realms of bio- and psycho-energetic fields. Because the body is a dense manifestation of spirit, it is the easiest to identify with, leading us to think that we *are* the physical body. In Patañjali's Yoga Sūtras, this is known as *asmitā* or egoism, misidentifying and mistaking one thing for another, in this case, the body as spirit and the temporal for the eternal.

Annamaya Kośa

The first sheath is known as the annamaya kośa, the sheath of the physical body. *Anna* refers to food, so sometimes this sheath is called "the food body." This is the kośa visible to the physical eye. We can see and touch this body that consists of the skeleton, muscles, organs, glands, et cetera. We can see its arterial and venous tributaries and its conduits of nerves, the brain and its interconnecting fibers. We can see the actions of the central nervous system on the striated muscles that carry out the brain's commands through the body's reflexes and locomotion. We can also see the nerves of the autonomic nervous system, which run along either side of the vertebrae and represent the polarities of constriction/dilation, the body's catabolic and anabolic processes, and the involuntary functions of respiration, digestion, and elimination.

Prāṇāmāya Kośa

Pra means "to bring forth" and *na* is the eternal cosmic vibration. *Prāṇa* is the life force that manifests through both the seen and unseen. In itself, prāṇa is not visible, but it can be sensed moving through every cell of our body and being. The pranic field, which is located within and around the physical sheath, was described by ancient seers (the rishi). According to the systems of yoga that acknowledge the subtle body, 72,000 nāḍīs or channels emanate from the *nabi* or navel plexus, spreading out like the rays of the sun. The nāḍīs, sometimes referred to as "subtle nerves," cannot be located and identified physiologically. The nāḍīs can, however, be felt and experienced through practices meant to clear and open the subtle channels. When this happens, the light and vibrations of the subtle energy field are revealed.

The nāḍīs correlate to the physical nerves but are not bound by the nerve impulses. The prāṇāmāya kośa governs the subtle currents that interact with many systems of our physical sheath. These currents are known as the five prāṇas: *Prāṇa prāṇa* regulates respiration and heart. *Apāna prāṇa* regulates the downward flow of the eliminative system and the downward movement of energy at the time of the birth and during a woman's moon cycles. *Samāna prāṇa* is the energy field that controls digestion assimilation and absorption. *Vyāna prāṇa* regulates the fluidity and mobility of blood, lymph, cerebrospinal fluid, etc. *Udāna prāṇa* governs metabolism and relates to words spoken and unspoken. (For more details, see The Five Prāṇas, page 254.)

Prāṇāmāya kośa is the subtle web connecting the endocrine glands and their corresponding cakras. The cakras, thought of as wheels or vortices of energy, can be accessed when the nāḍīs become clear and open and the endocrine glands are brought into balance through āsana and prāṇāyāma (which work on the subtle prāṇas that govern the physical glands).

There are seven major cakras, but I have experienced numerous sub-cakras or energy vortices that connect the major centers. The intelligence of these vortices does not suddenly awaken, but when consciousness becomes more sensitized, we begin to "feel" the prāṇāmāya kośa that that has always been present. As we transform the intellectual concept of prāṇāmāya kośa into experience, the energy currents of the subtle field become as real as the physical body, and we can recognize the interconnectedness between the visible and invisible aspects of life.

According to yoga philosophy, the physical body is a vehicle for an inner existence or soul. The subtle body or prāṇāyāma kośa surrounds the physical sheath through many energy channels and subtle vortices. Yoga practices, including āsana, activate the functions of the subtle as well as the physical body, working on many dimensional layers simultaneously.

Of the 72,000 nāḍīs, three are particularly important to yoga practices: iḍā, piṅgalā, and suṣumnā. Ida relates to the parasympathetic nervous system of the physical body. Piṅgalā relates to the sympathetic nervous system. Iḍā and piṅgalā represent the polarities of nature that manifest throughout subtle and physical anatomy. Piṅgalā nāḍī is associated with the right nostril and puruṣa, the masculine aspect that constricts and heats like the sun. Ida nāḍī is associated with the left nostril and prakṛti, related to the feminine aspect in that it cools and dilates, balancing to effects of piṅgalā nāḍī. Piṅgalā is known as Ha, one of the words for the sun. Ida is Tha or the moon. The two subtle currents of Ha and Tha are the basis of biological integration within āsana.

Iḍā and piṅgalā originate at the base of the spine and end at the third eye center at the apex of the nose. At the third eye center, these currents cross over to connect with the right and left hemispheres of the brain. In āsana we stand equally on our feet or sit equally on our buttock bones to balance iḍā and piṅgalā, which run respectively along the left and right sides of the spinal vertebrae. Doing so, we in turn align the pranic energies of right and left brain.

The objective of yoga is to align the polarities and bring the currents of iḍā and piṅgalā into the central channel of suṣumnā, which means "beyond." In ancient times, suṣumnā was said to be located in the area from the heart through the carotids and into the crown of the head, which when open reveals the knowledge of the cosmos. More recently, suṣumnā is associated with the central canal of the spinal cord. When the subtle channels of right and left are brought into balance, prāṇa is automatically pulled into the central channel of suṣumnā. Through the breath (especially during āsana) and the practice of prāṇāyāma, it is possible to direct and master these subtle currents to clear the channels so the light of illumination may reveal itself in the fulfillment of our own spiritual destiny. When the bio-energetic field or the Kuṇḍalinī force awakens, the iḍā and piṅgalā spiral around the suṣumnā nāḍī, activating the wheels or movement of the cakras.

In Sanskrit *ca* means "to go" and *kra* is from *kri* meaning "to do" or "to act." The word *cakra* refers to a wheel, which implies movement or momentum. The cakras are spinning vortices of energy that are vehicles from the physical to subtle realms of consciousness. Each of the seven major cakras is associated with physical nerves and glands, with an emotional or physical function, and also with the elements, and each has its own mantra. They are located at sequential intervals along the suṣumnā, the central nāḍī or energy line that forms a vertical path along the spine.

The first cakra, Mūlādhāra, correlates to the coccygeal nerve plexus at the base of the spine. *Mūla* means "base" and *dhāra,* is the "root support." Mūlādhāra is associated with the earth element and survival. Svādhiṣṭhāna, meaning "establishing one's own place within the eternal cosmic vibration," is located in the sacral or procreative plexus and is associated with sensuality, pleasure, and the water element. It relates to the reproductive endocrine glands. The third cakra, maṇipūra, is translated as "the city of jewels." This cakra relates to the solar plexus (the body's sun or storehouse of energy and light) and the element of fire. Its physical correlate is the adrenal glands. According to some yoga traditions, the 72,000 nāḍīs originate in the maṇipūra, which is the center of self-will, mental stamina, and emotional fortitude.

The heart cakra is anāhata, which means "unstruck sound" or "sound produced without friction." It is associated with love, compassion, and the air element. It relates on the physical plane to the thymus, the body's immune center and the gland that regulates the lymphatic system. At the throat, viśuddha cakra governs divine speech, creative intelligence, and spiritual expression. It relates to the ether element and the thyroid and parathyroid endocrine glands. Ājñā cakra is located within the brow at the apex of the nose. Ājñā means "command," as in answering the command of God and awakening to the higher calling of one's destiny. It is at this center that the inner guru reveals itself. Ājñā cakra is beyond the elements and beyond the earth plane. On a physical level it relates to the pituitary and pineal glands.

The seventh cakra, relating to the crown of the head, is sahasrāra, which means the "thousand-petaled lotus." Physically, it relates to the thalamus and hypothalamus glands within the upper region of the brain. It represents the communion with the Divine, and its opening gives the Yogin experiential knowledge of the cosmos.

Āsana and prāṇāyāma are connecting links to these subtle energy forms. During these practices, the life force or prāṇa travels through the subtle body and stimulates successive cakras to open and release their energy. Divine prāṇa can consciously or unconsciously awaken, and the esoteric energy systems are put into motion with consistent and steady practice of āsana and prāṇāyāma.

Mr. B. K. S. Iyengar once compared the skin of the outer arm and outer thigh to the physical body (annamaya kośa). At the same time, he compared the skin of the inner arm and inner thigh to the subtle body (prāṇāmāya kośa). The biceps (impacted by the outer arm) would relate more to the physical sheath, and the triceps to the subtle sheath. Thus, when we align both inner and outer legs and arms and balance upon the balls of the feet, we not only equalize the weight on the muscles and bones but simultaneously impact the annamaya and prāṇāmāya kośas.

variations on each. In Eastern cultures, "a thousand" means infinite. Thus, there are infinite ways in which the mind manifests and expresses itself through the gestures of the body. Even though we cannot see the mind, we can see it revealed through facial expressions, postural alignment, fluidity of movement, and the upliftment of the heart or the collapse of the chest.

The mental sheath also manifests as emotions. "E" is an Old English prefix that means to project outward. "Motion" is energy. So emotions project energy or motion outward. According to the Yoga Sūtras, emotions can be traced back to their origins, which are the vṛttis or thought waves.

Four parts of mind relate to the manomaya kośa: 1) Manas, the conscious mind; 2) buddhi, known as the overmind; 3) ahaṁkāra, the ego; and 4) citta, the subconscious mind. Manas is the part that gathers information through the sensory organs of sight, sound, smell, taste and touch. It is neutral in its experiences of life.

Cakra	Element	Prana Vayu	Bija Mantra	Associated Endocrine Glands	Associated Nerve Plexus
Sahasrara	Surya Vara	Entrance to Cosmic Consciousness	Silence where the sound returns	Thalamus, Hypothalamus	Cerebral Plexus
Ajna	Beyond the Elements	Omni-directional	AUM	Pituitary, Pineal Glands	Cavernous Plexus
Vishudha	Ether	Udana	HAM	Thyroid & Parathyroid	Pharyngeal Plexus
Anahata	Air	Prana	YAM	Thymus	Cardiac Plexus
Manipura	Fire	Samana	RAM	Adrenals	Solar Plexus
Svadhistana	Water	Vyana	VAM	Ovaries & Testes	Procreative Plexus
Muladhara	Earth	Apana	LAM	Perineum & Prostate	Coccygeal Plexus

Manomaya Kośa

Man means "to think" and refers to the mind. We cannot see "mind," but we can see the mind expressing itself through the body. Āsana includes eighty-four basic poses, but it is said that there are a thousand

Buddhi is from bodh meaning "to know." It is the part of mind that sees many perspectives simultaneously. When the sensory impressions enter into the vaults of the mind, buddhi (if operative) discriminates. Buddhi mind sees differences but does not compare those differences. It does not judge or criticize. It oversees the thoughts that arise out of the senses without attachment and aversions. It remains centered in the midst of polarities such as praise and blame, criticism or compliment. It is the blameless state of mind where intuition has an opportunity to flourish.

Buddhi mind is sometimes called the higher mind that sees all things as if from a mountaintop. It has a 360-degree view of life's situations and as a result is proactive rather than reactive. Buddhi mind, when faced with the anger of another, does not respond defensively or retaliate physically, verbally, or mentally. Buddhi mind is able to observe the pattern and pain that led to the expression of anger. It is the compassionate mind that transcends the need to defend and attack and seeks nothing for its separated self.

Ahaṁkāra literally means "I am doing." Aham is "I am" and kāra is from kri, meaning "to do" or "to act." The ahaṁkāra mind is contractive and self-serving, taking care of itself before others. When this part of the mind is prevalent, it territorializes and creates boundaries of separation, fueling life's conflicts with self and others. Ahaṁkāra reaches out beyond svadharma, competing and aggressively going beyond what is right for itself to achieve. We can see ahaṁkāra, in the collective ego of nations as they attack, protect, and defend, crossing the territorial boundaries of other states and peoples.

Ahaṁkāra is necessary in everyday life to maintain consciousness and individual identity, though it can sometimes trespass into the space of others through mental or verbal criticism or gossip. The ahaṁkāra mind is opposite of the buddhi mind. Ahaṁkāra contracts, while buddhi expands. When ahaṁkāra dominates, we feel as if we are performing and "doing" āsana. In buddhi mind, we feel as if a pose is being done through us. It can be difficult to transcend ahaṁkāra's contractive pull on consciousness so that we can lift to the transcendent state of the buddhi mind. We make our choices: Contraction is pain. Expansion brings peace of mind through transcendent awareness.

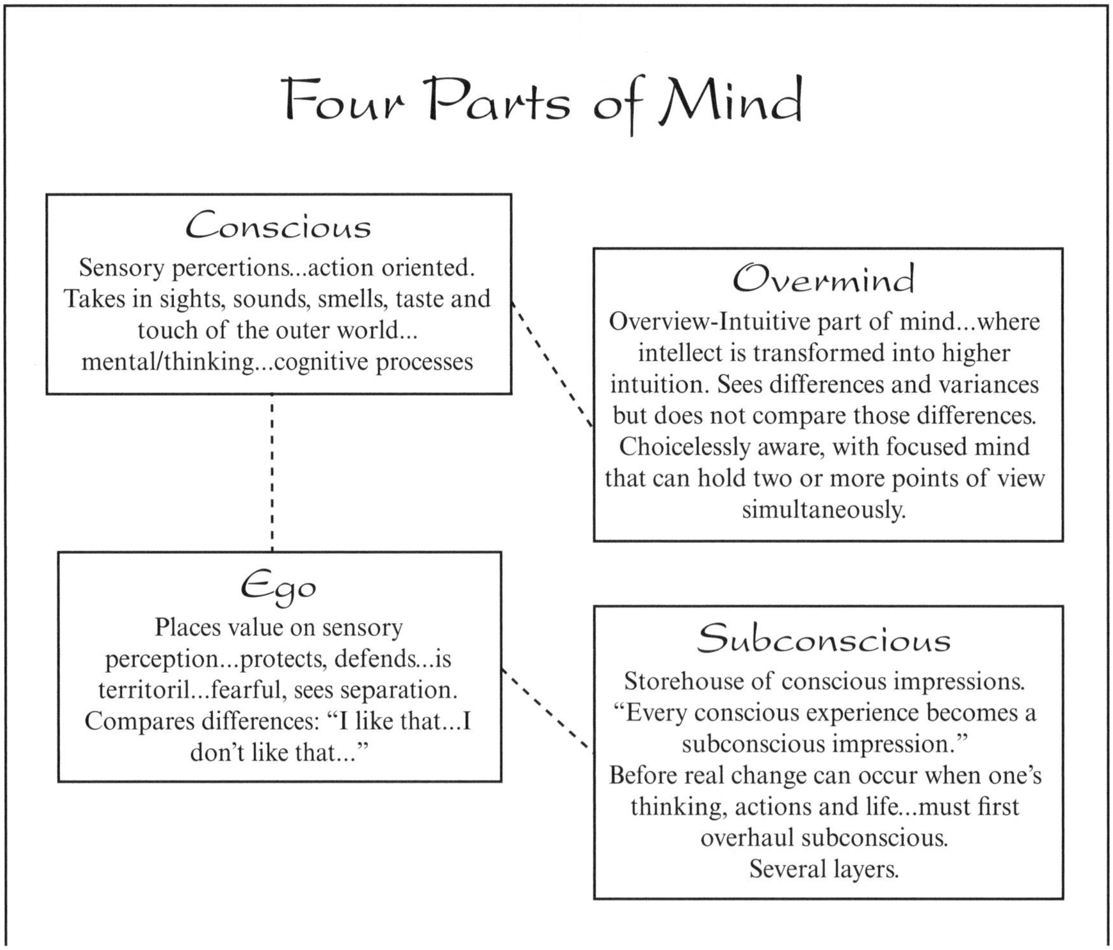

Four Parts of Mind
Conscious
Sensory percertions...action oriented. Takes in sights, sounds, smells, taste and touch of the outer world... mental/thinking...cognitive processes
Overmind
Overview-Intuitive part of mind...where intellect is transformed into higher intuition. Sees differences and variances but does not compare those differences. Choicelessly aware, with focused mind that can hold two or more points of view simultaneously.
Ego
Places value on sensory perception...protects, defends...is territoril...fearful, sees separation. Compares differences: "I like that...I don't like that..."
Subconscious
Storehouse of conscious impressions. "Every conscious experience becomes a subconscious impression." Before real change can occur when one's thinking, actions and life...must first overhaul subconscious. Several layers.

Cit means "to collect," and citta encompasses the entire mind, including the hidden parts we call the subconscious. In āsana, the front of the body correlates to the front brain, the conscious mind. The back of the body, the side we cannot see, relates to the subconscious. The conscious mind is like the tip of the iceberg visible above the surface of the water. The citta or subconscious is like the vast area of the iceberg that exists under the surface. It is this aspect of the citta mind that yoga is most concerned with. It is believed that if the subconscious is not in alignment, we cannot make changes on the conscious level of mind and, in turn, in our lives. No matter how many affirmations one might make, they will have little or no effect unless the subconscious is in agreement.

The impressions taken in—either through the lens of the buddhi or the lens of ahaṁkāra—will determine the condition of the waves of the mind. They may be turbulent or peaceful, or within the wide range between. As the mind filters the incoming impressions, it will determine which conscious experiences become subconscious impressions or saṁskāras. It is these impressions that become the modus operandi, that govern how we approach the series of events we call "life." The impressions can be positive, negative, or neutral. According to Eastern philosophy, they determine present and future life. Positive thought forms lead to a quiet and more peaceful mind. Negative thought forms can lead to a turbulent and restless mind, which is the opposite of yoga's intended purpose.

Imagine how a carriage traveling down the road relates to the four parts of mind. The road represents the polarities of opposites, virtue and vice. The carriage is the body, and the horses pulling the carriage are the five senses. The reins are manas. The driver may be ahaṁkāra (ego) or Atman, the individual soul. If the driver is Atman, the carriage will arrive safely. If the driver is ego, it may choose circuitous routes, taking the carriage over rocky roads that threaten to stop the journey. It may enter diversionary cul de sacs that lead away from the intended goal, which is self-realization or self-actualization.

We cannot see the mind, but we can observe it through the breath, which is the invisible link between mind and body. The breath will reflect which aspect of mind is most predominant. The way in which the mind influences the body reveals the interconnections between manomaya kośa, prāṇāmāya kośa, and annamaya kośa, showing the way the life force moves from the subtler planes to the denser physical plane. If the mind is turbulent, it can throw the prāṇas out of alignment in the prāṇāmāya kośa and in turn create imbalance in the annamaya kośa. When the prāṇāmāya kośa is out of balance, non-ease sifts into the annamaya kośa and the tissues of the physical body, where it becomes known as dis-ease or stress.

The manomaya kośa manifests through the five states of mind. Each of these states also relates to the breath, and in turn, the prāṇāmāya kośa. The five states of mind (described in detail in the Introduction, page 30) are: mūḍha (dull mind, shallow breath), kṣipta (scattered mind, erratic breath), vikṣipta (mind and breath alternate between scattered and calm), ekāgratā (calm mind and deep breath), and nirodhaḥ (heightened awareness).

When the mind is in a state of nirodhaḥ, the thought waves are calm, and the breath appears as to be stopped. However, this is the essence of prāṇāyāma where the in-breath and out-breath feed into one another. In this state, we are no longer breathing, but breath is. The mind is in a samādhi state of deep internal awareness. This is the very essence of yoga described in the second sūtra, Yogas citta vṛtti nirodhaḥ, or "Yoga is to still the turbulence of the waves that arise within the field of the mind."

Vijñanamaya Kośa

Vi means "to negate" and jñana (or gnana) refers to knowledge. Vijñanamaya kośa can be thought of as the sheath that transcends the thinking mind. This is the level of being where intellect is transformed into intuition. In this kośa, there is a sense of knowing—or remembering—what we have never forgotten. When one operates in the vibratory frequency of this sheath, there is faith and spiritual understanding.

Vijñana nāḍī is the subtle channel that moves from the heart to the higher brain. This nāḍī physiologically relates to the carotid arteries that run along the sides of the neck, protected by the strong sternocleidomastoid muscles. This area is one the most complex in the entire body. Shoulderstand helps to clear and open vijñana nāḍī, which allows prāṇa to flow unobstructed from the heart center into the brain. In other words, the vijñana nāḍī unites the mind and heart. This is interesting because the vijñanamaya kośa is where intellect is transformed into higher intuition.

Suṣumnā, the central energy channel correlating to the spinal cord, was once said to be located in the carotids, which correspond to the subtle channel of vijñana nāḍī. It is believed that when prāṇa becomes balanced in the iḍā and piṅgalā (of the prāṇāmāya kośa) and in the sympathetic and parasympathetic nervous systems (of the annamaya kośa), it is automatically drawn into the vijñana nāḍī, which then opens the crown cakra, where the knowledge of the cosmos is revealed.

The vijñanamaya kośa is where the right brain becomes active. Its role is to bring knowledge in as a holographic sense of knowing (rather than the sequential and compartmentalized thinking associated with the left brain). Holographic knowledge is felt and experienced in every cell of one's being, leading to great faith in the unseen. This is the sattvic or serene state. It is bhakti, the devotional path where we offer all life's activities to the Divine. It is a form of Īśvara Praṇidhāna, the surrender to God or Self. It is, according to the Yoga Sūtras, the Buddhi aspect of mind. The buddhi or overmind does not compare or judge people but holds all beings equally in its consciousness. It loves with equanimity and holds great compassion. Vijñanamaya kośa transcends the thinking mind to experience true nonattachment in the midst of a sense of immense love of all humanity. When in the presence of someone in vijñanamaya kośa, one feels comfortable and unconditionally loved.

In this kośa, one's conscience becomes highly sensitized, like the ball of the eye, to those things it may have been immune to at one time. As children, we may do or say things that are hurtful to others, that we may not do as we grow and evolve into greater sensitivity. We may no longer play games of killing ants or bullying others. We not only restrain our unkind words, we also restrain our unkind thoughts. We feel others' journeys as ours and understand the motivation behind their words and actions at a deeper level than ever before. We assign no blame but hold all in our heart with compassion, feeling them as one with ourselves.

In vijñanamaya kośa, we can practice āsana like a little kitten carried by its mother. All we have to do is let go and loosen the nape of the neck, which is symbolic of letting go of the ego that separates us from the awareness of the Universal Source. Āsana becomes a devotional offering of one part of the body to another, the offering the individual to the universal. Eventually, there may come a time when it feels as if the two parts of the body merge as one. We no longer have the separative consciousness of knowing what's upper and what's lower, back and front, top and bottom. Instead, we feel as if All Is. This is the merger that brings us into the experiential awareness of ānandamaya kośa.

Ānandamaya Kośa

In this sheath we feel oneness with the creative source and divine intelligence. In Sanskrit, the prefix ā is a long vowel sound that serves to enhance or emphasize the word parts that follow. Nanda means "happiness" (like Nandi, the bull that is the vehicle of Lord Shiva, lord of all yogis). Ānanda, therefore, means "superlative happiness" or bliss. Ānandamaya kośa can be compared to the various samādhi states described in the Yoga Sūtras. It is the mergence into a rapturous blissful state of consciousness—even for a few moments.

In ānandamaya kośa, we no longer know who we are, where we are, or even what we are—all merges into a blissful feeling that transcends time and space. The senses turn inward, and the fluctuations of the mind waves cease. It is as though one pierces the clouds to bathe in the light of the sun that is always shining. Ānandamaya kośa is above the individual and collective pains of this world. First, however, one experiences the vijñanamaya kośa to understand the collective pain of humanity before being able to expand beyond. One of the great yoga masters has said that we must first experience attachment before we can experience true detachment: "Until then, all is indifference."

Āsana and the Kośas

In the practice of āsana, if we focus on muscles, we will strengthen the muscles. But we can we use the body (annamaya kośa) to transcend the physical, mental, and emotional pains that keep us locked into individuated consciousness. When we practice āsana with breath awareness, we transform breath into prāṇa, and we access prāṇāmāya kośa. Practicing āsana this way affects every muscle fiber, organ, and system of the annamaya kośa (the physical body) and all the channels and vortices of the prāṇāmāya kośa (the subtle body).

Because breath is the invisible link between the body and mind, self-observation will reveal the mind's hidden depths. We come to understand the mind and the thought waves that produce emotions in manomaya kośa. This relates to dhāraṇā or concentration, the sixth limb of Aṣṭāṅga Yoga that Patañjali outlines in the Yoga Sūtras.

When āsana and prāṇāyāma are practiced as bhakti, a devotional offering to all of creation and its source, the heart cakra awakens, and we remember our eternal connection to the Divine. We transform intellect into intuition in vijñanamaya kośa, which would relate to dhyāna or meditation, as it is described in the Yoga Sūtras. Dhyāna is the state where subject and object merge and become one, like oil being poured in an uninterrupted flow from one vessel into another.

If dhyāna is sustained, the yogin enters into the first state of samādhi, which is related to Ānandamaya kośa. When we practice an āsana with the remembrance of our eternal connection, we enter into yantra of that āsana. Here, we realize that we are already one with the source of all forms, and we experience the blissful liberation of Divine Union that is yoga.

The Five Prāṇas

Pra means "to bring forth," and na is the Eternal Cosmic Vibration. Prāṇa, the life force, is influenced by thought and emotion, which may cause it to fall out of alignment, which in turn can cause dis-ease or nonease. The practices of Yoga—including prāṇāyāma, āsana, and meditation—are meant to preserve and, if necessary, realign and balance prāṇa.

Like breath-centered āsana, prāṇāyāma is a way to open the portals to receive the light of illumination. The suffix ya adds emphasis, as in "Yeah, really do it!" Ma refers to the worldly measurement of day and night, and all the polarities they represent: sun/moon, masculine/feminine, sympathetic/parasympathetic, and piṅgalā/iḍā. The purpose of prāṇāyāma is to clear the nāḍīs, the channels of the subtle body that correlate to the nervous system, and the vortices of subtle energy known as cakras.

There are five main types of prāṇa, which relate to the endocrine glands on the physical level and to the five lower cakras on the subtle level. The five prāṇas can also be brought into balance through the repetition of the corresponding bīja or seed mantra that is inherent within each cakra. These mantras have no meaning but are pure vibration. The five prāṇas (also known as vāyus) are prāṇa, apāna, udāna, samāna, and vyāna.

Prāṇa Prāṇa

Centered in the cardiac region, prāṇa prāṇa controls respiration, the health of the heart, and the thymus gland, which is associated with immunity and the lymphatic system. Unlike the circulatory system, the lymphatic system has no pump of its own, so lymph flow relies on the movement of the muscles, the heartbeat, and the expansion and contraction of the lungs. Lymph gives energy to the lower intestine and helps to balance the entire body.

Prāṇa prāṇa relates to the element of air and the sense of touch. It helps us begin to sensitize and refine consciousness, relating to intuition and intensifying the ability to "feel" what another is experiencing or even thinking.

Since movement stimulates lymphatic circulation, all āsanas would influence prāṇa prāṇa , but it is particularly affected by āsanas that stimulate the nerve roots coming off the thoracic region of the spine, including backbends such as Uṣṭrāsana, (Camel Pose), Bhujaṅgāsana (Cobra Pose), Dhanurāsana (Bow Pose), Matsyāsana (Fish Pose), and Ūrdhva Dhanurāsana (Upward-Facing Bow Pose).

The bīja mantra for this area is *yam*, which stimulates and regulates the cardiac plexus and anāhata cakra.

Apāna Prāṇa

This prāṇa relates to mūlādhāra cakra and the earth element. It is associated with the olfactory nerves and is responsible for the sense of smell. Primarily, it is responsible for the eliminative functions of the body. Apāna prāṇa governs the small and large intestines, the rectum, and the excretion of urine. It is responsible for the downward flow of blood during the menstrual cycle, which is why it is recommended that women do not practice yoga āsanas that invert the body during the their moon cycles. Constipation indicates that apāna prāṇa is deficient; to balance this condition, one would work with the downward pull of gravity in the coccygeal plexuses.

The seed syllable that lies within the subtle areas of mūlādhāra cakra is *lam*. This bīja mantra can be repeated and chanted to increase energy or śakti in this region, and to ground one's mind and emotions when there is excessive vata. Āsanas to help regulate and balance this apāna prāṇa include standing poses, forward bends, and sitting practices with a downward sweep of attention.

Samāna Prāṇa

Located in the navel or solar plexus region at the midline of the body, samāna prāṇa regulates digestion. This prāṇa may become blocked by poor posture with anterior compression and by stress and anxiety held in the diaphragmatic region. Samāna prāṇa controls the balance and health of the digestive process and the organs of digestion such as the liver, gallbladder, stomach, pancreas, and even the spleen. It regulates the kidneys and the adrenal glands, the little nightcaps that sit perched upon the kidneys. In Western medicine, the kidneys and the adrenals are considered to be separate. In Chinese medicine, they are one and the same. What affects one, impacts the other.

This prāṇa relates to the element of fire, which corresponds to the eyes and the sense of sight. It is associated with maṇipūra cakra and its bīja mantra, which is *ram. Ra* is the sun, and this prāṇa is related to the solar plexus region, the storehouse of energy, light, and warmth on physical and subtle levels of being. Twisting āsanas work with samāna prāṇa to help balance digestive problems. This would include supine twists, such as Jaṭhara Parivartanāsana ; seated twists, such as Marīcyāsana and Parivṛtta Jānu Śīrṣāsana (Revolved Head-to-Knee Pose); and twisting variations of standing poses like Ardha Candrāsana or Parivṛtta Trikoṇāsana (Revolved Triangle).

Udāna Prāṇa

Located in the region of the throat, udāna prāṇa controls the health of the thyroid and parathyroid glands. Through the thyroid, it is responsible for the metabolic and catabolic process of the body, and through the parathyroids, the metabolism of calcium. Udāna prāṇa relates to viśuddha cakra, the ears, and the sense of sound. Viśuddhi is associated with the element of ether (akāśha or space), and it is the last cakra holding our consciousness on the physical plane. When this center awakens, it is said that the goddess Saraswatī dances on the tongue and one's words have the power to manifest and to heal—that is, the words will not only be heard but will also be "felt." The bīja for this cakra is *ham,* a mantra that has the power to release negativity and negative thinking. This particular bīja is spoken once on an exhalation, not chanted repeatedly like the other bijas.

Vyāna Prāṇa

This prāṇa springs out of the second cakra, svādhiṣṭhāna cakra, associated with the water element and the sense of taste. Vyāna prāṇa is the regulator of the currents that course throughout the physiological being, including the blood flow and the synapses of the nervous system. It regulates any free-flowing energy that may be sluggish. It also relates to the lymphatic circulation, the synovial fluid within the joints, and the cerebrospinal fluid (CSF) that is pumped between the spinal cord and the brain. Science has finally concurred that CSF is pumped up against the gravitational field in accordance with the movement of the sacrum, which is the home of svādhiṣṭhāna cakra. This pelvic or procreative plexus is also where vyāna prāṇa is said to originate, within the area of the procreative organs.

Because vyāna prāṇa is responsible for nerve conduction and the circulatory currents of all fluids, including the flow of the heart and blood vessels from the aorta to the tiniest capillaries, it is the prāṇa that balances the entire system. Vyāna prāṇa nourishes, renews, and regenerates the nervous system, increasing sensory impulses. It is responsible for clearing and strengthening blood vessels and creating new lymphatic vessels.

Vyāna prāṇa is associated with the second cakra's bīja sound, *vam.*

The Prāṇas and the Breath

The five prāṇas of the subtle body manifest in the physical body as the breath. We can observe the prāṇas by becoming sensitive to the way breath circulates around the circumference and center of the nostrils. Over the years, I have found that it is possible to determine where prāṇa is deficient or overactive in the organs and glands by observing the subtlety of the breath as it brushes against the rims and center of the nostril. To practice this particular form of prāṇāyāma requires concentration (dhāraṇā) upon the breath. This focuses and quiets the mind.

The observation of the five prāṇas increases one's sensitivity to the way the breath enters and leaves the gateways of the nostrils. First, we observe whether the breath is flowing through the right and left nostrils equally. If, for example, the breath is more prevalent in the right nostril, it means the left hemisphere of the brain is more active. This indicates a dominance of the fire element, which suggests a greater stimulation of maṇipūra cakra or samāna prāṇa. This would also reflect stimulation of the adrenal glands because the right nostril corresponds to the sympathetic nervous system. When the breath predominates in the right nostril, it can also reflect constriction in the blood vessels or even high blood pressure. Constriction is one of the functions of the sympathetic nervous system, which relates to piṅgalā nāḍī.

As we further refine our observations of the breath, we may, for example, notice that the breath is less prevalent on the upper left outside edge of the nostrils. In this case, the fire element and samāna prāṇa may be diminished, and the digestive organs may be deficient in prāṇa. This could relate to the digestive organs on the left side of the body, such as the pancreas, the spleen, and the left aperture of the stomach. If the breath feels diminished at the inner corner of the left nostril, which relates to the element of air, there may be deficient or imbalanced prāṇa within the heart or region of the left lung.

Breath observation is a fascinating self-diagnostic tool. It helps us tune into the subtle energy field, and it can be a powerful practice for concentration and meditation that not only balances the prāṇas but expands awareness from the gateways of the nostrils to the gateway of universal consciousness.

The Prāṇas and the Cakras

When they placed pressure on one finger or another, students have felt a corresponding ley line to the points of prāṇa within the nostril and, in turn, the prāṇa activated within the subtle centers of the cakras. The breath eventually becomes so refined that it does not create friction upon the membranes and passes eventually through the very center of the nostrils without moving a hair or disturbing the membranes within the nostrils. This is the practice of ahiṁsā (nonviolence) that quiets the waves of the mind, which is the essence of all yoga.

It can be a fascinating self-study to trace the pranic currents and see how one part of the body interrelates with another, increasing self-awareness and revealing the secrets of the universal ley lines through the energy field of the body. Eventually, we may be able to diagnose illness in the pranic field before it manifests from the subtle energy body into the tissues of the physical body. For this reason, yoga is called a preventative rather than a curative. Yoga practices detect the prāṇas as they go out of alignment with one another, and they can bring the prāṇas back into alignment before the imbalance sifts down into the physical tissues.

Pra	To Bring Forth, going forward, force behind it
Na	The Eternal Cosmic Vibration
Ya	Yes, Really, Accentuates
Ma	Mother Nature, to measure (time, distance, the polarities of sun/moon, etc.)
Prāṇāyāma	Accentuates bringing forth the Eternal Cosmic Vibration into this world of duality.

Physics of the Five Main Prāṇas	
Udāna	Upward, levity
Apāna	Downward, gravity
Samāna	Center, spins
Vyāna	Movement or Locomotion (allows earth to move around sun)
Prāṇa	Drives them all

Prāṇa as an outward expression of āsana	
Sitting	Samāna Prāṇa
Standing	Apāna Prāṇa
Inverted	Prāṇa Prāṇa
Circuitous	Vyāna Prāṇa

The Bandhas

The bandhas, often referred to as "locks," are muscular constrictions of the body that direct or redirect prāṇa from the lower to upper cakras. They are meant to encase the prāṇa within the central energy channel of the suṣumnā, which correlates to the physical spinal column and the central canal of the spinal cord. In some cases, this will awaken the bio- or psycho-nuclear energy that the ancients call kuṇḍalinī.

For several years, I studied and practiced intense bandhas with a Himalayan master of prāṇāyāma. Years later, I asked Mr. Iyengar why he didn't teach the bandhas. His look was one of astonishment, as if to say, "Don't you know?" His gaze softened as he muttered, "Because the bandhas are in āsana." Those few words changed the course of my practice.

Now I understand why Mr. Iyengar was insistent that we lift the buttocks and tailbone to reach for the light in Adho Mukha Śvānāsana or Prasārita Pādottānāsana or Uttānāsana. Doing so creates a natural mūla bandha, the lock that reverses an excessive downward flow of prāṇa. The excessive downward pull of energy—which can result in such ailments as heavy menstruation, miscarriage, irregular elimination, uterine or abdominal prolapse, and even depression and fatigue—could be reversed in āsana.

I found it exciting to discover that mūla bandha was not merely a muscular contraction of the anal or sphincter muscles, but that it could happen effortlessly and spontaneously with an adjustment of the angles of certain poses. As I made these adjustments while practicing āsana, I could feel pranic energy mildly reverse its course, rising to an area just behind the navel or solar plexus. It felt as though prāṇa was organically and naturally pushing through the granthi (psychic knot) at the navel center in order to travel upward to the heart.

This is where the relationship between the bandhas becomes important. If we were simply to tighten our muscles to create mūla bandha, this would intensify the energy in maṇipūra cakra, the navel center that harnesses the energies of the sun. This region is known as the solar plexus, the body's generator of light, energy, and warmth. The solar plexus is a storehouse for the digestive fires of agni, helping us digest both food and emotions. If agni is low, we may not be able to handle everything coming at us in life. As a result, mucus buildup may occur, leading to colds and other ailments.

The navel plexus is also an area of self-will. Overemphasizing mūla bandha can direct prāṇa upward to this plexus, where it can get stuck and over-accumulate. This can lead to a sense of defensiveness and emotional armoring, as well as to an increase of willfulness and egoistic aggressions. Instead of bringing us closer to the essence of yoga and the realization of the oneness of all life forms, this can actually result in a growing sense of separation.

To offset this pranic coagulation, we focus on the next lock, uḍḍīyāna bandha, which is used to redirect prāṇa up toward the heart center. This bandha is described as the great bird Uḍḍīyāna, which (through the redirection of prāṇa) flies upward toward the heart plexus. Uḍḍīyāna bandha is a major contraction of the abdominal and digestive organs in a heroic effort to draw the prāṇa up from the coccygeal plexus and solar plexus against the downward gravitational pull to the area behind the heart center.

Engaging uḍḍīyāna bandha, however, can be problematic. It can increase blood pressure and put strain on the heart. It can even, through its forceful muscular action, increase vata imbalance and depress the eliminative function of the apāna prāṇa flow associated with mūlādhāra, the root cakra.

Instead of creating mūla bandha and uḍḍīyāna bandha through muscular contraction, which I found trapped and created more imbalance of the pranic currents, I learned to relax, align, and elongate the spine, in turn lengthening the midline of the front of the body. Doing this allowed for an organic and effortless upliftment within the āsana. This gave space for the flow of apāna prāṇa, which is responsible for elimination, and samāna prāṇa, responsible for digestion. This movement, which might be more accurately thought of as a "non-movement," seemed to bring the prāṇa naturally and effortlessly to the heart plexus. I felt no strain on the heart or lungs, and the granthi of the solar plexus seemed to unravel, allowing the prāṇa to rise freely to the heart plexus.

When the bandhas are practiced this way—without straining the musculature and with no strain showing on the face—the prāṇas seek their own balance. All I did was to give them space through breathing and elongation. When we do this in āsana, the prāṇas find their own place, settling into areas previously deprived by the muscular overexertion that can lead to pranic coagulation and bodily compression.

Using the breath is important when moving into a pose, holding a pose, or exiting a pose. I have found it important to move only on an exhalation, while relaxing and softening the abdominal and pelvic muscles to allow the prāṇa to find its own course. It was miraculous to discover the intelligence that the pranic currents have when we don't block or interfere with their course.

It takes sensitivity and discernment to distinguish mūla bandha from uḍḍīyāna bandha. The best postures for learning an organic unfoldment of these bandhas are Uttānāsana, Prasārita Pādottānāsana, Adho Mukha Śvānāsana, Śīrṣāsana, Halāsana (from Viparīta Karaṇī), and forward bending from a seated pose such as Jānu Śīrṣāsana or Paścimottānāsana.

Traveling up the spinal column, the next bandha is jālandhara. Jāla refers to a web or network, and dhāra is support. This bandha is commonly referred to as the chin lock. It is often employed during breath retention, in particular aṅtara kumbhaka or, as the ancients called it, stambha vṛtti, which describes establishing a steadiness of the mind waves through retention of both the inhalation and exhalation. Aṅtara means "internal" or "inward," and kumbha is a pitcher or jar. The jar is symbolic of our lungs. We can fill and hold in, or we can empty and hold out.

In deep prāṇāyāma practices, one usually does not retain the inhalation for a very long time. The retention begins with an exhalation. According to Patañjali's Yoga Sūtras, the prāṇāyāma of kevala kumbhaka is found on the exhalation, not on the inhalation. Kevala means "isolated and absolutely pure."

The action of jālandhara bandha is not simply to lower the chin to the chest (which often causes students to collapse the shoulders). It is an intense lift of the spine, which requires moving the skin down the back and up the neck simultaneously. Doing this actually creates a slight backbend as the spine comes into the front body to lift the heart center toward the softly descending chin. This extends the cervical spine from C7 to the base of the skull, elongating the ligament at the back of the neck, and elongating the carotid sinuses and arteries on the sides of the neck. Through the cervical stimulation of the parasympathetic nervous system, jālandhara bandha preserves the dilation of the blood vessels. This helps prevent the blood pressure from rising during the retention of the inhalation. The best poses in which to learn jālandhara bandha are Sasangāsana (Rabbit Pose), Sālamba Sarvāṅgāsana (Shoulderstand), Eka Pāda Sarvāṅgāsana (One-Legged Shoulderstand), Halāsana (Plow Pose), and Karṇa Pīdāsana (Ear Pressure Pose).

The chin lock is one of the most difficult practices in yoga. It is an intense movement and requires dedicated practice to develop the necessary elongation of the neck and spine. When the head and chest are in the appropriate position, meditation (dhyāna) occurs spontaneously. The senses turn inward, and the eyes automatically are drawn toward the back of the skull, which brings consciousness from the external to the internal realms of Self. For this to occur there can be no tension in the throat, the neck, or the face. The tension is held in the active uplift of the spine, which frees prāṇa to flow upward.

The essence of the chin lock is to contain the prāṇa within the octaves of the spinal nerve plexuses, which brings the prāṇa into the central canal known as suṣumnā. It is here that the goddess Kuṇḍalinī is aroused from her sleep and arises, winding her way through the subtle centers. If this energy is unobstructed, it brings illumination. However, pranic or psychic blocks can cause energy to back up in the system, leading to a variety of undesirable conditions. But, as I often ask students, why would we want to do this anyway? We are not living in societal isolation in the high Himalayas, subsisting on a frugal diet of a couple of glasses of milk a day.

I must say that after years of practicing prāṇāyāmas with the bandhas in the traditional manner, I no longer practice this way. Instead, I practice the prāṇāyāma and bandhas within āsana. By adjusting the hands, we can adjust the breath within the nostrils, and as we become more subtle, we can even feel the five prāṇas and their corresponding cakras within the rims of the nostrils. Within various postures, we can alternate or balance the breath and in turn balance the hemispheres of the brain by equalizing pressure between the hands, the elbows, the buttock bones, the shoulders, and the feet.

The mind is far more subtle than the fingers. I prefer practicing non-digital prāṇāyāma, using the mind to alternate pranic currents of right and left to bring about the alignment of the polarities of the body. When the breath flows through both nostrils simultaneously, this reflects balance between the two major divisions of the autonomic nervous system, the parasympathetic (which dilates) and sympathetic (which stimulates), and respectively, between the two hemispheres of the brain.

Adho Mukha Śvānāsana (Downward-Facing Dog Pose) is ideal for developing an awareness of mahā mudra, the "great seal" created by practicing three bandhas simultaneously. In this āsana, a natural mūla bandha occurs when the tailbone rises enough to organically and spontaneously bring the prāṇa up from the root cakra. Then, with elongation, breathing, and the total passivity of the navel plexus, prāṇa can flow effortlessly to the heart center. When the spine comes in like a backbend on the exhalation, the chest lifts to the chin. As the chest comes to the chin, the head and neck extend out and then relax, and the chin bows gently, offering to the altar of the heart. The pose becomes a prayer that unties the knots, allowing prāṇa to find its own path. We need to trust prāṇa's intelligence and allow it to seek out passages that have newly opened so that the Divine Light may enter.

A Heart Full of Gratitude

When the heart is so full, it is difficult to find words to express gratitude. I am grateful to all who have helped shape my life, which has been dedicated to finding a way of serenity and peace in the midst of all the poses of yoga and life. Many yoga teachers and students who have studied with me throughout the years encouraged me to put these teachings into a written form, "to leave the legacy." I thank them for holding the vision and working to help make this happen. I also honor my beloved teachers, many of whom are now in Mahā Samadhi, no longer on the earth plane. My deepest gratitude to:

—Patañjali, the father of yoga, who compiled existing teachings and continues to inspire and illumine those who endeavor to seek a way to traverse life's hurdles to understand and realize their existing Oneness with the Divine

—Thomas H. David, whose pioneering efforts led to chiropractic licensing in the State of California. A man ahead of his time, he was a visionary of natural health modalities. His school of naturopathy, his natural healing methods, and his work with Dr. Bates saved patients' vision and lives. His work was a boon to the people of his time and era. I am proud to be his daughter and student.

—Gyda C. David, a licensed physical therapist and one of the first reflexologists in the nation, who was my teacher, guru, guide, and also my mother. She introduced me to my first yoga teachers and gave me invaluable spiritual support. Her clairvoyant knowledge of the body was an inspiration that I have continued to share with yoga students and teachers throughout these many years.

—Dr. Bhagad Singh, who became my first yoga teacher when I was fifteen years old. He taught prāṇāyāma and the secrets of life through a gesture of the hand. His presence and fullness of Being began my course on the path of yoga.

—Master Kirpal Singh, who privately initiated my mother and our family into the secrets of Shabda Yoga. He was a living example of the Christ-like masters who once walked upon the face of the earth.

—Dr. Haridas Chaudhuri, disciple of Sri Aurobindo Gosh and the founder of the California Institute for Integral Studies. For years, Dr. Chaudhuri was a fulcrum for my spiritual exploration. He taught me how to integrate existing teachings in a coherent web of understanding.

—Swami Vishnudevananda, founder of Sivānanda yoga centers in the U.S., Canada, India, and the Bahamas. His love for his master, Sri Swami Sivānanda Saraswatī of Rishikesh, India, continues be an inspiration of devotion, vision, and selfless service.

—Sant Keshavadas, a great Hindu saint and well-known bhakti yogi who inspired me to open the heart and bring love and devotion to my teachings and my life in service to humanity

—Swami Satchidananda, founder of Integral Yoga and Yogaville, who traveled the world to participate in interfaith dialogue as a way of bringing peace to conflict situations. Swamiji was both inspiration and support for launching yoga into the world and applying its universal qualities to bring warring factions together in peace dialogues.

—Ma Yoga Śakti, a disciple of Sivānanda devotee Swami Satyananda. He was the first ordained to teach the depths of Yoga Nidrā, and Mataji was the first swami from India that our family hosted in our home in the U.S.

—Dr. David Teplitz, a disciple of Ramana Maharshi and a truly great Sanskrit teacher. A linguist and choral director, he infused within me an infinite love of Sanskrit and its deep Tibetan resonance, which clears the subtle channels so that the sounds of creation can flow through one's Being.

—Swami Nadabrahmananda, from the Sivānanda ashram in Rishikesh, India, taught me the spiritual essence of sound through Indian music and the rhythms of the universe through the tabla drums and the stringed instrument of the veena.

—Swami Hridayananda, a doctor and disciple of Swami Sivānanda Saraswatī. She built the first hospital at the Sivānanda ashram in Rishikesh, India, and was a major inspiration through her example as a woman, wife, mother, grandmother, and renunciate.

—S. N. Goenka, my Vipassana meditation teacher for several years, who brought the Hiniyana system of Buddhism to the U.S. He was always an example of meditative stillness, calm, equanimity, and compassion.

—Swami Bhimesan, a political science major from India, studied with the great masters of Durgā worship in the high Himalayas. Swamiji took care of Master Sivānanda during the last four years of the master's life. He lived with my family for over two years, blessing our home with his presence and performing Durgā pujas five times a day. He helped host many other swamis and masters who visited and stayed in our home.

—Baba Hari Dass, the silent saint who founded Mount Madonna Center, has inspired me throughout the years through his condensation of philosophy into the smallest common denominator that pierces mind and heart like an arrow of awakening and understanding.

—Swami Veda Bharati, a scholar of scriptures whose very presence conveys the deeper teachings and experience of yoga. He teaches through his translations and interpretations of Patañjali's Yoga Sutras, as well as through his deep meditative silence.

—Swami Jyotirmayananda Saraswatī, a disciple of Master Sivānanda, initiated me and gave me the name Rama, which has lasted more than four decades. He taught me the organizational simplicity of the Yoga Sutras and how they can be integrated into daily life, in which we don't just study the sutras but live them.

—Mr. B. K. S. Iyengar, who inspired me to trust my inner experiences of the convergence of asana with Eastern philosophy and my belief that we cannot separate the body from scripture. He gave the world the gift of alignment, not just within our poses but also within our lives, which we can change through the practice of asana.

—Mr. T. K. V. Desikachar, son of the great Krishnamacharya and nephew of Mr. B. K. S. Iyengar. Throughout the years, Mr. Desikachar has inspired me by his unique integration of yoga philosophy in daily life. When I wanted to quit teaching he was insistent that I continue, strongly urging me to write and leave a legacy for future generations of teachers. His family now carries on the teaching tradition.

—Ronald Eugene Vernon, who turned me upside down for my first headstand and encouraged me to teach my first class. As the teaching grew and consumed our married life and family in the flame of yoga, he continued to open our home to visiting teachers and swamis, and he supported scores of gurus and devotees from a variety of paths. His moral and financial support helped me to help so many others to begin and strengthen their organizations in spreading the light of yoga.

—My children, Adrian, Erin, and Andrea who received the teachings of yoga through osmosis when the Great Ones held satsangs in our home. I commend them for their patience and understanding, especially for those times when I could not be with them even while I was teaching or conducting meditation and yoga classes in our home. Today, their lives and their love and caring help to assuage any guilt I felt those years when I was called upon to serve the macrocosmic family of humankind.

—My heart is filled with gratitude for the Universal Spirit that continues to guide me, lifts me when I have fallen, and is patient in the hills and valleys of life's experiences.

I honor and acknowledge the following for their direct effort and continuing moral support:

—Kathleen Bryant, who helped transcribe, edit, and organize interviews taped fifteen years ago. A special thanks to her for holding the vision of possibilities, and her endless patience and many hours of work in bringing this book into the published form.

—Ruth Hartung (Sraddhasagar), founding director of Seven Centers Yoga Arts in Sedona, Arizona. I thank her for her vision and faith in the teachings and for her unwavering perseverance in bringing these writings forth to preserve the teachings for yoga teachers in the years to come. She is the Śakti that has made this project happen.

—Ana Hansen, who exemplifies and teaches the true heart of yoga. Her precision, grace, and serenity have supported and encouraged me, and she gave me the momentum and organization to finish these writings. Her editing skills and insights were invaluable far more than she may ever know.

—Mira Michelle Murphy, my youngest child, whose love and innate wisdom of yoga, Āyurveda, and natural healing supports and sustains me and so many others when faced with life's challenges. My heart is filled with gratitude for her moral support and participation as a model for this book as well as her continued commitment to carry on the work.

—Joan Giguirre Thompson, a quiet presence on earth who has always been on the forefront of transformational visionary change. She heals through her wisdom, beauty, and presence. She opened her heart and home for a handful of teachers to gather for one week to ask questions, the answers of which formed the foundation of this book.

—Joy Lindsey, whose vision of possibilities was the motivating force and inspiration to put the teachings into a written form. She gathered together the handful of teachers for recording my commentaries on asana and philosophy that became the original basis of this book.

—Marybeth Marcus, founder and director of Desert Song Yoga in Phoenix, Arizona, was one of the teachers who gathered for the interviews and recordings. A teacher of teachers, she is a continual light of integrity, compassion, and inspiration for current and future generations of yoga teachers.

—Zoreh Afsarzdeh, founder and director of High Desert Yoga in Albuquerque, New Mexico, who also gave a week of her time to meet many years ago and be part of the interviews that became the original transcript for this book. A teacher of teachers, she too prepares and supports future generations to carry the light of the eternal flame of yoga into darkened corners of our world.

—Ginny Beal, a yoga teacher and my friend in yoga and life. She believes in and sustains the continuance of my teachings. Her vision, love, and ideas have lifted my spirit when it was wavering. She has organized and inspired me to continue to share yoga and is a continual source of strength, light, wisdom, and encouragement. She makes it happen.

—Connie Reynolds, founder and director of the Yoga College in Sioux City, Iowa, for her weeks of transcribing interviews in the midst of a busy teaching schedule. Her heart, love, and continually unfolding knowledge of yoga will ignite and light the path of students for generations to come.

—Dr. Cynthia Russell for her dedication to transcription and living with my voice in her ear. Her intuitive understandings of the teachings permeate not just the head but every cell of her Being.

—Friederike Almstedt, a dedicated student of Yoga and Sanskrit, for her scholarly assistance in the final work of adding the diacritical marks to the Sanskrit in this manual.—Kristi Hook, whose love and creativity is bringing forth ever-new insights, clarity, and dedication to interpreting this work for generations of Light Beings to come. Kristi carries the flame of yoga to inspire the teachers of today and tomorrow.

—Barbara Kittel, whose love and nonjudgmental support sustains me on whatever life adventures may arise. Her work in teaching and healing is on the forefront of future modalities.

—Melissa Spamer and Christopher Neal, for their hours of work designing illustrations for this book, which they fit into a schedule of studying, international travel and teaching, getting married and honeymooning. They are gifted artists, teachers of teachers, and healers with backgrounds in Āyurveda, Chinese medicine, and yoga.

—Rev. Max Lafser, my husband, whose ageless wisdom expands far beyond the pulpit of his Unity church. He touches my heart and the hearts of thousands of others who are inspired by his words and presence. I thank him for his patience, understanding, and nurturing during this time of bringing my teachings into the written form. Even though he does not formally practice yoga, he *is* yoga.

—A special note of gratitude for the support of my friends and colleagues throughout the years and a heartfelt tribute to the true teachers of yoga… the students.

These writings are the outgrowth of my half-century of studies as well as the study of the inner self. They have organically arisen from within me through deep practices, self observation, and the discovery of yoga scriptures that support the inner experiences.

I humbly offer them to the reader and future generations of yoga students and teachers. Each generation is a springboard for the next. As Khalil Gibran in The Prophet speaks of the bow launching the arrows of the future generations, he reminds us that we are to let our bending be in gladness. For even as the great archer "loves the arrow that flies, so He loves also the bow that is stable."

May the blessings of the masters be with you as you continue your eternal journey upon the path to the pathless land of Yoga.

Love to you always,

Rama

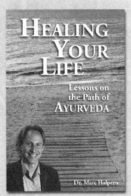

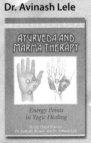

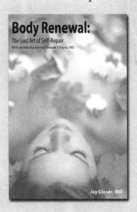

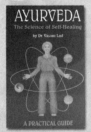

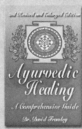

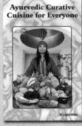

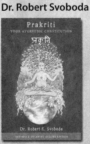

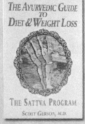

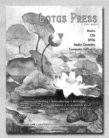

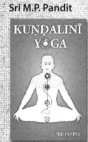

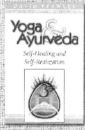

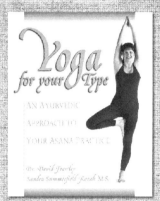

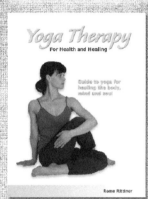

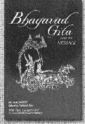

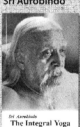

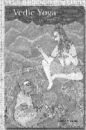

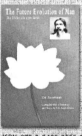

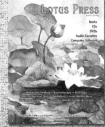